a LANGE medical book

Molecular Basis of
Medical Cell Biology

First Edition

By

Gerald M. Fuller, PhD
Professor of Cell Biology
University of Alabama School of Medicine
Birmingham, Alabama

Dennis Shields, PhD
Professor of Developmental & Molecular Biology
Albert Einstein College of Medicine
Bronx, New York

Appleton & Lange
Stamford, Connecticut

Notice: The authors and the publisher of this volume have taken care to make certain that the doses of drugs and schedules of treatment are correct and compatible with the standards generally accepted at the time of publication. Nevertheless, as new information becomes available, changes in treatment and in the use of drugs become necessary. The reader is advised to carefully consult the instruction and information material included in the package insert of each drug or therapeutic agent before administration. This advice is especially important when using, administering, or recommending new or infrequently used drugs. The authors and publisher disclaim all responsibility for any liability, loss, injury, or damage incurred as a consequence, directly or indirectly, of the use and application of any of the contents of this volume.

Prentice Hall International (UK) Limited, *London*
Prentice Hall of Australia Pty. Limited, *Sydney*
Prentice Hall Canada, Inc., *Toronto*
Prentice Hall Hispanoamericana, S.A., *Mexico*
Prentice Hall of India Private Limited, *New Delhi*
Prentice Hall of Japan, Inc., *Tokyo*
Simon & Schuster Asia Pte. Ltd., *Singapore*
Editora Prentice Hall do Brasil Ltda., *Rio de Janeiro*
Prentice Hall, *Upper Saddle River, New Jersey*

ISSN: 1094-6543

Acquisitions Editor: John P. Butler
Development Editor: Amanda M. Suver
Production Editor: Karen W. Davis
Art Coordinator: Eve Siegel

ISBN 0-8385-1384-0

90000

9 780838 513842

PRINTED IN THE UNITED STATES OF AMERICA

To our families:

Mark, Kevin, and Tracy Fuller

Toni, Jacqueline, Rebecca, and Matthew Shields

Contents in Brief

Contents

10. Cell Signaling Pathways: Communication Via Enzyme-Linked & Enzyme-Associated Receptors

Preface

In the past 20 years, the knowledge gained from molecular and cell biology has completely revolutionized our way of thinking about how cells work and our ability to manipulate their function. Recombinant DNA technology—in concert with the Genome Project, which is enabling us to determine the complete DNA sequences of bacteria, yeast, and mammals, including humans—is changing our understanding of genetic diseases. Native and modified genes can now be readily introduced into different cells, including the embryos of flies (*Drosophila melanogaster*), worms (*Caenorhabditis elegans*), frogs (*Xenopus laevis*), and mice (*Mus* spp.), and the effects of these mutations on individual cells or indeed on the development of the whole organism can be analyzed in cellular and molecular detail. As we approach the new millennium, the introduction of new genes into organisms has profound implications for the physician, because our ability to understand, diagnose, and treat diseases has changed fundamentally.

We are on the verge of introducing genes into cells to correct defective genetic functions and to target specific drugs to cancer cells, thereby killing only those cells whose growth is uncontrolled. Furthermore, our knowledge of the complex signaling networks and interactions that regulate cell growth and development has expanded enormously in the past five years. These discoveries are leading to new diagnostics and treatment modalities for disorders—such as cancer, diabetes, cardiac disease, and genetic defects—that were previously inconceivable or were confined to the realms of science fiction. To take full advantage of the new therapeutic interventions, the modern physician must understand the molecular details of cell function, communication, development, and growth.

The aim of this book is to present these details in a precise, straightforward, and succinct fashion, which will enable medical students, physicians, and advanced undergraduates to fully understand the cellular and molecular basis of disease processes. To achieve this goal, we have attempted to describe mammalian cells in terms of their molecular architecture and biochemical function. As each organelle system is described, we have related its function to specific diseases. For example, we now have a detailed molecular and cellular understanding of cystic fibrosis, a hereditary disease affecting approximately 1 in 2000 individuals. In this disease, a complex membrane protein that normally resides on the plasma membrane and functions in chloride transport has a single amino acid change. This alteration dramatically affects the protein's cellular localization because the mutated protein cannot fold correctly in the endoplasmic reticulum (ER). Consequently, instead of its normal transport to the cell membrane, the protein is retained in the ER and degraded in the cytoplasm.

We have attempted to integrate such knowledge derived from recent research exploiting such diverse organisms as yeast cells, fruit flies, nematodes, and mice to present a comprehensive overview of modern cell biology as it relates to understanding human disease. In the early chapters, we discuss the fundamental principles of cell organization and the basic molecules that constitute organelles. In the later chapters, we discuss the function of individual organelles, the organization of the cytoskeleton, intracellular protein transport and secretion, signal transduction, cell signaling, and growth regulation. Although each chapter builds on previous material, we have tried to ensure that chapters can be readily understood on their own; thus each one presents a comprehensive overview of the material that will enable readers to rapidly review individual topics. This book will therefore be a valuable aid to students preparing for medical board examinations.

The idea of the book was developed from our being course leaders in cell biology at our respective universities. We felt that most medical students would have had more than a "smattering" of cell biology, and indeed many have been exposed to more comprehensive text than ours. Our goal is to refresh in students' memories the concepts of modern cell biology and to show how these concepts apply to cell function in a medical or disease context. We hope we have done this. Many important molecular details had to be glossed over in keeping with the original plan of having a text that could be revised frequently and integrated into the teaching of histology at an affordable price.

ACKNOWLEDGMENTS

We wish to acknowledge the generous contributions from other authors and their texts. We are especially appreciative of the generosity of several of the Appleton & Lange authors: Drs. Walter X. Balcavage, William F. Ganong, Eric R. Kandel, Robert K. Murray, and their respective coauthors. In addition, we acknowledge the aid of two of the gold standard texts of modern cell biology, *Molecular Biology of the Cell*, by Dr. Bruce Alberts and colleagues, and *Molecular Cell Biology,* by Dr. Harvey Lodish and coauthors. The textual organization of these books contributed much to the way we put our chapters together.

On a personal note we wish to acknowledge very special individuals who helped each of us in countless ways. Mr. Nelson L. Fuentes, at the University of Alabama, and Ms. Elyse Rizzo, at Albert Einstein College of Medicine, were especially important in keeping the authors on track and in organizing each of the chapters. We also thank Ms. Amanda Suver for taking on the task of editing and working through some difficult administrative problems.

Gerald M. Fuller, PhD
Dennis Shields, PhD

Birmingham
September, 1997

Different Cell Phenotypes & How They Form

1

THE EVOLUTION OF A SCIENTIFIC DISCIPLINE

Early cell biologists referred to themselves as **cytologists.** These scientists were mostly concerned with cell structure (morphology), and their discipline focused on sectioning tissues and staining tissues and cells. They examined the structures within cells by using different types of stains and fixation embedding procedures and then extrapolated the function of the cells by observing their structure. This approach was remarkably accurate for the time, but as the tools and techniques changed so did the cell biologist. Cytologists and microanatomists became **cell biochemists** and **cell molecular biologists.** Physical and molecular biochemistry led the way to understanding the three-dimensional conformation of molecules that control cell activity. The application of electron beams in the development of the electron microscope became as important in creating images of cells as were light waves. As techniques in immunology developed and the understanding of how an antibody recognized its antigen increased, cell biologists found that antibodies could pinpoint molecules within a cell. The use of antibodies has allowed the cell biologist to probe the interior of the cell in ways never before thought possible. Today, therefore, cell biologists use antibodies to localize, quantitate, and determine the interactions of even tiny amounts of a protein within cellular compartments. It is difficult to judge any one major leap in biochemistry, genetics, immunology, embryology, or physical chemistry as the most crucial technological advance in cell biology. If there were one achievement equal to the microscope (of any variety), however, it might be the use of antibodies to identify, localize, and follow the fate of regulatory proteins within the cell.

A new horizon in cell biology emerged when it was shown that individual types of mammalian cells could be grown in the laboratory with a technique referred to as **tissue and cell culture.** This technology has been used to grow cells from all organs of the body, including skin, liver, kidney, pituitary glands, muscle, and even some types of cells from the nervous system. The development of this technology has led the way to the design of experiments that mimic environmental conditions of the cell. With the use of cell culture technology, normal physiologic conditions of the body can be subtly altered. The responses of the cell may therefore be examined in ways that were impossible with cells still in the animal. Step by step, cell type by cell type, new information has been gathered about how cells communicate with one another. The importance of **extracellular matrix molecules** to cell growth and communication has been firmly established through the use of cell culture systems. Information about cell division, the molecules that control it, cell aging, and differences between tumor cells and normal cells has begun to unfold. By combining antibodies with cells on a tissue culture plate, cell biologists have been able to define molecules that were missing, defective, or overactive during changes in cell "social behavior."

Since the late 1970s, **molecular biology** has provided the cell biologist with powerful tools to explore the chemistry and regulation of individual genes and has completely changed how a cell can be studied. Cloning, sequencing, manipulating, and expressing genes in tissue culture cells are as routine today as making specific antibodies was only a decade ago. Now, so we can fully understand how a protein functions, it is usually cloned and then made in huge quantities with the use of prokaryotic or eukaryotic cells. The chemistry of the protein, including its three-dimensional configuration, can therefore be examined in detail. Any individual molecule can be isolated, and its innermost structure determined. Not only can one make a rare molecule in amounts never before possible, but the molecule can be genetically inserted into a cell and the response to its "overexpression" examined. By knowing exactly which molecules are involved in a cell function, the cell biologist can take the function apart, molecule by molecule, and determine the details of each interaction in a way never even dreamed of only 2 or 3 decades ago. Further, for the past 10 years it has been possible to introduce genes into mice—the so-called transgenic mice—and study their function. This technology has paved the way for creating animals that manifest a particular genetic defect and studying its phenotype during development as well as in adult animals. In addition, by targeting particular oncogenes to specific cells, it has been possible to produce tumors in these cells that can then be studied both in the whole animal as well as in tissue culture.

We would indeed be remiss if we failed to emphasize how much has been learned of human cell function by studying less complex organisms. We cite here four different types of organisms and how each has been especially useful. Our list, however, is by no means exhaustive. First, yeast cells have been especially useful in elucidating the molecular events of the cell cycle because they can be genetically manipulated and easily grown in the laboratory. The **kinases** and **cyclins,** which are subunits of proteins whose synthesis and degradation increase and decrease during the cell cycle, are the major molecules that drive a cell through the cycle. The study of these molecules has been instrumental in developing our current knowledge of how mammalian cells progress through the cell cycle. Yeast cells have also been a major cellular model for advancing our understanding of the molecular basis of secretion: the pathways of intracellular vesicle trafficking, protein sorting, and organelle biogenesis are now understood in some detail as a result of using yeast cells.

Two completely different invertebrate organisms, *Caenorhabditis elegans* (a small nematode) and *Drosophila melanogaster* (the fruit fly), have served as powerful models for studying cell development, organogenesis, programmed cell death, and the molecular genetics of cell behavior. Informed physicians will immediately recognize the importance of new information about cell function, derived from the nematode or fruit fly, and how it could easily have a direct bearing on their understanding of human cellular behavior. Indeed, the importance of fruit flies in contributing to our understanding of early development and embryogenesis was recently recognized by the awarding of the Nobel Prize to Christine Nusslein-Volhard, Eric Wieschaus, and Edward Lewis (1995).

In summary, all eukaryotic cells use similar molecules to carry out cell function; thus, we are all related and likely share common origins. The greater our understanding of simple systems, the more we know about ourselves.

MAMMALIAN CELL PHENOTYPES

Although not all mammalian cells look or behave alike, they share identical genetic material. We now know that the 200 or so different cellular phenotypes within the human body are determined by which

genes are expressed and by the signals that control when a particular gene or set of genes is expressed. In this chapter, we discuss the many different cellular phenotypes in the mammalian body and how they are socially and functionally arranged. We then turn our attention to the basic mechanisms that control gene expression and the locations in the cell that are most sensitive to regulatory events. Finally, we consider how cells in adult tissue replenish themselves during adult life.

The Systematic Organization of Cells in Tissues

The term **tissue** (L. *texere,* to weave) was coined by the French surgeon Bichat to describe his concept of the different "textures" of the human body. On the basis of his extensive studies of cadavers, Bichat proposed that the body is composed of many different materials woven together to form a variety of fabrics or tissues. His observations were indeed correct. It was later recognized, however, that there are actually only four basic types of cells: epithelial, connective, muscle, and nervous. Within each of these basic tissues are many subtypes that exhibit different morphologic and functional phenotypes.

We do not describe here the details of each basic tissue; that task is properly reserved for histology. It is valuable, however, to describe briefly the characteristics of each fundamental cell type before discussing the molecular events that occur within these cells.

Cells of the epithelium. The exterior of the body and nearly all the internal surfaces are covered by a continuous sheet of cells known as the epithelial membrane, which is composed of epithelial cells. This tissue exhibits close cell-to-cell contact and forms strong, tight connections that are impervious to the passage of fluids (Figure 1–1). Epithelial cells are polarized, as they have distinct surfaces (apical and basolateral). These cells also have a broad range of specializations, and one of their more prominent features is the propensity to secrete fluids produced by the cell. These substances can be directly secreted to the cell surface, or the epithelial cells can form ducts or channels through which copious amounts of material are released for lubrication. Certain types of epithelial cells secrete directly into the blood stream; these cells are usually located near capillary networks (see Chapter 2).

Cells of connective tissue. The most basic role of connective tissue cells is to support, connect, and nourish cells in other tissues. Many cell types within this category produce substantial quantities of extracellular matrix material (Figure 1–2). The organization of this matrix is proteinaceous, as it contains various types of collagens and other structural proteins, such as fibronectin, laminin, and vitronectin (see Chapter 8). One of the more obvious specializations of connective tissue is that it produces unique types of

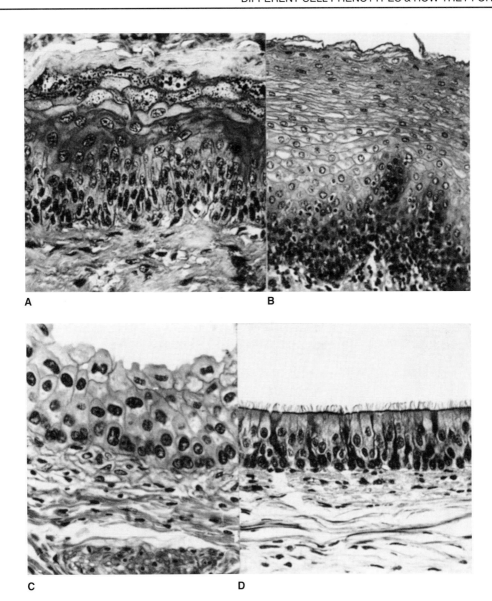

Figure 1–1. Types of epithelial tissue. These photomicrographs show four types of complex epithelial tissue: stratified squamous keratinized epithelium (A), stratified squamous nonkeratinized epithelium (B), transitional epithelium (C), and ciliated pseudostratified columnar epithelium (D). All slides were stained with hematoxylin and eosin. × 500. (From Junqueira LC: *Basic Histology,* 8th ed. Appleton & Lange, 1995, p. 62, with permission.)

collagen and other matrix molecules. One important structural element of connective tissue cells is the **basement membrane;** most epithelial cells are supported on this structure. Although the basement membrane is mostly composed of materials derived from connective tissue cells, other cell types contribute to its structure in certain instances (Figure 1–3).

The **fibroblast** is a relatively undifferentiated connective tissue cell. It is a precursor cell that forms other types of connective tissue cells, including adipocytes (fat cells), smooth muscle cells, and bone- and cartilage-producing cells. Certain fibroblastic cells of connective tissue specialize in the production, modification, and remodeling of bone and cartilage. These cells are known as osteoblasts, osteocytes, chondroblasts, and chondrocytes. The manufacture of bone and cartilage is a dynamic process that typically occurs throughout the lifetime of an organism. Blood cells, including erythrocytes, monocytes, neutrophils, basophils, eosinophils, and platelets, are derived from

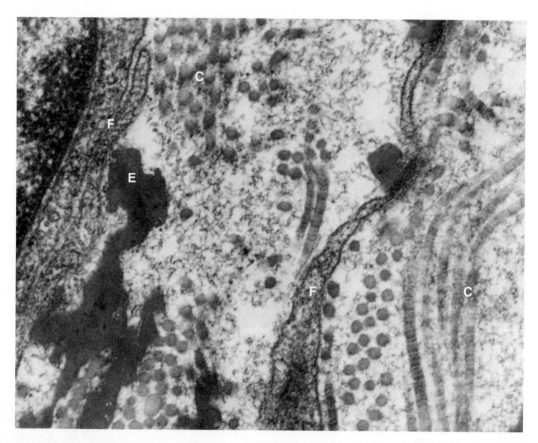

Figure 1–2. Connective tissue matrix. In an electron micrograph, various elements of the matrix are visualized. The matrix consists of proteins and cells embedded in ground substance. Collagen (C) and elastic (E) fibers and fibroblast cells (F) are visible. The granularity of the ground substance is an artifact of the fixation procedure used in preparing the sample. × 100,000. (From Junqueira LC: *Basic Histology,* 8th ed. Appleton & Lange, 1995, p. 89, with permission.)

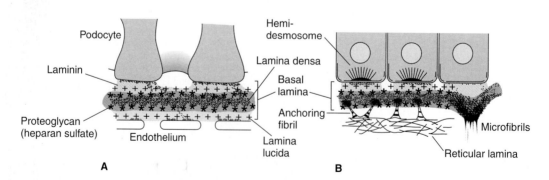

Figure 1–3. Types of basement membranes. This thick basement membrane (A) connects an epithelial and an endothelial cell layer. It is formed by fusion of the basal laminae of the two layers. A thick central lamina densa (darker colored zone) has a lamina lucida (lighter colored zone) on either side. Such basement membranes are found in the kidney glomerulus (shown here) and in the pulmonary alveoli. The more common type of basement membrane (B) forms the boundary between an epithelial cell layer and connective tissue. It is formed by association of the cell's basal lamina and the reticular lamina of the connective tissue. Note anchoring fibrils composed of type VII collagen, which bind the basal lamina to collagen. Microfibrils perforate the basal lamina, binding it to elastic fibers in connective tissue. (From Junqueira LC: *Basic Histology,* 8th ed. Appleton & Lange, 1995, p. 63, with permission.)

connective tissue cells. These cells are produced in the myeloid tissue of the inner compartment of bones, called the bone marrow.

Cells of muscle tissue. The third basic tissue is muscle. Although cells in this tissue are specialized for contraction, their outward appearance is usually quite distinct (and dissimilar from one another). There are four categories of contractile cells: skeletal or striated muscle cells, cardiac (heart) muscle cells, smooth muscle cells (derived from fibroblasts), and myoepithelial cells (derived from ectoderm).

Skeletal muscle cells usually have a highly elongated shape and are often referred to as muscle fibers. A single muscle fiber (cell) is a syncytium that contains many nuclei with a common cytoplasm. New muscle fibers develop from the fusion of myoblasts (Figures 1–4 and 1–5). Cardiac muscle cells, like striated muscle cells, form a syncytial structure. The contractile proteins (myosin, actin, and other structural proteins) are aligned in an orderly arrangement called a **sarcomere** (see Chapter 7). Smooth muscle

cells do not form syncytial connections. Rather, they align into long bundles, and their contraction is much slower and more prolonged than that of striated or cardiac cells. These cells, which are important components of blood vessels, participate in directing blood flow, especially in the microcirculation (capillary beds). Myoepithelial cells also lack striations and are derived embryologically from ectoderm rather than from mesoderm, which is the embryonic origin of the other muscle cells. These contractile cells regulate the responses of certain sensory cells, such as the iris, sweat glands, milk, and other glands that respond to sensory information (Figure 1–6).

Cells of nervous tissue. Nerve cells, the fourth major class of basic tissue, are characterized by their "irritability" and capacity to conduct electrical impulses. These cells constitute the master communication network of the body. The neuron is divided into three large groups: unipolar, bipolar, and multipolar. These groups reflect the number of processes that arise from the cell body (Figure 1–7). The simplest,

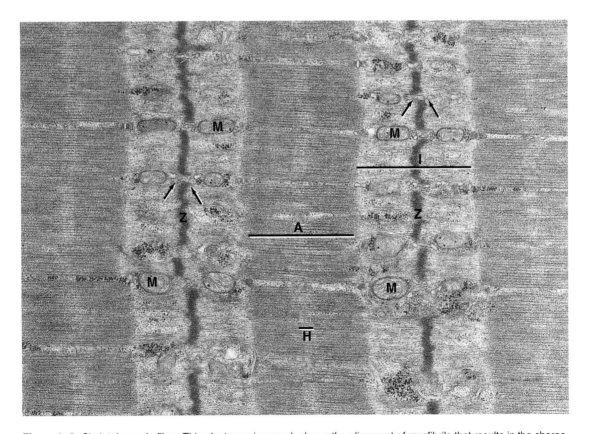

Figure 1–4. Skeletal muscle fiber. This electron micrograph shows the alignment of myofibrils that results in the characteristic striated morphology of this type of cell. The sarcomere, the contractile unit of the fiber, is delineated by adjacent Z lines (Z), which bisect the I band (I). Within the sarcomere is an electron-dense A band (A) bisected by an electron-lucent H band (H). Mitochondria (M) are also visible. Rat; × 24,280. (Reproduced, with permission, from Berman I: *Color Atlas of Basic Histology.* Appleton & Lange, 1993, p. 72. Courtesy of M Snow.) See also Figure 7–12 for additional details.

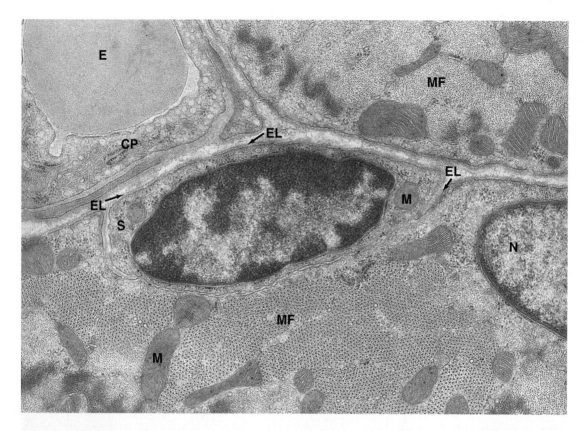

Figure 1–5. Skeletal muscle satellite cell in cross section. This electron micrograph of a skeletal muscle satellite cell shows that it (S) lies completely within the external lamina (EL) of the muscle fiber (MF) at the bottom of the micrograph. (N = nucleus of muscle fiber; M = mitochondria; CP = cell process of capillary endothelial cell; E = erythrocyte.) Rat; × 25,600. (Reproduced, with permission, from Berman I: *Color Atlas of Basic Histology.* Appleton & Lange, 1993, p. 72. Courtesy of M Snow.)

the unipolar neuron, has a single primary process with many branches; one branch serves as the axon, and the others function as dendrites. Most unipolar neurons are found in invertebrates. The bipolar neuron has two major identifiable processes: a dendritic process with many branches that convey information from the periphery to the cell body and an axon that conveys information from the cell body to other neurons. The axons of neurons terminate at neuronal junctions called **synapses.** Electrical impulses are transferred from one neuron to the next by secretion of chemical substances called **neurotransmitters,** which are released at the synaptic junction. Bipolar neurons communicate signals to the central nervous system (CNS) through neuron relay systems. Multipolar neurons are predominant in the CNS of vertebrates. These cells have a single axon, but they have a complex array of dendritic connections. For example, a multipolar axon of a spinal motor cell possesses a moderate number of dendrites, approximately 10,000. Approximately 2000 of these dendritic con-

nections occur at the cell body, whereas approximately 8000 connections occur on the dendritic tree. A Purkinje cell in the cerebellum is a much larger multipolar neuron and has as many as 150,000 dendritic contacts.

A second major class of nervous system cells is composed of the **glial cells.** There are approximately 10–50 times more glial cells than neurons in the CNS of vertebrates. The three main types of glial cells are oligodendroglial cells, Schwann cells, and astrocytes. Glial cells perform several major functions in the CNS, including:

1. support elements for neurons and separate and insulate neurons from one another;
2. produce myelin, which is an insulating sheath necessary for certain types of neurons;
3. serve as scavenger cells to clear cellular debris;
4. help form the impervious cellular barrier between the brain and capillaries, called the blood-brain barrier.

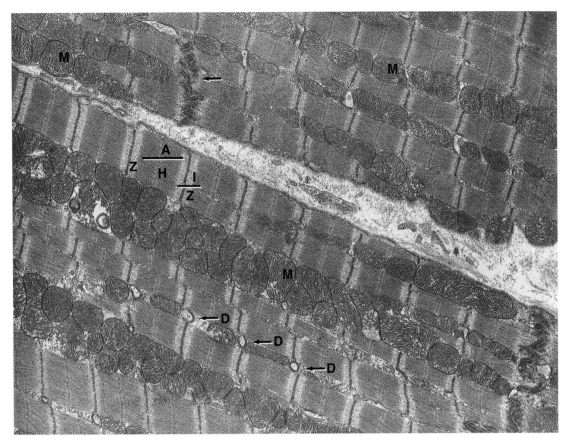

Figure 1–6. Cardiac muscle. This low-power electron micrograph of cardiac muscle illustrates its characteristic features. As in other skeletal muscle, a sarcomere is delineated by adjacent Z lines (Z). Note the intercalated disk (arrow), which is a unique feature of cardiac muscle morphology. (I = I band; A = A band; H = H band; M = mitochondria; D = diads of tubular system.) Rat; × 5500. (Reproduced, with permission, from Berman I: *Color Atlas of Basic Histology.* Appleton & Lange, 1993, p. 77. Courtesy of J-P Brunschwig.)

Glial cells participate in other important roles within the CNS, and these functions are still being discovered and documented.

Different Phenotypes of Cells of the Four Basic Tissues

We have very briefly listed and commented on the four basic types of cells that comprise the tissues of the body. Like the carbon atom of organic chemistry, these cells have been modified in almost unimaginable ways to form phenotypes far removed from the original basic structure of the progenitor cells. This same concept of building and modifying the basic structure of the cell is fundamental to the differentiation and formation of specialized function. A compendium of some 200 distinctly different cell types was recently compiled from histology texts. The cells of each category were identified and examined with the use of light and electron microscopy. This catalog

of human cells has a particularly useful focus: It lets us see in a relatively small space a variety of cellular phenotypes that have been developed to carry out myriad cellular tasks (Table 1–1).

For more on the structure of cells that play a key role in human health and disease, the reader is referred to in *Color Atlas of Basic Histopathology*, by Clara Milikowski and Irwin Berman, Appleton & Lange, 1997.

REGULATION OF GENE EXPRESSION: BRIEF OVERVIEW

With very few exceptions, each cell in the human body contains precisely the same complement of genes (thought to be between 100,000 and 300,000). Cells differ so greatly from one another because different combinations of genes are expressed in

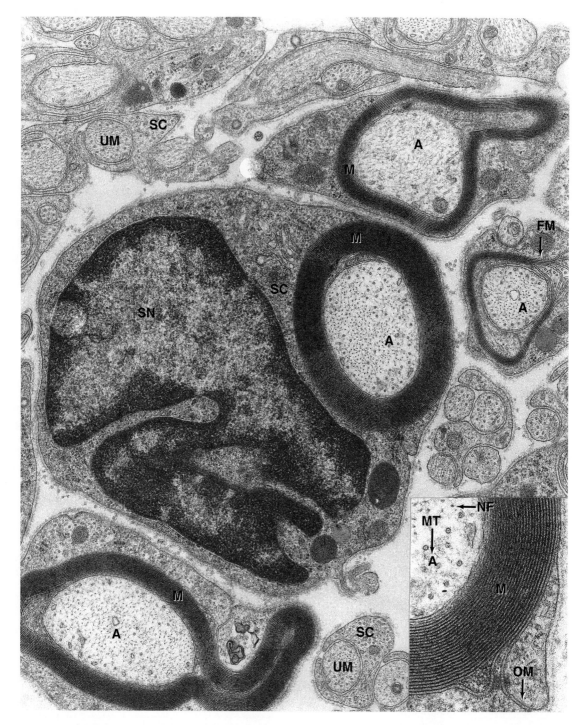

Figure 1–7. Peripheral nerve fibers. This electron micrograph shows myelinated and unmyelinated nerve fibers. (SN = Schwann cell nucleus; SC = Schwann cell cytoplasm; M = myelin sheath; FM = forming myelin sheath; UM = unmyelinated axon.) Rat; × 28,420. The inset micrograph shows a partial view of a myelinated axon in cross section. (OM = outer mesaxon; M = myelin sheath; NF = neurofilaments; MT = microtubules.) Rat; × 69,580. (Reproduced, with permission, from Berman I: *Color Atlas of Basic Histology.* Appleton & Lange, 1993, p. 68. Courtesy of M Bartlett Bunge.)

Table 1–1. Adult human cell types.[1]

Keratinizing epithelial cells
  Keratinocyte of epidermis (= differentiating epidermal cell)
  Basal cell of epidermis (stem cell)
  Keratinocyte of fingernails and toenails
  Basal cell of nail bed (stem cell)
  Hair shaft cells
    Medullary
    Cortical
    Cuticular
  Hair-root sheath cells
    Cuticular
    Of Huxley's layer
    Of Henle's layer
    External
  Hair matrix cell (stem cell)
Cells of wet stratified barrier epithelia
  Surface epithelial cell of stratified squamous epithelium of cornea, tongue, oral cavity, esophagus, anal canal, distal urethra, vagina
  Basal cell of these epithelia (stem cell)
  Cell of urinary epithelium (lining bladder and urinary ducts)
Epithelial cells specialized for exocrine secretion
  Cells of salivary gland
    Mucous cell (secretion rich in polysaccharide)
    Serous cell (secretion rich in glycoprotein enzymes)
  Cell of von Ebner's gland in tongue (secretion to wash over taste buds)
  Cell of mammary gland, secreting milk
  Cell of lacrimal gland, secreting tears
  Cell of ceruminous gland of ear, secreting wax
  Cell of eccrine sweat gland, secreting glycoproteins (dark cell)
  Cell of eccrine sweat gland, secreting small molecules (clear cell)
  Cell of apocrine sweat gland (odoriferous secretion, sex-hormone sensitive)
  Cell of gland of Moll in eyelid (specialized sweat gland)
  Cell of sebaceous gland, secreting lipid-rich sebum
  Cell of Bowman's gland in nose (secretion to wash over olfactory epithelium)
  Cell of Brunner's gland in duodenum, secreting alkaline solution of mucus and enzymes
  Cell of seminal vesicle, secreting components of seminal fluid, including fructose (as fuel for swimming sperm)
  Cell of prostate gland, secreting other components of seminal fluid
  Cell of bulbourethral gland, secreting mucus
  Cell of Bartholin's gland, secreting vaginal lubricant
  Cell of gland of Littré, secreting mucus

Cell of endometrium of uterus, secreting mainly carbohydrates
Isolated goblet cell of respiratory and digestive tracts, secreting mucus
Mucous cell of lining of stomach
Zymogenic cell of gastric gland, secreting pepsinogen
Oxyntic cell of gastric gland, secreting HCl
Acinar cell of pancreas, secreting digestive enzymes and bicarbonate
Paneth cell of small intestine, secreting lysozyme
Type II pneumocyte of lung, secreting surfactant
Clara cell of lung (function unknown)
Cells specialized for secretion of hormones
  Cells of anterior pituitary, secreting
    Growth hormone
    Follicle-stimulating hormone
    Luteinizing hormone
    Prolactin
    Adrenocorticotropic hormone
    Thyroid-stimulating hormone
  Cell of intermediate pituitary, secreting
    Melanocyte-stimulating hormone
  Cells of posterior pituitary, secreting
    Oxytocin
    Vasopressin
  Cells of gut and respiratory tract, secreting
    Serotonin
    Endorphin
    Somatostatin
    Gastrin
    Secretin
    Cholecystokinin
    Insulin
    Glucagon
    Bombesin
  Cells of thyroid gland, secreting
    Thyroid hormone
    Calcitonin
  Cells of parathyroid gland, secreting
    Parathyroid hormone
    Oxyphil cell (function unknown)
  Cells of adrenal gland, secreting
    Epinephrine
    Norepinephrine
    Steroid hormones
      Mineralocorticoids
      Glucocorticoids
  Cells of gonads, secreting
    Testosterone (Leydig cell of testis)
    Estrogen (theca interna cell of ovarian follicle)
    Progesterone (corpus luteum cell of ruptured ovarian follicle)
  Cells of juxtaglomerular apparatus of kidney
    Juxtaglomerular cell (secreting renin)
    Macula densa cell
    Peripolar cell
    Mesangial cell
    (Uncertain but probably related in function; possibly involved in secretion of erythropoietin)

Epithelial absorptive cells in gut, exocrine glands, and urogenital tract
  Brush border cell of intestine (with microvilli)
  Striated duct cell of exocrine glands
  Gall bladder epithelial cell
  Brush border cell of proximal tubule of kidney
  Distal tubule cell of kidney
  Nonciliated cell of ductulus efferens
  Epididymal principal cell
  Epididymal basal cell
Cells specialized for metabolism and storage
  Hepatocyte (liver cell)
  Fat cells
    White fat
    Brown fat
  Lipocyte of liver
Epithelial cells serving primarily a barrier function, lining the lung, gut, exocrine glands, and urogenital tract
  Type I pneumocyte (lining air space of lung)
  Pancreatic duct cell (centroacinar cell)
  Nonstriated duct cell of sweat gland, salivary gland, mammary gland, etc (various)
  Parietal cell of kidney glomerulus
  Podocyte of kidney glomerulus
  Cell of thin segment of loop of Henle (in kidney)
  Collecting duct cell (in kidney)
  Duct cell of seminal vesicle, prostate gland, etc (various)
Epithelial cells lining closed internal body cavities
  Vascular endothelial cells of blood vessels and lymphatics
    Fenestrated
    Continuous
    Splenic
  Synovial cell (lining joint cavities, secreting largely hyaluronic acid)
  Serosal cell (lining peritoneal, pleural, and pericardial cavities)
  Squamous cell (lining perilymphatic space of ear)
  Cells lining endolymphatic space of ear
    Squamous cell
    Columnar cells of endolymphatic sac
      With microvilli
      Without microvilli
    "Dark" cell
    Vestibular membrane cell
    Stria vascularis basal cell
    Stria vascularis marginal cell
    Cell of Claudius
    Cell of Boettcher
  Choroid plexus cell (secreting cerebrospinal fluid)
  Squamous cell of pia-arachnoid
  Cells of ciliary epithelium of eye
    Pigmented
    Nonpigmented
  Corneal "endothelial" cell

(continued)

Table 1–1 (cont'd). Adult human cell types.[1]

Ciliated cells with propulsive function
Of respiratory tract
Of oviduct and of endometrium of uterus (in female)
Of rete testis and ductulus efferens (in male)
Of central nervous system (ependymal cell lining brain cavities)
Cell specialized for secretion of extracellular matrix
Epithelial
Ameloblast (secreting enamel of tooth)
Planum semilunatum cell of vestibular apparatus of ear (secreting proteoglycan)
Interdental cell of organ of Corti (secreting tectorial "membrane" covering hair cells of organ of Corti)
Nonepithelial (connective tissue)
Fibroblasts (various—of loose connective tissue, of cornea, of tendon, of reticular tissue of bone marrow, etc)
Pericyte of blood capillary
Nucleus pulposus cell of intervertebral disc
Cementoblast/cementocyte (secreting bonelike cementum of root of tooth)
Odontoblast/odontocyte (secreting dentin of tooth)
Chondrocytes
Of hyaline cartilage
Of fibrocartilage
Of elastic cartilage
Osteoblast/osteocyte
Osteoprogenitor cell (stem cell of osteoblasts)
Hyalocyte of vitreous body of eye
Stellate cell of perilymphatic space of ear
Contractile cells
Skeletal muscle cells
Red (slow)
White (fast)
Intermediate
Muscle spindle–nuclear bag
Muscle spindle–nuclear chain
Satellite cell (stem cell)
Heart muscle cells
Ordinary
Nodal
Purkinje fiber
Smooth muscle cells (various)
Myoepithelial cells

Of iris
Of exocrine glands
Cells of blood and immune system
Red blood cell
Megakaryocyte
Macrophages and related cells
Monocyte
Connective-tissue macrophage (various)
Langerhans cell (in epidermis)
Osteoclast (in bone)
Dendritic cell (in lymphoid tissues)
Microglial cell (in central nervous system)
Neutrophil
Eosinophil
Basophil
Mast cell
T lymphocyte
Helper T cell
Suppressor T cell
Killer T cell
B lymphocyte
Immunoglobulin M
Immunoglobulin G
Immunoglobulin A
Immunoglobulin E
Killer cell
Stem cells and committed progenitors for the blood and immune system (various)
Sensory transducers
Photoreceptors
Rod
Cones
Blue sensitive
Green sensitive
Red sensitive
Hearing
Inner hair cell of organ of Corti
Outer hair cell of organ of Corti
Acceleration and gravity
Type I hair cell of vestibular apparatus of ear
Type II hair cell of vestibular apparatus of ear
Taste
Type II taste bud cell
Smell
Olfactory neuron
Basal cell of olfactory epithelium (stem cell for olfactory neurons)
Blood pH
Carotid body cell
Type I
Type II
Touch
Merkel cell of epidermis

Primary sensory neurons specialized for touch (various)
Temperature
Primary sensory neurons specialized for temperature
Cold sensitive
Heat sensitive
Pain
Primary sensory neurons specialized for pain (various)
Configurations and forces in musculoskeletal system
Proprioceptive primary sensory neurons (various)
Autonomic neurons
Cholinergic (various)
Adrenergic (various)
Peptidergic (various)
Supporting cells of sense organs and of peripheral neurons
Supporting cells of organ of Corti
Inner pillar cell
Outer pillar cell
Inner phalangeal cell
Outer phalangeal cell
Border cell
Hensen cell
Supporting cell of vestibular apparatus
Supporting cell of taste bud (type I taste bud cell)
Supporting cell of olfactory epithelium
Schwann cell
Satellite cell (encapsulating peripheral nerve cell bodies)
Enteric glial cell
Neurons and glial cells of central nervous system
Neurons (huge variety of types—still poorly classified)
Glial cells
Astrocyte (various)
Oligodendrocyte
Lens cells
Anterior lens epithelial cell
Lens fiber (crystallin-containing cell)
Pigment cells
Melanocyte
Retinal pigmented epithelial cell
Germ cells
Oogonium/oocyte
Spermatocyte
Spermatogonium (stem cell for spermatocyte)
Nurse cells
Ovarian follicle cell
Sertoli cell (in testis)
Thymus epithelial cell

[1]From Alberts B et al: *Molecular Biology of the Cell,* 3rd ed. Garland, 1994, p. 1188, with permission.

specific cell types. Both repression and activation of genes occur during development; often, both are maintained throughout the life of the differentiated cell. Moreover, during cell development, many genes become irreversibly shut down; these genes therefore lose competence for transcription and are never expressed in that cell type.

In addition to these more or less permanent modifications, the expression of many genes within specific cell types is regulated. For example, the rate at which transcription of the messenger ribonucleic acid (mRNA) of that gene occurs can be transiently increased or decreased by the action of proteins that bind to regulatory regions of the gene. The activity of these regulatory proteins is in turn controlled by receptors located either within the cell or on the cell surface. These different receptors recognize specific molecules, such as steroid hormones, peptide growth factors, and neurotransmitters, and relay molecular messages into the cell that controls the regulatory proteins for deoxyribonucleic acid (DNA; see Appendix A).

The two major functional regions of template DNA are the coding and regulatory regions. Messenger RNA is transcribed from DNA (encoding a protein) by the action of the enzyme RNA polymerase II. The regulatory region of the gene usually lies upstream of the coding region. Because these DNA regulatory elements reside near the coding region and are linked to it, they are called *cis*-**regulatory elements.** In contrast, the transcription of regulatory proteins that bind to these elements are called ***trans*-regulatory elements** because they often encode genes that are not linked to the gene being regulated.

The regulatory region of a structural gene consists of a proximal region called the **promoter.** This region is close to the transcription start site and, in most instances, contains a region of approximately eight base pairs, which includes several adenine (A) and thymidine (T) nucleotides. This region, which is usually referred to as the **TATA box,** is also surrounded by a region rich in guanine (G) and cytosine (C).

The TATA box and adjacent DNA elements in the promoter are involved in positioning the RNA polymerase in the region in which transcription of mRNA begins. The TATA box is occupied by a complex of other proteins called the TATA box–binding proteins. These proteins are thought to interact directly with RNA polymerase II, and their binding is directed to a region of DNA adjacent to the site at which transcription starts. In addition, other DNA regulatory modules are often near the TATA box. These modules include the CAAT box and the G-C–rich modules that may facilitate the initial binding of the polymerase. Another DNA regulatory region is called the **enhancer region.** The enhancer elements can be located within a few hundred base pairs of the promoter but are usually found far away from the gene they help regulate. Each individual control element of the enhancer region is usually 7–20 base pairs long and functions as a binding site for proteins that control whether a gene will be transcribed by RNA polymerase II. It is interesting that the enhancer elements are neither sequence nor orientation specific.

Enhancer or promoter DNA sequences to which cell-specific regulatory proteins bind are called response elements. The cyclic adenosine monophosphate (cAMP) response element therefore consists of the sequence ACGTCA; this sequence recognizes cAMP response element binding proteins, which are activated by phosphorylation under the control of cAMP-dependent protein kinase (see Chapter 9). Other specific response elements have been identified. For example, intracellular steroid hormone receptors, growth hormone, and other proteins bind to specific DNA sequences that control the transcription of genes downstream of the binding of these proteins.

Some genes—the so-called constitutively expressed genes—have regulatory proteins that are always bound to their promoter regions, thereby permitting basal levels of transcription. On the other hand, the promoter regions of some genes are bound by regulatory proteins only intermittently, which permits the gene to be induced or repressed by appropriate transcriptional regulators. Whether the RNA polymerase II binds and transcribes a gene, and how often it does so in any given period, is determined by transcriptional regulators that bind to different segments of the promoter and enhancer regions.

Transcription factors that bind gene-control regions typically have three functional domains:

1. a DNA-binding domain, which contains many basic residues that permit the protein to recognize and bind selectively to a specific DNA sequence;
2. an activator domain, which is often acidic and permits the protein to contact and activate basal transcriptional machinery (TATA box–binding proteins and RNA polymerase II);
3. one or more ligand-binding or phosphorylating domains, which are required to activate the transcription factors.

Because DNA transcription factors are key regulators of gene expression, their biochemical properties have been the subject of intense examination. We now recognize three major families:

1. Helix-turn-helix proteins. This group of DNA binding proteins are most commonly homodimers. Each subunit contains a protein alpha helix motif that fits into the major groove of the DNA helix. This is the "recognition helix." In some instances, the remaining portion of the protein backbone will fold out of the major DNA helix and surround it, and a second helix motif will fit into the major groove on the next turn of

the DNA. When these proteins fit into the DNA site, they affect the conformation of the DNA and make it either more accessible for transcription (and would be "inducers") or less accessible (and would be "repressors").

2. Zinc finger proteins. This group is so named because a stretch of approximately 23 amino acids that contain alternating cystines and histidines forms a finger-like projection whose structure is maintained by the binding of a zinc ion. The proteins interact with the DNA through the loop region. Glucocorticoid, estrogen, vitamin A, progesterone, thyroid, and retinoic acid receptors each contain two zinc fingers.

3. Amphipathic helical proteins. This group includes two subgroups: helix-loop-helix proteins and leucine zipper proteins (see Chapter 9).

Gene regulatory proteins that contain a leucine zipper motif can form either homodimers, in which each of the subunits are identical, or heterodimers, in which the subunits are not alike. Because heterodimers form from two different proteins with different DNA binding specificities, the ability of certain transcription factors to form functional dimers greatly expands the repertoire of DNA-binding proteins and, hence, gene control. The formation of heterodimers, and even oligomers, of DNA binding proteins (ie, combinatorial control) is one of the most important mechanisms used by eukaryotic cells to control gene expression. It is also important that not all transcription factors can form heterodimers. Otherwise, the cross-talk and specificity for gene control could become incomprehensible to the cell.

Clearly, the principal event in the cell for regulating its behavior and morphology is at the level of gene transcription. This event, however, is not the only opportunity to manage the phenotype of a cell. As determined from many types of studies, several other events can be crucial for controlling gene expression. For example, in addition to transcribing the gene to make an mRNA template, the cellular machinery must process the gene's message; that is, introns must be eliminated, and other components added to the transcript to ensure that the mRNA is functional. After the mRNA is processed, it must be transported from the nucleus into the cytoplasm. Once in the cytoplasm, the mRNA must be translated. The mechanisms of translating mRNA involve a larger number of regulatory molecules, and loss or inactivity of any of these molecules would have a strong influence on the cytoplastic expression of that gene product. Within the cytoplasm, the mRNA can be targeted for rapid degradation or it can be protected by other cytoplasmic proteins; thus, the stability and half-life of the mRNA is a potential site for gene regulation. The final gene product, the protein, must also be functional (active) to reflect the activity of the gene.

SUMMARY

In this chapter, we introduced the four basic types of tissue found in eukaryotes. Within each class, there is extensive cell specialization that is reflected by the cell's phenotype. We showed how the 200 or so different types of cells in the human body can be grouped according to function. The many different morphologic forms are the result of the specific differentiated genes being expressed. We also introduced the concept of how eukaryotic genes are regulated at the transcriptional level. We discussed gene regulatory sites, including the responsive elements in the promoter and enhancer regions. In addition, the basic structure of transcription factors and their various functional domains were presented. External signals received by the cell often stimulate the transcription of genes that control other transcription factors, which in turn "open up" sets of structural genes that lead to the differentiated phenotype of the cell. This tier of gene control is often followed during development. There are particularly sensitive places in the cell where a gene product can be controlled in addition to its transcription.

Molecular Architecture & Functional Components of the Cell Membrane

2

IMPORTANCE OF MEMBRANES IN CELL FUNCTION

Variations in Membranes

This chapter examines the structural and functional properties of cell membranes, in particular the plasma membrane, with a view toward understanding how the membrane carries out its many functions. On the basis of our discussion in Chapter 1 of the more than 200 types of cells found in the human body, it is evident that no single structural form of the plasma cell membrane exists. Rather, the membrane takes on a number of forms depending on the structural and functional role of the cell (Table 2–1).

The cell membrane is defined as *a barrier that surrounds the cytoplasm and marks the boundary of the cell.* However, we know that the membrane is far more than a barrier between the cytosol and the extracellular milieu. The membrane contains molecules that transmit signals from outside the cell into the cytoplasm, as well as to intracellular organelles (Figure 2–1).

Proteins and Lipids

All cell membranes are a complex mixture of proteins and lipids. Three important concepts about membrane structure are

1. **They are *not* homogeneous.** The composition of the membranes surrounding intracellular organelles and the plasma membrane all differ from one another.
2. **Many membrane components are in a state of constant dynamic flux.** Consequently, the membrane is an ever-changing mosaic. Moreover, some parts of a membrane change faster than other parts.
3. **Membrane components are *highly* asymmetric.** The proportions and types of lipids of the inner and outer leaflets are different. Membrane proteins are arranged in the lipids in a highly asymmetrical fashion and have well-defined extracellular and intracellular domains.

When examining a cell that has been prepared for **light microscopy,** we can observe the edge of the cell delineated by the plasma membrane. This snapshot of the membrane, however, does not reveal certain important variations in its structure (Table 2–2). For example, the plasma membrane has specialized areas; each has a unique morphology and performs a specific biomolecular task. Also, the surfaces of most cells that are attached to other cells or to the extracellular matrix have different properties, as we will discuss later in this chapter. A good example of the multispecificity of cells: epithelial cells that form linings in the skin and capillaries.

The diverse morphology of mammalian cells is often a reflection of the complex cytoskeletal network of structural proteins that lie beneath the membrane and within the cytoplasm. The main components of the cytoskeleton—including actin filaments, microtubules, and intermediate filaments—are described in Chapter 7; it is important here to note that these structural elements also help to form the shape of the surface membrane.

In cells that migrate on surfaces or through extracellular spaces, cytoskeletal proteins undergo polymerization and depolymerization as part of motility. Consequently, the membrane also undergoes significant changes. *It is important to understand that this process is made possible by the flexibility and dynamics of the molecules that make up the plasma*

Table 2–1. Major intracellular organelles and their functions. Only the major functions associated with each organelle are listed. In a number of instances, many other pathways, processes, or reactions occur in the organelle.[1]

Organelle or Fraction[2]	Marker	Major Functions
Nucleus	DNA	Site of chromosomes Site of DNA-directed RNA synthesis (transcription)
Mitochondrion	Glutamic dehydrogenase	Citric acid cycle, oxidative phosphorylation
Ribosome[2]	High content of RNA	Site of protein synthesis (translation of mRNA into protein)
Endoplasmic reticulum	Glucose-6-phosphatase	Membrane-bound ribosomes are a major site of protein synthesis Synthesis of various lipids Oxidation of many xenobiotics (cytochrome P450)
Lysosome	Acid phosphatase	Site of many hydrolases (enzymes catalyzing degradative reactions)
Plasma membrane	Na^+ - K^+ ATPase 5′-Nucleotidase	Transport of molecules in and out of cells Intercellular adhesion and communication
Golgi apparatus	Galactosyl transferase	Intracellular sorting of proteins Glycosylation reactions Sulfation reactions
Peroxisome	Catalase Uric acid oxidase	Degradation of certain fatty acids and amino acids Production and degradation of hydrogen peroxide
Cytoskeleton[2]	No specific enzyme markers[3]	Microfilaments, microtubules, intermediate filaments
Cytosol[2]	Lactate dehydrogenase	Enzymes of glycolysis, fatty acid synthesis

[1]Reproduced, with permission, from Murray RK et al: *Harper's Biochemistry,* Appleton & Lange, 1996, p. 9.
[2]An organelle can be defined as a subcellular entity that is membrane-limited and is isolated by centrifugation at high speeds. According to this definition, ribosomes, the cytoskeleton, and the cytosol are not organelles. However, they are considered in this table along with the organelles because they also are usually isolated by centrifugation. They can be considered subcellular entities or fractions. An organelle as isolated by one cycle of differential centrifugation is rarely pure; to obtain a pure fraction usually requires at least several cycles.
[3]The cytoskeletal fractions can be recognized by electron microscopy or by analysis by electrophoresis of the characteristic proteins that they contain.

membrane. This point cannot be overemphasized because it forms the basis for understanding the functional responses of cells. Before continuing, students who would like to review the biochemistry of cellular lipids and proteins are referred to a recent standard biochemistry text.

Important Membrane Functions

Membranes control the intracellular environment of the cell. A major functional property of the membrane is that it forms a barrier around the cytoplasm, and this barrier controls the molecules that flow in and out of the cell. To a large extent, this process results from the impermeability of the lipids of the membrane to water and other hydrophilic molecules. Membranes possess proteins that form channels and pores that are involved in highly selective transport of molecules into and out of the cell.

Membranes permit and facilitate communication between and within cells. The membrane is where molecular information is received, transduced, and relayed into the cell (Table 2–3). Cell behavior is regulated by its immediate neighbors and by mole-

cules produced by cells farther away. For example, normal cells growing in a tissue culture plate stop dividing when the surface of the dish is completely covered with cells and all cells are touching each other. This phenomenon is called **density-dependent inhibition (DDI) of growth.** Conversely, mutant cells that have lost the ability to receive the DDI signal continue to grow and form layer after layer of cells. Cells that display this behavior form tumors.

The relay of electrical signals between nerve cells occurs at the membrane, as does information that allows cells to form close communication with one another, eg, in the formation of neuronal networks. It is now recognized that the ebb and flow of specific markers on the cell surface is critical in cellular differentiation and in the formation of assemblies of cells that make tissues and organs. In the early stages of embryogenesis, a cell typically *associates* (binds) and *disassociates* with various other cells. This process is regulated at the cell surface by molecules called **homotypic markers,** which play important roles in tissue formation. These same markers appear on cells that are actively engaged in tissue repair fol-

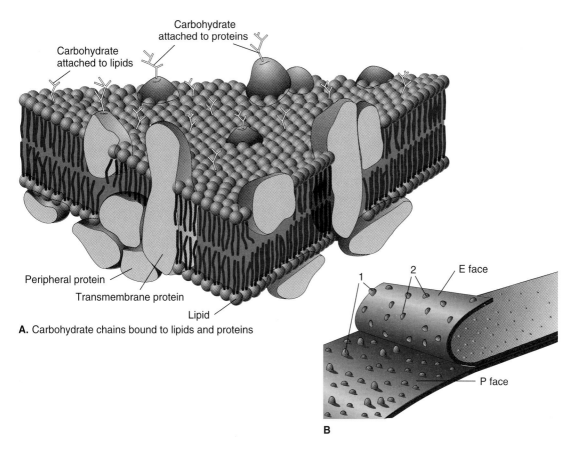

A. Carbohydrate chains bound to lipids and proteins

B

Figure 2–1. (A) Fluid mosaic model of membrane structure. The membrane consists of a lipid bilayer (hydrophilic surfaces, hydrophobic core) and associated proteins. Integral proteins are embedded in the lipid. Proteins that completely span the bilayer are called transmembrane proteins. Peripheral proteins are loosely bound to the cytoplasmic surface. Many lipids and proteins on the external surface have oligosaccharide chains that are exposed to the extracellular environment. (B) When a membrane is freeze fractured, it splits into two lipid layers along the weakest plane of the bilayer, where the hydrophobic tails interact (E = extracellular face; P = protoplasmic face). Most of the membrane particles (1) remain attached to the P face. They are thought to represent proteins or protein aggregates. Few particles remain attached to the E face. For each particle, there is a corresponding depression (2) on the opposite surface. (Modified and reproduced, with permission, from Krstić RV: *Ultrastructure of the Mammalian Cell.* Springer-Verlag, 1979.)

Table 2–2. Enzymatic markers of different membranes.[1]

Membrane	Enzyme
Plasma	5′-Nucleotidase Adenylyl cyclase Na⁺-K⁺ ATPase
Endoplasmic reticulum	Glucose-6-phosphatase
Golgi complex	Galactosyltransferase
Inner mitochondrial membrane	ATP synthase

[1]Membranes contain many proteins, some of which have enzymatic activity. Some of these enzymes are located only in certain membranes and can therefore be used as markers to follow the purification of these membranes. (Reproduced, with permission, from Murray RK et al: *Harper's Biochemistry,* Appleton & Lange, 1996, p. 487.)

Table 2–3. Transfer of material and information across membranes.[1]

Cross-membrane movement of small molecules
  Diffusion (passive and facilitated)
  Active transport
Cross-membrane movement of large molecules
  Endocytosis
  Exocytosis
Signal transmission across membranes
  Cell surface receptors
  1. Signal trasduction (eg, glucagon → cAMP)
  2. Signal internalization (coupled with endocytosis, eg, the LDL receptor, insulin receptor)
  Movement to intracellular receptors (steroid hormones; a form of diffusion)
Intercellular contact and communication

[1]Reproduced, with permission, from Murray RK et al: *Harper's Biochemistry,* Appleton & Lange, 1996, p. 487.

lowing injury. By characterizing homotypic markers and determining the biomolecular signals that regulate their expression, researchers have gained a better understanding of tissue formation and repair.

Membranes allow for tissue formation by forming cell-cell contacts. Many proteins embedded in the membrane have large carbohydrate structures covalently linked on the external face of the cell. These **glycoproteins** frequently terminate in sialic acid residues and give the external cell surface an overall negative charge. The carbohydrate side chains on these glycoproteins and **glycolipids** are important in cell-cell contact. These carbohydrate residues form specific surface antigens, thereby making the membrane surface very immunogenic. The structure of these cell surface antigens is under strict genetic control and is used by the immune system to distinguish between **self** and **non-self.** All cells in an individual bear similar cell surface antigens, and these differ from the surface antigens in any other individual.

Clinical Implications: Blood Transfusion & Graft Transplantation

Among other things, the compatibility of cell surface antigens determines the success of blood transfusion or graft transplantation. The most important surface antigens that determine the success of blood transfusion are the **blood group antigens.** Their antigenic behavior is due to the precise structure of the carbohydrate moieties of the glycoproteins and glycolipids on the erythrocyte surface.

A second set of antigens called transplantation or **histocompatibility antigens** determines the individuality of cell surfaces. Unlike the blood group antigens that define the antigenicity of body fluids as well as cell surfaces, histocompatibility antigens are restricted to the cell surface. The antigenic determinants are polypeptide chains of a group of transmembrane proteins coded for directly by the **major histocompatibility complex** (MHC) on the mammalian genome.

Thus, through histocompatibility and blood group antigens, the plasma membrane of mammalian cells express the genetic individuality of the cell. This complex is invaluable in the defense of the organism, as we will see later. Specifically, the immune response of a T lymphocyte is activated by contact with a cell surface antigen (Ag) that is presented to the T cell by an MHC molecule (Figure 2–2).

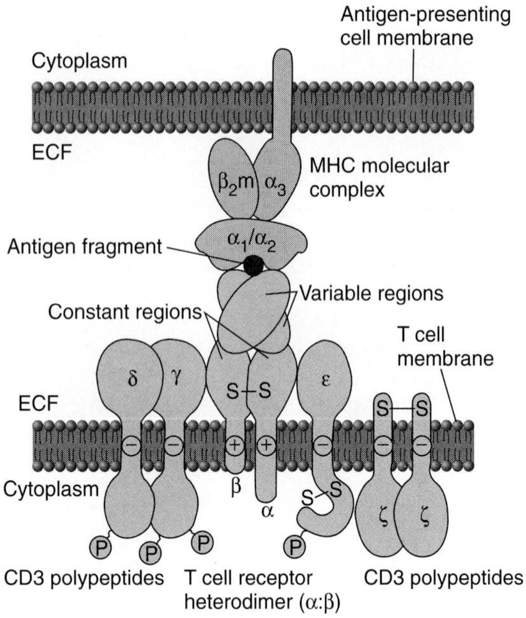

WHERE & HOW MEMBRANES ARE MADE

Location

Protein synthesis occurs principally in two locations: the cytosol and the membrane of the endoplas-

Figure 2–2. Interaction between an antigen-presenting cell (top) and a T lymphocyte (bottom). The MHC protein complex and antigen fragment bind to the α and β subunits of the T cell receptor. The associated CD3 polypeptides on the T cell are part of the receptor complex and may be involved in signal transduction. (ECF = extra-cellular fluid.) (From Krensky AM et al: T-lymphocyte-antigen interactions in transplant rejection. N Engl J Med 1990;332:510. Modified and reproduced by permission of *The New England Journal of Medicine.*)

mic reticulum (ER). Proteins destined to be released into the cytoplasm—for eventual residence in the cell's interior—are synthesized on **ribosomes** located in the **cytosol.** In fact, all ribosomes reside in the cytosol; however, before they attach to a messenger ribonucleic acid (mRNA), ribosomes exist as the two major ribosomal particles, the 40S and 60S **ribonucleoprotein complexes.**

When mRNA is released into the cytoplasm from nuclear pores, an initiation complex is formed in which the 40S particle forms a complex with the mRNA. Once this complex is formed, the 60S particle associates to give a functional ribosome that immediately begins to translate the mRNA into a nascent polypeptide.

When the ribosome encounters a nucleotide sequence that encodes an amino acid sequence which signals that the protein undergoing translation will be a membrane protein or will be secreted from the cell, the protein synthesizing machinery stops reading the mRNA—until it can move to the surface of the ER membrane.

Results from studies of protein synthesis that involve polyribosomes associated with the ER ("membrane-bound ribosomes") suggest that all **integral proteins** are made on the ER membrane, including proteins destined for the plasma membrane. Cellular organelles involved in the synthesis and processing of proteins are shown in Figure 2–3. (Additional details of protein synthesis are provided in Chapter 3.)

Membrane lipids are also manufactured in the ER and are transferred to the plasma membrane. The process of transferring proteins and lipids from the ER to the plasma membrane occurs through **transport vesicles;** the mechanism by which this occurs is discussed in greater detail in Chapters 3 and 4.

An important corollary to the concept that components of the plasma membrane are synthesized in the ER is that these components are transported in a membrane form, ie, the **membrane vesicle.** Thus, it is important to keep in mind that *membranes originate only from preexisting membranes.* Although most of the emphasis in this chapter is on the structure and function of the plasma membrane, it should be emphasized that other organelle membranes of the cell have the same appearance; however, they possess a protein and lipid composition that differs significantly from that of the plasma membrane and the membranes of other cellular organelles.

TYPES & FUNCTION OF MEMBRANE LIPIDS

Table 2–4 lists the major types of membrane lipids, and Table 2–5 shows how lipid unsaturation is related to membrane fluidity, as described below.

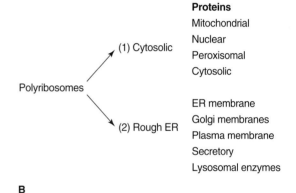

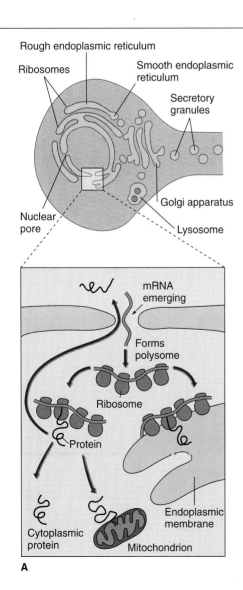

Figure 2–3. Organelles responsible for protein synthesis and processing. (A) Enlargement of a nuclear pore shows mRNA molecules emerging from the nucleus and attaching to ribosomes, forming polysomes. Three classes of proteins are synthesized, with protein class determined by information encoded in the mRNA. (B) The two distinct branches of protein processing are based on the site of protein synthesis (cytosolic or membrane-bound polyribosomes, 1 and 2, respectively.) Note that the mitochondrial proteins in 1 are encoded by nuclear genes. (ER = endoplasmic reticulum.) (Modified and reproduced, with permission, from (A) Kandel ER, Schwartz JH, Jessell TM: *Essentials of Neural Science and Behavior.* Appleton & Lange, 1995, p. 59, and (B) Murray RK: *Harper's Biochemistry,* 24th ed. Appleton & Lange, 1996, p. 491.)

Table 2–4. Principal lipids found in biological membranes. The percentage composition is that of the individual lipids, calculated on the basis of total membrane lipid content.[1]

Principal Membrane Lipids	Net Charge on Head Group	Percentage Composition (range)
Phosphoglycerides	0 to –2	50–90%
Phosphatidylcholine	0	40–60%
Phosphatidylethanolamine	0	20–30%
Phosphatidylserine	–1	5–15%
Cardiolipin	–2	0–20%
Phosphatidylinositol	–1	5–10%
Sphingomyelin	0	5–20%
Cholesterol	0	0–10%

[1]Reproduced, with permission, from Balcavage WX, King MW: *Biochemistry: Examination & Board Review,* Appleton & Lange, 1995, p. 104.

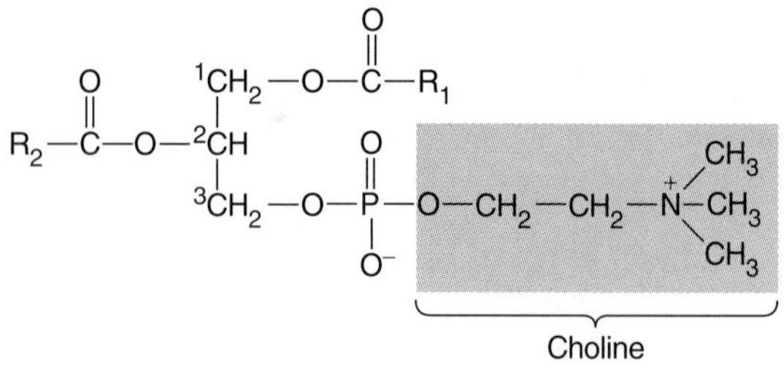

Glycerolphospholipids

The phosphoglycerides are the major class of lipids in biologic membranes. As the name implies, phosphoglycerides contain a glycerol backbone plus esterified fatty acids and alcohols in addition to phosphate. Most polar lipids have a similar overall structure with minor variations. The fatty acyl chains have structural variations, notably, double bonds that impart distinct properties to the **protein-lipid bilayer.** Because carbon atoms involved in a double-bond configuration are not free to rotate, the atoms occupy a fixed position that causes *bends* in the otherwise straight all-trans hydrocarbon chain. This *kink* prevents close packing of the lipid tails and thereby affects the viscosity or fluidity of the membrane.

The length of the acyl chain also has a biologic consequence: *shorter chains are less capable of packing into more rigid structures,* and hence tend to make the membrane less viscous. Thus, both the

Figure 2–4. Structure of phosphatidylcholine.

length of the acyl chain and the number of double bonds play an important role in affecting the fluidity of the membrane.

Sphingolipids

The second major type of membrane lipid are the **sphingolipids,** which are derivatives of C18 amino alcohols. The most common sphingolipids are the **ceramides,** which contain either a phosphatidylcholine (Figure 2–4) or phosphatidylethanolamine. Although sphingomyelins lack the glycerol backbone of phosphatidylglycerol, the overall conformation of the two types of lipids is quite similar. Myelin, the lipid material that surrounds and insulates many nerves, is composed mostly of sphingomyelin (Figure 2–5, Table 2–6).

Glycosphingolipids: Clinical Correlates

Glycosphingolipids are a large subfamily of sphingolipids that contain arrays of sugars linked in the C-X position. The simplest sphingoglycolipids are the **cerebrosides,** which contain a single simple carbohydrate, eg, galactose or glucose. The cerebrosides are present in the membranes of the central ner-

Table 2–5. Relationship of lipid unsaturation to membrane fluidity.[1]

1.	With a constant fatty acyl chain length and constant temperature, the greater the number of double bonds the more fluid the membrane.
2.	With a constant number of double bonds and constant temperature, the longer the acyl chain length the less fluid the membrane.
3.	With any combination of chain length and double bonds, the greater the temperature the more fluid the membrane.

[1]Reproduced, with permission, from Balcavage WX, King MW: *Biochemistry: Examination & Board Review,* Appleton & Lange, 1995, p. 106.

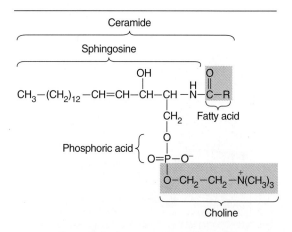

Figure 2–5. Structure of sphingomyelin.

Table 2–6. Disorders associated with abnormal sphingolipid metabolism.[1]

Disorder	Enzyme Deficiency	Accumulating Substance	Symptoms
Tay-Sachs disease	Hexosaminidase A	G_{M2} ganglioside	Mental retardation, blindness, early mortality
Gaucher's disease	Glucocerebrosidase	Glucocerebroside	Hepatosplenomegaly, mental retardation in infantile form, long bone degeneration
Fabry's disease	α-Galactosidase A	Globotriaosylceramide or Ceramide trihexoside (CTH)	Kidney failure, skin rashes
Niemann-Pick disease	Sphingomyelinase	Sphingomyelin	Mental retardation, hepatosplenomegaly
Krabbe's disease; globoid leukodystrophy	Galactocerebrosidase	Galactocerebroside	Mental retardation, myelin deficiency
Sandhoff-Jatzkewitz disease	Hexosaminidase A and B	Globoside or G_{M2} ganglioside	Same symptoms as Tay-Sachs, progresses more rapidly
G_{M1} gangliosidosis	G_{M1} ganglioside: β-galactosidase	G_{M1} ganglioside	Mental retardation, skeletal abnormalities, hepatomegaly
Sulfatide lipodosis; metachromatic leukodystrophy	Arylsulfatase A	Sulfatide	Mental retardation, metachromasia of nerves
Fucosidosis	α-L-Fucosidase	Pentahexosylfucoglycolipid	Cerebral degeneration, thickened skin, muscle spasticity
Farber's lipogranulomatosis	Acid ceramidase	Ceramide	Hepatosplenomegaly, painful swollen joints

[1]Reproduced, with permission, from Balcavago WX, King MW: *Biochemistry: Examination & Board Review,* Appleton & Lange, 1995, p. 88.

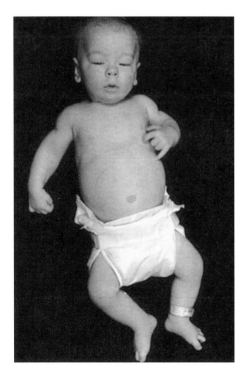

Figure 2–6. Child with GM_1 gangliosidosis. (Reproduced, with permission, from Oski FA et al (editors): *Principles and Practice of Pediatrics,* 2nd ed. Lippincott, 1994.)

vous system and are involved in insulating the neuron. A second member of the sphingoglycolipid family are the **gangliosides,** which have more than 60 different members. This family is distinguished by its complex carbohydrates, which function in several ways. Their complex head-groups extend well beyond the surface of the cell and act as specific receptors for various molecules.

Gangliosides are specific determinants of cell-cell recognition, so they likely play an important role in cell growth and differentiation of tissues. Dysfunction in ganglioside metabolism can lead to an autosomal recessive disorder called gangliosidosis (Figure 2–6).

The well-known blood group antigens A, B, and O are due to specific arrangements of carbohydrates on glycolipids within the plasma membrane of cells. As stated, the plasma membrane undergoes a huge amount of turnover; thus, the cell must be able to degrade the complex glycolipids. In certain human diseases, the enzymes required to degrade these glycolipids are either missing or dysfunctional. When this occurs, the cell cannot break down glycolipids. This leads to the accumulation of glycolipids in the cell and ultimately causes cell death. The group of diseases caused by an inability to degrade complex glycolipids are called the **mucopolysaccharidoses,** of

Table 2–7. The mucopolysaccharidoses.[1]

Type	Lysosomal Enzyme or Biochemical Defect	Clinical Sample	Inheritance
Hurler, type IH	α-L-Iduronidase	WBC	AR
Scheie, type IS	α-L-Iduronidase	WBC	AR
Hunter, type II	Iduronosulfatase	S	XL
Sanfilippo A, type IIIA	Heparan-N-sulfamidase	WBC	AR
Sanfilippo B, type IIIB	α-N-Acetylglucosaminidase	S	AR
Sanfilippo C, type IIIC	Acetyl-CoA:α-glucosaminide N-acetyltransferase	WBC	AR
Sanfilippo D, type IIID	N-Acetylglucosamine-6-sulfatase	WBC	AR
Morquio A, type IVA	N-Acetylgalactosamine-6-sulfatase	SF	AR
Morquio B, type IVB	β-Galactosidase, specific for keratan sulfate	SF	AR
Maroteaux-Lamy, type VI	Aryl sulfatase B	WBC	AR
Sly, type VII	β-Glucuronidase	WBC	AR

[1]Reproduced, with permission, from Seashore MR, Wappner RS: *Genetics in Primary Care & Clinical Medicine,* Appleton & Lange, 1996, p. 241.
AR = autosomal recessive; XL = X-linked; S = serum; SF = cultured skin fibroblasts; WBC = leukocytes.

which Hunter syndrome, Hurler syndrome, and Sanfilippo syndrome are the most notable (Table 2–7).

For more on genetic diseases associated with abnormalities of membrane lipids, consult *Genetics in Primary Care and Clinical Medicine,* Appleton & Lange, 1996.

Cholesterol

Cholesterol is the third major class of membrane lipids. This steroid serves a number of roles in membrane function (Figure 2–7). The polar OH group gives the molecule a weak amphipathic character, whereas its fused ring structure is hydrophobic and intercalates with the acyl chains of the other lipids. The insertion of this portion of the cholesterol molecule into the hydrophobic domains of the other lipids has the effect of reducing the "packing together" of the unsaturated acyl chain. This keeps the interior of the bilayer less viscous and hence slightly more fluid. The resulting fluidity facilitates the lateral movement of lipids within the plane of the lipid bilayer.

A somewhat opposite effect is attributed to the OH-region of the steroid, which is located nearer the head-groups of the other lipids. The OH-region serves as a "cementing together" of the hydrophilic regions of the membrane. When this occurs, it makes the membrane less permeable to small molecules. Most membrane phospholipids contain one or more *cis* double bonds in their acyl chains. This makes it difficult to pack together, the chains are more flexible, and hence the membrane is less viscous at ambient temperatures.

This flexibility permits cavities to form, which in turn facilitates the movement of small water-soluble molecules, eg, glucose. The presence of cholesterol helps to seal the membrane more tightly near the hydrophilic domain and at the same time fill the cavities formed from the kinked *cis* double bond in the acyl chain. Although it can readily flip-flop across the bilayer, cholesterol tends to accumulate in the outer leaflet—this also thickens the bilayer. The physical and chemical properties of cholesterol are critical to its role in membrane permeability (Figures 2–8 and 2–9).

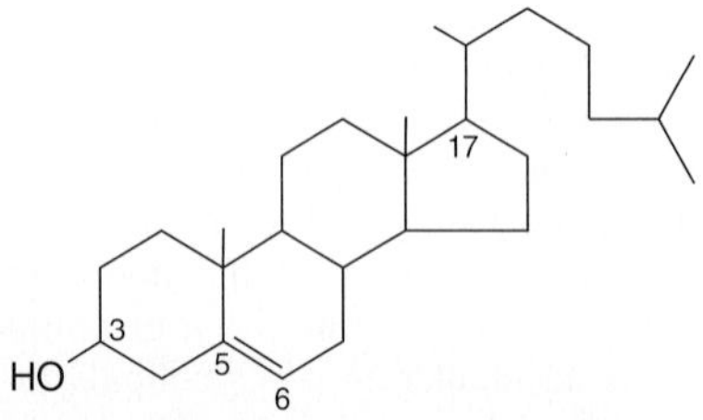

Figure 2–7. Structure of cholesterol.

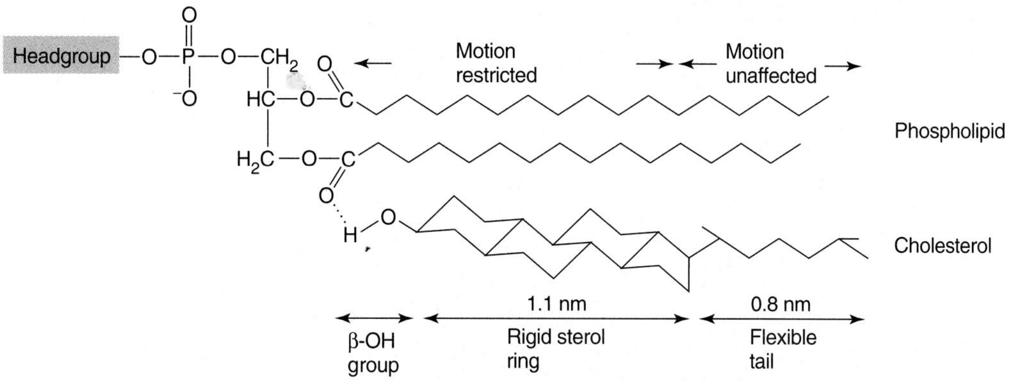

Figure 2–8. Insertion of cholesterol into a phospholipid bilayer. The diagram shows the alignment of a cholesterol molecule with a phospholipid that is part of a lipid bilayer. (Modified from Houslay MD, Stanley KK: *Dynamics of Biological Membranes.* John Wiley & Sons, 1983, p. 72. Copyright © 1983 John Wiley & Sons. Reprinted by permission of John Wiley & Sons, Ltd.)

FUNCTIONAL PROPERTIES OF LIPIDS

The following architectural features of lipid molecules determine the structure and function in the membranes of eukaryotic cells.

Amphipathic Nature of Lipids

The **amphipathic character** of membrane lipids helps to determine the lipid bilayer. Two well-defined domains exist for phospholipids. One comprises the phosphate head-group with its substitutions. This domain has chemical features that make it soluble in water, hence it is described as **hydrophilic.** In contrast, the acyl chains that protrude away from the glycerol backbone are quite apolar and, thus, insoluble in water. For this reason, they are said to be **hydrophobic.** The property of having both a hydrophilic and hydrophobic region in the same molecule is called **amphipathic.**

If one were to place pure phosphatidylcholine in water, the hydrophilic region would be readily soluble, but the hydrophobic domains would be forced out of the water into the air, a little like raised hair on

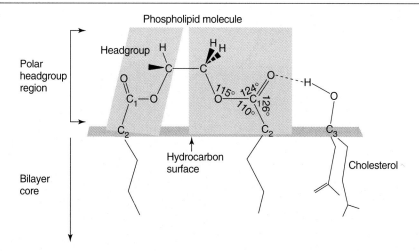

Figure 2–9. Interaction of cholesterol and phospholipid. A cholesterol molecule and a phospholipid molecule interact at the interface between the hydrophilic and hydrophobic portions of the membrane. This diagram shows hydrogen-bond formation between the carbonyl group of the phospholipid and the β-hydroxyl group of the cholesterol. (Modified and reproduced, with permission, from Huang CH: A structural model for the cholesterol-phosphatidylcholine complexes in bilayer membranes. Lipids 1977;12:348. Published by the American Oil Chemists' Society.)

the scalp. It is possible to drive the lipid into the water environment, but the amount of energy (thermal or chemical) required to do this would be quite large. The reason is because water is a polar solvent, and its molecules move at random. To force water molecules into an ordered structure around the apolar acyl chains of the lipid for it to be dissolved in the solution would demand the expenditure of energy. Since this does not happen under physiologic conditions, other events occur that demand much less energy. The apolar regions of the lipid associate with one another and position themselves away from the aqueous environment. This movement of the lipid leads to the formation of two basic types of macromolecular structures (Figure 2–10).

Micelle Arrangement

The **micelle** arrangement can form as either a single or double layer of lipids. The monomolecular arrangement is often the form taken by lipoproteins. The other major form that lipids assume in an aqueous environment is a **bimolecular leaflet,** which is the arrangement utilized in the formation of the membrane bilayer. It should be remembered that *formation of the bilayer occurs spontaneously, and the cell maintains this structure by thermodynamic forces—not by covalent bonds.*

Membrane Lipids Form Special Fluid

The viscosity properties of membrane lipids makes

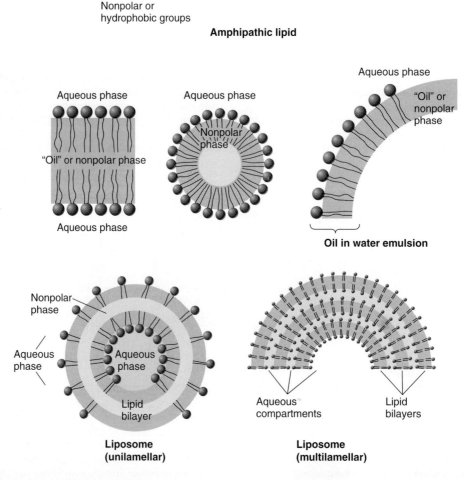

Figure 2–10. Formation of lipid membranes, micelles, emulsions, and liposomes from phospholipid molecules based on their amphipathic nature. (Modified and reproduced, with permission, from Murray RK: *Harper's Biochemistry,* 24th ed. Appleton & Lange, 1996, 157.)

them especially suited to perform membrane functions. Several chemical factors contribute to the viscosity of lipids in the bilayer, in particular:

- The number of hydrocarbons (CH_2) in the acyl chain
- The number of double-bonds in the chain
- The amount of cholesterol located in the bilayer.

The longer and more saturated the acyl chains are, the more likely they are to form close associations, ie, to pack tightly together. This results in a more rigid and less fluid bilayer. It should be noted that the fluidity of the membrane resides to a large extent within the hydrophobic domain. The hydrophilic regions containing the polar head groups of the lipids, however, are not nearly so flexible. How does this occur? The polar groups tend to "organize" to some extent the water molecules that surround them, and this leads to a cementing together of the polar groups. Thus, indirectly and somewhat paradoxically, the associations between water molecules in biologic fluids contribute to the structural maintenance and integrity of the membrane—in this instance, the interaction of water molecules with the polar head-groups of the lipid bilayer.

Although one might imagine that different types of lipids are randomly associated in the membrane, that is not the case. This fact enables the lipids of the membrane to provide regions for specific cellular functions. For example, lipids with saturated acyl chains can accumulate at a particular location in the membrane of a cell, thus making that particular region stiffer and less fluid. In fact, this condition is found at membrane sites that serve to attach the cell to its substrate or to other cells. Moreover, each side of the bilayer has a different lipid composition. Thus, not only can there be packing and accumulation of certain lipids at particular locations of the membrane, but particular regions of each side of the bilayer can exist. This in turn makes the bilayer a type of **lipid mosaic** (Figure 2–1). These phenomena demonstrate that lipids in the bilayer participate in a variety of cellular functions and, at the same time, play a key structural role in the formation of membranes that enclose the cell and its organelles.

Movement Within Plane of Membrane Bilayer

Individual lipids can move within the plane of the membrane. One of the earliest clues that the lipids of a membrane are active came from studies using electron spin resonance (ESR) spectroscopy: A **spin label** was used—a specially tagged lipid containing a nitroxyl group with an unpaired electron. With this labeling technique, investigators demonstrated that a lipid molecule moves rapidly within the plane of the membrane. Calculations of the kinetics of this movement indicate that a single molecule can traverse the

length of a typical eukaryotic cell in about 5–10 seconds. Thus, in a typical mammalian cell membrane, lipids are in constant motion, and they are continually exchanging places. Moreover, individual lipids rotate on their long axis in addition to their lateral movement. Within the lipid bilayer, individual molecules are free to *move within the plane of the membrane* unless they confront some barrier, which often occurs, as we will discuss later in this chapter.

Movement of individual lipids within the bilayer specifically refers to movement within one leaflet of the bilayer. The questions arises: Can lipids on the outer leaflet trade places with lipids on the inner leaflet? The answer is yes, but if this were to occur by simple diffusion, the process would take a very long time and not be of much value to the cell. Thus, for all practical purposes, the **flip-flop** of lipids from one leaflet to the other does not occur by the mechanisms that have been detected for lateral movement.

The amphipathic property of the lipid explains why simple flipping from one side of the bilayer to another is unduly difficult. For a membrane lipid to "flip-flop" requires that for a brief period of time, the polar region must pass through the apolar domain and vice versa. This requires too much energy for the cell to expend in an unassisted process. Keep in mind that lipid flipping across leaflets is not a trivial pursuit on the part of the cell, since maintaining a selected lipid composition on each side of the membrane is extremely important for cell structure and function. Several mechanisms are involved in the movement of lipids from one side of the bilayer to the other.

If one compares the total lipid composition in hepatocytes with that in erythrocytes, differences in the relative proportion of each type of lipid in the membrane are apparent. It is not clear why the membrane lipid proportion varies depending on the cell type, but it may relate to the biological functions of that cell or organelle. Also, the ratio of lipids and proteins can vary widely within different types of membranes. For example, the protein-lipid ratio in mitochondrial membranes is much higher than in the Golgi apparatus or endoplasmic reticulum, in large part because many mitochondrial energy-developing enzymes are, themselves, membrane proteins. In this case, membrane lipids appear to serve more as mortar for the proteins than in other organelles, in which membrane lipids serve additional functional roles.

Translocation & Impact on Cell Function

The search for the mechanism(s) responsible for translocating a lipid from the inner to the outer leaflet has been quite active. The translocation of lipids depends on the nature of the lipid, accounting for the difficulty in determining the mechanism(s) responsible for such translocation.

Lipids are synthesized and added to only one side of the leaflet. Uncharged or neutral lipids can cross the membrane by virtue of lipid solubility without requiring a special process. It has been shown, for example, that in hepatocytes a phospholipid exchange protein is involved in binding the phospholipid from one side of a leaflet and inserting it into another membrane compartment. In addition, it has been shown that a mixing of lipids can occur in the formation of vesicles from one membrane and their fusion to another membrane. Whether this is a major mechanism for developing asymmetry of the lipids in each leaflet is not known.

The inner leaflet (directed to the cytoplasm) has a higher proportion of phosphatidylserine, which carries a net negative charge, thus making the inner surface more negative than that of the external face. Similarly, the phosphatidylinositol is located almost exclusively on the inner leaflet, which is logical because this lipid is involved in a signal transduction pathway that carries a signal into the cytoplasm (Chapters 9 and 10). Glycolipids such as gangliosides and cerebrosides are found exclusively in the outer leaflet. It is generally thought that lipids bearing carbohydrate side-chains are almost always located in the leaflet that faces away from the cytoplasm.

From these examples it is clear that the asymmetric arrangement of the lipids in each leaflet is an important arrangement for cell function, and specific mechanisms exist to maintain this asymmetry. It should be clear from the foregoing discussion that membrane lipids constitute a critically important component of biological membranes and must be considered in all aspects of biological function.

SPECIALIZED MEMBRANE LIPIDS IN CELL SIGNALING

Eicosanoids

Eicosanoid (Greek eikos = 20) is a term applicable to any C_{20} fatty acid (Table 2–8). A large number of oxygenated eicosanoids are formed biosynthetically from **arachidonic acid,** the most commonly occurring C_{20} polyunsaturated fatty acid found in mammalian membranes. Oxygenated eicosanoids fall into two groups. The first includes the **prostaglandins** (or prostanoids) and the thromboxanes. The second includes the hydroxy and hydroperoxy fatty acids and the third are the **leukotrienes.** Prostaglandins and thromboxanes are the products formed following cyclooxygenase rearrangement of arachidonic acid. The second group are called **lipoxygenase** products, since leukotriene formation is catalyzed by one of a number of related deoxygenases called lipoxygenases. These two families of compounds are hormone-like mole-

Table 2–8. Properties of significant eicosanoids.[1]

Elcosanoid	Major Site(s) of Synthesis	Major Biological Acitivities
PGD_2	Mast cells	Vasodilation
PGE_2	Kidney, spleen, heart	Vasodilation, enhancement of the effects of bradykinin and histamine, induction of uterine contractions, and of platelet aggregation, maintaining the open passageway of the fetal ductus arteriosus
PGF_2	Kidney, spleen, heart	Vasoconstriction, smooth muscle contraction
PGH_2		Precursor to thromboxanes A_2 and B_2, induction of platelet aggregation and vasoconstriction
PGI_2	Heart, vascular endothelial cells	Inhibits platelet aggregation, induces vasodilation
TXA_2	Platelets	Induces platelet aggregation and vasoconstriction
TXB_2	Platelets	Induces vasoconstriction
LTB_4	Monocytes, basophils, neutrophils, eosinophils, mast cells, epithelial cells	Induces leukocyte chemotaxis and aggregation
LTC_4	Monocytes and alveolar macrophages, basophils, eosinophils, mast cells, epithelial cells	Component of SRS-A[2], induces vasodilation and bronchoconstriction
LTD_4	Monocytes and alveolar macrophages, eosinophils, mast cells, epithelial cells	Predominant component of SRS-A[2], induces vasodilation and bronchoconstriction
LTE_4	Mast cells and basophils	Component of SRS-A[2], induces vasodilation and bronchoconstriction

[1]Reproduced, with permission, from Balcavage WX, King MW: *Biochemistry: Examination & Board Review,* Appleton & Lange, 1995, p. 205.
[2]SRS-A = Slow-reactive substance of anaphylaxis.

cules; they have profound albeit short-lived influence, and they are effective at very low concentrations.

Prostaglandin Biosynthesis: Clinical Correlates

Prostaglandins are formed only in bursts in response to certain stimuli (Figure 2–11).

The essential prerequisite for prostaglandin formation is the availability of its precursor fatty acid, arachidonic acid. This precursor molecule is normally found esterified at the sn-2 position of membrane phosphoglycerides. After the application of a stimulus to a cell, prostaglandins are detected within 10–20 seconds. Synthesis proceeds for 1–5 minutes

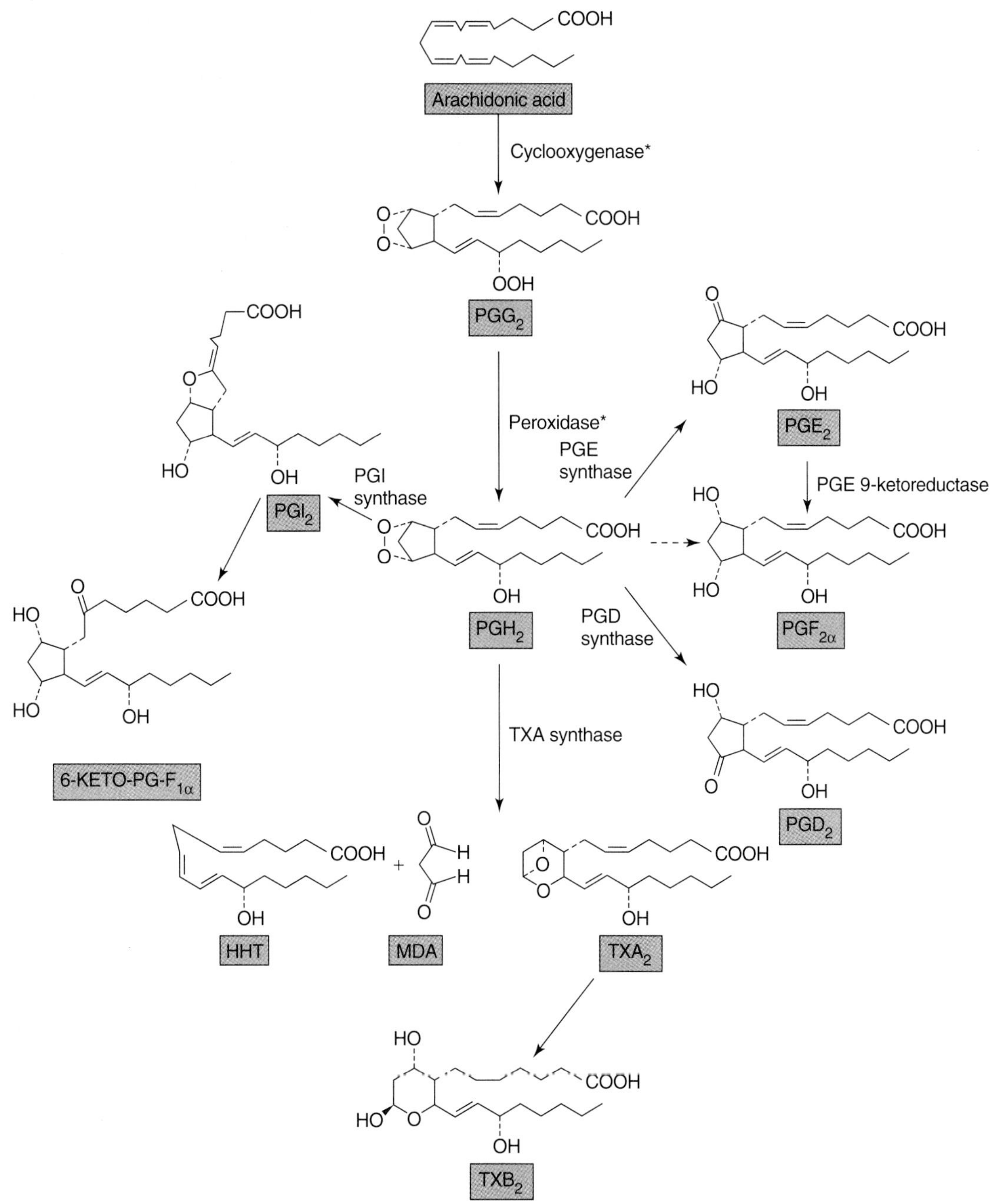

Figure 2–11. Biosynthesis of prostaglandin and thromboxane. The names of specific compounds are given in boxes. Asterisks indicate that both cyclooxygenase and peroxidase steps are catalyzed by the single enzyme prostaglandin endoperoxidase (PGH) synthase. (Modified and reproduced, with permission, from Katzung BG: *Basic & Clinical Pharmacology,* 6th ed. Appleton & Lange, 1995, p. 293.)

and then stops. The pathway of arachidonic acid release and metabolism is shown in Figure 2–12. Among the physiologic stimuli of arachidonic acid release are hormones such as angiotensin II, bradykinin, and epinephrine.

On the other hand, any process or factor causing a generalized effect on cellular membranes and resulting in the turnover of phospholipids fits into the category of pathologic stimuli. Examples include mechanical damage, ischemia, and membrane-active venoms such as the bee venom melittin. Blood platelets have been shown to release larger quantities of prostaglandins when they undergo physiologic aggregation as an initial step in a clotting reaction.

Platelets: Arachidonate Formation

In the platelet, arachidonate is derived primarily from two phospholipids, phosphatidylinositol and phosphatidylcholine. Treatment of platelets with thrombin or collagen causes the formation of diglyco-phosphatidylinositol-specific phospholipase C. This phospholipase C is probably activated as a result of stimuli-induced Ca^{2+} mobilization. Once the arachidonic acid has been cleaved from the lipid, cyclooxygenase initiates the cascade and converts arachidonate into prostaglandins that are rapidly synthesized and released from cells. The prostaglandins then act on ectoreceptors found on the outside of the plasma membrane.

Leukotriene Pathway

The leukotriene pathway involving lipoxygenases leads to the formation of small molecules that participate in inflammatory responses and allergic reactions. These substances are produced at very low levels but exert their action at 10^{-10} M; they are more than 10,000 times more potent than histamine.

The **peptidoleukotrienes** are involved in the respiratory system—where they control the diameter of the bronchioles—and in mucus secretion by goblet cells located in the airways. These lipid products, derived from the lipids of the membranes, reinforce the importance of understanding (1) the type of lipid in the membrane, (2) where it is located, and (3) how it is involved in a variety of important biological responses.

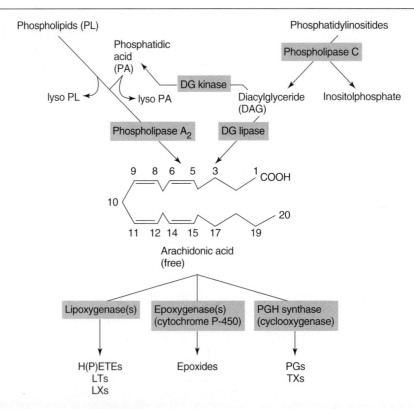

Figure 2–12. Pathways of arachidonic acid release and metabolism. (Modified and reproduced, with permission, from Katzung BG: *Basic & Clinical Pharmacology,* 6th ed. Appleton & Lange, 1995, p. 291.)

Prostaglandins & Leukotrienes: Clinical Correlates

Prostaglandins and leukotrienes are involved in:

1. The inflammatory response and the development of inflammatory abnormalities such as rheumatoid arthritis and lesions of the skin (eg, psoriasis).
2. Production of pain and fever.
3. Induction of blood coagulation (by augmenting platelet aggregation).
4. Regulation of blood pressure by affecting vasodilation and relaxation of smooth muscle cells and small arteries and veins.

5. Regulation of uterine contractions during labor.
6. Regulation of sleep and wake cycles.

Some major cellular mast cell mediators of acute inflammation, including prostaglandins, thromboxane A, and leukotrienes, are listed in Figure 2–13.

Phosphoinositides

Another critically important class of membrane lipids are the phosphoinositides. This family of lipids is intimately involved in relaying certain signals into the cell (discussed in Chapter 9). Inositol-containing phospholipids are ubiquitous components of all eukaryotic cells and constitute 2–8% of the total lipid.

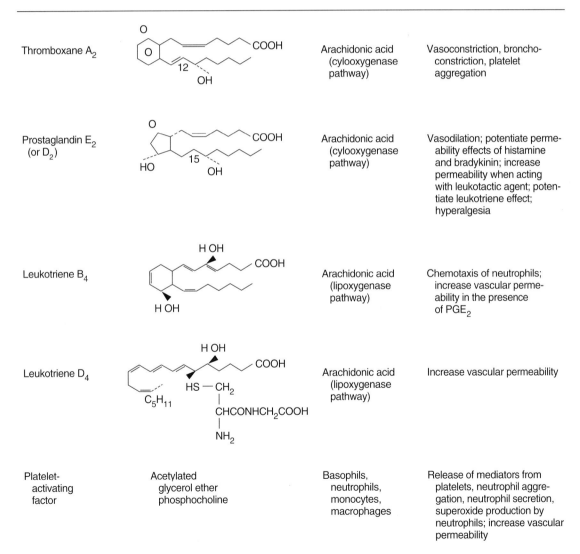

Figure 2–13. Mediators of mast cell function. The names, structures, and biological activities of important compounds that regulate (stimulate) mast cells are shown. (Modified and reproduced, with permission, from Sell S: *Immunology, Immunopathology, & Immunity,* 5th ed. Appleton & Lange, 1996, p. 215.)

There are three major forms of inositol-containing phospholipids:

1. Phosphoinositol-phosphate (PI)
2. Phosphoinositol-4-phosphate (PIP)
3. Phosphoinositol-4,5-phosphate (PIP$_2$)

Phosphoinositol-phosphate accounts for about 80% of the PI found in the membrane. The inositols are synthesized in the endoplasmic reticulum by a series of enzymatic reactions. In the formation of the different phosphorylated forms of inositol, a separate kinase is used. A phosphate is added to specific hydroxyl groups on the inositol ring. During a signaling event, another family of membrane-associated proteins are activated. These latter proteins are specific lipases that cleave the inositol head-group from the lipid.

This cleavage process results in the formation of two highly reactive molecules:

1. The phosphorylated inositol, which at this stage has three phosphates linked in positions 1, 4, 5 (it is called IP$_3$). This small hydrophilic molecule binds to internal receptors that open calcium channels to allow Ca to move into the cytosol.
2. The bound lipid moiety diacylglycerol (DAG) from which IP$_3$ is cleaved is also a very reactive species, but it remains in the lipid bilayer. DAG appears to move within the plane of the membrane to a position next to a kinase enzyme that recently associated close to the inner face of the lipid (in reaction to the presence of increased intracellular calcium ions).

Phosphatidylinositol metabolism in cell membranes is illustrated in Figure 2–14.

A more detailed discussion of signaling and information processing occurs in Chapter 9. Here we want to emphasize the critical importance of lipids and their position in the membrane: The lipid bilayer acts

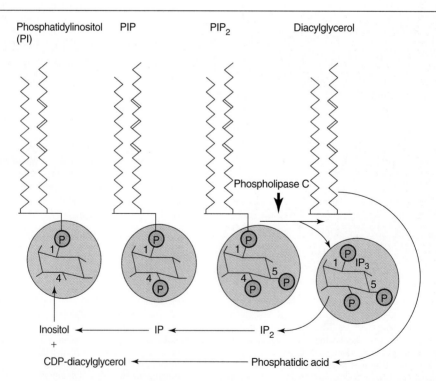

Figure 2–14. Membrane metabolism of phosphatidylinositol. Phosphatidylinositol (PI) is phosphorylated to form first phosphatidylinositol 4-phosphate (PIP) and then phosphatidylinositol 4,5-*bis*phosphate (PIP$_2$). The enzymes phospholipase Cβ_1 and β_2 catalyze the breakdown of PIP$_2$ to inositol 1,4,5-triphosphate (IP$_3$) and diacylglycerol. Subsequent steps produce inositol and CDP-diacylglycerol, which complete the metabolic cycle. (CDP = cytosine diphosphate.) (Modified, with permission, from Berridge MJ: Inositol triphosphate and diacylglycerol as second messengers. Biochem J 1984;220:345.)

not only as a physical barrier but also as an essential source for receiving, interpreting, and responding to incoming information that is critical to cell function.

PROTEIN-LIPID MOSAIC

Proteins contribute approximately 50% of the mass of most cell membranes. A breakthrough in understanding how membrane proteins associate with membrane lipids occurred when Dr Jon Singer and then-graduate-student Garth Nicholson demonstrated that the bulk of membrane proteins are embedded in a more or less perpendicular arrangement (Singer and Nicholson, 1972). These observations led to the proposal of the **protein-lipid mosaic model** of membranes (Figure 2–1). Hundreds of studies have con-

firmed and expanded the original Singer-Nicholson model. The protein-lipid mosaic is now unequivocally accepted as a representation of how these two classes of molecules are arranged in a cell membrane.

MEMBRANE PROTEINS: PHYSICAL & CHEMICAL PROPERTIES

The red blood cell (RBC) has been an especially useful model to study the architecture and topology of membrane proteins and lipids in a biological membrane. Information in Figure 2–15 outlines how RBCs are isolated and their membranes purified.

Although many specialized features of membrane proteins are not found in RBC membranes, RBCs have proved to be an excellent and easily accessible way to study the structure and function of membranes. The following principles of protein structure and function have been deduced using the membrane of RBCs.

Thermodynamic Principles

Many of the same thermodynamic rules that form lipid micelles or the lipid bilayer also apply to the folding of polypeptides: The R-groups or **side groups** of amino acids in a protein provide a major driving force for dictating how a protein will fold into its functional conformation. Recall that there are 8–10 different amino acids with side chains that are nonpolar and thus are more likely to partition away from the aqueous environment, whereas the opposite occurs with amino acids that have hydrophilic side groups.

The folding of the linear polymer of amino acids into a large three-dimensional structure occurs, in part, because of thermodynamic energy required to expose hydrophobic groups in a hydrophilic environment. Thus, regions of a polypeptide containing stretches of hydrophilic amino acids will fold into the middle of the molecule.

Although rules of protein folding are more involved than just the tucking of side chains into or away from the bulk aqueous phase, it is the hydrophobic interactions that provide an important driving force in protein folding. Correct folding of a protein, however, is not a spontaneous process driven by thermodynamics; rather, it involves catalysis by chaperone molecules (Chapter 3). A genetic alteration of changing even a single amino acid at a given position in a protein often leads to changes in its three-dimensional structure and consequently alterations in its functional activity. As will be discussed, genetic defects in membrane proteins can have profound effects on cell function.

Membrane Proteins Are of Two Basic Types

Using the red cell membrane as a model, re-

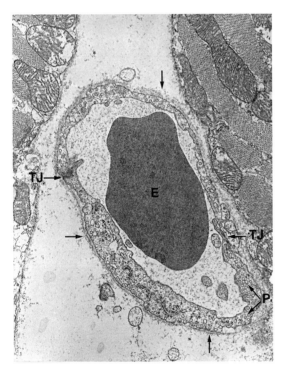

Figure 2–15. The erythrocyte (red blood cell). (Modified and reproduced, with permission, from Berman I: *Color Atlas of Basic Histology.* Appleton & Lange, 1993, 151.)

Circulating erythrocytes lose their nuclei and other organelles during maturation in bone marrow, and because erythrocytes are so numerous in peripheral blood (approximately 10^6/mL), they can be separated easily from other blood cells. When washed erythrocytes are placed in water, they swell and lyse. After hemoglobin and other intracellular proteins are removed, a preparation of pure plasma membrane remains.

searchers observed that there are two types of membrane proteins. One type, called **peripheral** proteins, is associated with the membrane mainly by ionic interaction. That is, if one treats a membrane preparation with a buffer containing high concentrations of salt, certain types of proteins can be extracted from the membrane and inserted into the buffer. Examples of peripheral proteins are fibronectin (located on the external surface of most cell types except circulating blood cells) and spectrin (located on the inner surface of most cell membranes, but especially present in RBCs).

The second type of membrane protein is known as **integral** proteins. These proteins are either buried in the lipid bilayer or transmembrane, meaning they pass through the lipid bilayer completely. To isolate and study integral proteins, one must remove them from the lipid using either organic solvents (such as acetone or alcohols) that extract the lipids or detergents that dissolve the lipids. Most membrane proteins are integral proteins.

One of the first integral proteins to be completely purified and its amino acid sequence determined was a 28-kDa protein called glycophorin A. Examination of its amino acid sequence revealed a *linear* sequence of some 24 amino acids that contain almost total hydrophobic side chains. The sequence begins and ends with the charged amino acid arginine (ARG^+-Val-Gln-Leu-Ala-His-His-Phe-Ser-Glu-Pro-Glu-Ile-Thr-Leu-Ile-Ile-Phe-Gly-Val-Met-Ala-Gly-Val-Ile–Gyl-Thr-Ile-Leu-Leu-Ile-Ser-Thr-Gly-Ile-ARG^+). A number of experiments were carried out showing that glycophorin spanned the membrane and that the hydrophobic sequence described above was the spanning domain. Although the sequence of the membrane-spanning region shows that apolar amino acids are the most numerous (even though a few "charged" residues are also present), these substituents are almost always neutralized by interacting with a residue with an opposite charge (ie, $-His^{(+)(-)}Glu-$). It is also important to emphasize that in the hydrophobic milieu within the membrane, the apolar amino acids fold into an alpha-helical configuration that maximizes the thermodynamic parameters of the bilayer. These and other observations of the orientation of glycophorin provide unequivocal evidence that the proteins of the bilayer actually span the lipid leaflet and that this type of protein is, like that of phospholipids, **amphipathic,** having major domains that are hydrophobic and others that are hydrophilic.

Integral Proteins Move Within the Plane of the Membrane

Previously we described experiments demonstrating that individual lipid molecules move within the plane of their leaflets. Using a similar approach, researchers have shown that integral membrane proteins also move within the plane of the membrane. When researchers fused a mouse cell with a human cell and then measured whether human surface antigens could migrate to the mouse part of the fused cell, they observed that membrane proteins indeed *could* migrate to different locations on the cell surface. This finding has provided the basis for understanding a number of events of cell behavior, including clustering of receptors, endocytosis, and phagocytosis—all of which involve the movement of proteins that are embedded in a lipid bilayer (see Figure 2–19).

Are protein movements random, like icebergs floating in the ocean, or are there directed movements, and if so, how do they occur? The answer is that many proteins do move significant distances; however, because they are associated in different ways with the proteins of the cytoskeleton, not all proteins are able to move within the membrane. Despite that many proteins have associations with the cytoskeleton, a surprisingly large number have been shown to undergo slow lateral diffusion. This movement is likely due to the dynamics of the structural components of most cells that are forming and breaking down continually.

INTEGRAL PROTEINS

As indicated earlier, membrane proteins are operationally grouped into two general types: those that are associated with the lipid bilayer and those that are integrated within the lipid leaflets. We will consider the lipid-integrated proteins first.

Single-Pass Transmembrane (Monotopic) Proteins

The single-pass transmembrane proteins represent a large group that traverse the membrane only once, ie, *there is only one membrane-spanning region in the protein's polypeptide chain.* **Glycophorin** is a good example of the single-pass transmembrane protein. A large number of monotopic proteins are receptor proteins that have a recognition-binding domain in the extracytoplasmic domain of the protein, linked to a single transmembrane domain that passes through the lipid bilayer. The cytoplasmic region of the receptor usually contains the catalytic or "activation" domain. In some cases, receptors are composed of more than one polypeptide, and each subunit of a receptor may contain a single membrane pass domain.

Multipass Transmembrane (Polytopic) Proteins

A number of membrane proteins have more than one membrane-spanning domain. These membrane-spanning regions are **threaded** through the bilayer by a mechanism described in Chapter 4. For our purposes here, it is important to note that most multipass (polytopic) membrane proteins belong to a group of receptor molecules that are unique because they activate a special information signaling pathway. Moreover, various forms of membrane proteins have evolved to carry out this function. The details of how this signal cascade is initiated are presented in Chapter 9.

Lipid-Linked Membrane Proteins

Some membrane proteins are linked into the bilayer by forming an amide linkage between the amino terminal residue (usually it must be glycine) and the carboxyl group of a long-chained fatty acid (most often the fatty acid is either myristic or palmitic acid). The protein tethered in this way can face either the cytoplasmic side or the external face of the membrane.

A second type of lipid-linked protein is formed by a thioester linkage between cysteine and special type of isoprene structure. These structures are related to cholesterol. The cysteine residue that forms this type of linkage consists of four amino acids from the end of the protein chain. After the formation of the thioester linkage, the three terminal residues are

cleaved off and the new carboxyl-terminal amino acid is methylated (Figure 2–16).

Carbohydrate-Linked Proteins

Some membrane proteins are attached to the lipid bilayer through the formation of a carbohydrate-to-protein link. This occurs through a phosphoester link. The lipid is glycosylphosphoinoside, which is pre-formed in the membrane, then a specified protein is attached to this membrane anchor. Such proteins are said to be linked by a **glycerolphosphoinoside (GPI) anchor.** Several types of proteins are linked into the membrane though a GPI anchor; some are receptors, others appear to serve as cell surface recognition domains. We will encounter GPI-linked membrane proteins in later chapters.

PERIPHERAL PROTEINS

As stated, the second major type of protein associated with the cell membrane—peripheral proteins—are not embedded or tethered into the lipid bilayer.

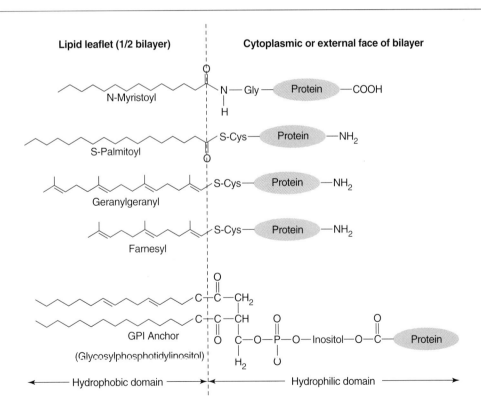

Figure 2–16. Protein linkages within membranes. Some proteins are linked to the lipid bilayer by their amino terminal residue (usually glycine), whereas others are linked at the carboxyl terminus. Some linkages occur through the formation of a thioester bond with the SH– group of the cysteine positioned four residues from the carboxyl terminus. After a thioester bond forms, the remaining carboxyl-terminal residues are removed as the last step of linkage. Many other proteins are tethered to the membrane through a carbohydrate link, as depicted by the GPI-linked protein.

Rather, they are associated mainly by strong ionic interactions. Moreover, peripheral proteins are strongly associated with integral proteins in what is called a **protein-protein** interaction within the membrane. Two important examples of peripheral proteins are

- Spectrin, which is found on the inner surface of the cell
- Fibronectin, which is located on the external face of the membrane.

The clinical significance of these key peripheral proteins is addressed in the next section and in Chapter 7.

MEMBRANE CYTOSKELETON

Thus far, we have focused on the types of molecules involved in forming the membrane bilayer. For information concerning the arrangement of proteins within the membrane, we have again used a detailed analysis of the erythrocyte membrane (Figure 2–1).

When mature RBCs are repeatedly washed—ie, centrifuged, resuspended in isotonic saline, and allowed to swell in water to effect lysis—**membrane "ghosts"** can be isolated by centrifugation. If the membrane ghosts are solubilized in a negatively charged ionic detergent such as sodium dodecyl sulfate (SDS), the proteins can be separated on polyacrylamide gels and stained. After this electrophoretic procedure, a banding pattern like that shown in Figure 2–17 is obtained. This pattern indicates the various proteins that form the erythrocyte membrane skeleton.

Erythrocyte Cytoskeletal Proteins

Note that the gel contains eleven bands that are strongly stained. By convention, the bands are numbered beginning with the slowest (and largest) migrating units:

- Bands 1 and 2 represent the large polypeptides of the protein spectrin (240 and 220 kDa)
- Bands 2.1 and 2.2 are ankyrins (210–200 kDa)
- Band 3 is the major anion exchange protein (93 kDa)
- Band 4.1 is a member of a family of proteins that associate with spectrin and actin in the membrane skeleton
- Band 4.2 is N-myristolyated and associates with band 3 and with ankyrin
- Band 4.9 is an actin-bundling protein
- Band 5 is actin (43 kDa)

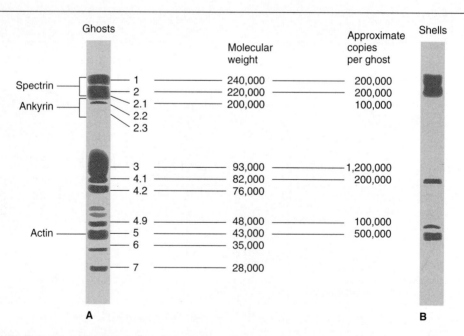

Figure 2–17. Electrophoresis of erythrocyte preparations. The protein band pattern on the left (A) was made from a preparation of red-cell ghosts. The band pattern on the right (B) was made from shells—ghosts treated with 1% Triton X-100 detergent in hypotonic buffer. In comparing the two bands, note that the shells have lost the Band 3 integral membrane protein and some peripheral proteins. The shells have retained the cytoskeletal proteins, including spectrin, ankyrin, and actin. (Modified and reproduced, with permission, from Branton D, Cohen CM, Tyler J: Interaction of cytoskeletal proteins on the human erythrocyte membrane. Cell 1981;24:24.)

The function of the other two bands (35 kDa and 28 kDa) is not yet known.

Glycophorin is not shown on this gel because of its high content of carbohydrate, and the type of protein stain used does not detect this. Two of the proteins of the RBC ghost (band 3 and glycophorin) are integral, ie, they are embedded into the membrane. Both these components are involved in forming the meshwork of membrane skeleton.

Spectrin Cytoskeleton

The structural arrangements that make up the spectrin membrane skeleton involve almost all the proteins shown on the SDS gel. Spectrin forms a tetramer in which adjacent α and β monomers encircle each other; then another α and β associate in a head-to-head arrangement that produces a thin (approximately 100 nm) filament. The ends of spectrin filaments form short connections with actin and tropomyosin. Two other cytoskeletal proteins, band 4.1 and adducin, associate with the actin-spectrin junction and help anchor the longer spectrin filaments to band 3, which is firmly embedded in the bilayer. The protein ankyrin (band 4.1) has two binding sites, one for the cytoplasmic region of band 3 and the other for the spectrin β chain near the center of the tetramer. The associations of band 3, spectrin, ankyrin, band 4.1, actin, tropomyosin, and adducin form a complex that provides the structural rigidity that keeps the erythrocyte in its biconcave disk from.

Genetic alterations of any proteins that are part of the complex can significantly alter the shape of the red blood cell; clinical abnormalities can result (Table 2–9).

Structural Model for Eukaryotic Cell Membranes

Although the information described above is derived from studies of the erythrocyte, it has been established that spectrins, ankyrins, actins, and other structural proteins are present in nearly all other cell types. These proteins are considered operational components of the membrane cytoskeleton. Thus, what has emerged from the detailed analysis of the erythrocyte is a conceptual picture of all eukaryotic plasma membranes. Variations in the number and types of proteins associated with the membrane cytoskeleton do occur; however, a membrane structural motif exists for all cells, and it involves many of the proteins that are found in the erythrocyte.

Table 2–9. Genetic abnormalities in hereditary red cell skeleton defects.[1]

Clinical Presentation	Molecular Defect	Inheritance	Map Location
Hereditary spherocytosis, classical (MIM 182870)	Deficient spectrin	AD	14q22–q23.2
Hereditary spherocytosis, classical (MIM 182900)	Deficient ankyrin	AD	8p11.2
Hereditary spherocytosis, classical (MIM 109270)	Insertion, band 3 protein	AD	17q21–qter
Hereditary spherocytosis, classical (MIM 182870), (MIM 182900)	Deficient spectrin-protein 4.1 binding	AD	—
Hereditary spherocytosis, severe	Deficient α-spectrin	AR	1q21
Hereditary spherocytosis, severe	Deficient protein 4.1	AR	1p36.2–p34
Hereditary spherocytosis, severe	Deficient β-spectrin	AR	14q22–q23.2
Hereditary elliptocytosis (MIM 182860)	Deficient α-spectrin	AD	1q21
Hereditary elliptocytosis (MIM 182870)	Deletion β-spectrin	AD	14q22–q23.2
Hereditary elliptocytosis (MIM 141700)	Deficient ankyrin	AD	8p11.2
Hereditary elliptocytosis (MIM 130500)	Insertion protein 4.1	AD	1p36–p34
Hereditary elliptocytosis (MIM 130500)	Deficient protein 4.1	AD	1p36–p34
Acanthocytosis, ovalocytosis (MIM 109270)	Deleted protein band 3		
Hereditary elliptocytosis, Melanesian (MIM 109270)	Deleted protein band 3	AD	17q21–q22
Pyropolkilocytosis (MIM 266140)	Several RBC membrane proteins	AR	—
Ovalocytosis (MIM 166900)	Several RBC membrane proteins	AD	—

[1]Reproduced, with permission, from Seashore MR, Wappner RS: *Genetics in Primary Care & Clinical Medicine*, Appleton & Lange, 1966, p. 70.

MEMBRANE FACES OF POLARIZED CELLS

Most types of cells in higher organisms are organized in patterns that are much more complex than simple cell aggregates; higher order eukaryotic cells undergo extensive movement, rearrangement, and shuffling until prescribed sets of **cell-cell associations** are achieved. These associations often involve many different types of cells, including epithelial cells, muscle cells, nerve cells, and cells of connective tissue.

One of the principal features of this organization is the establishment of precise sides of the cell. For example, in the simplest arrangement in which epithelial cells adhere to each other, three different surfaces form. The **basal surface** is the face that attaches to an acellular matrix. The faces attached to other cells and to the acellular substrate are known as the **basolateral** surface. A third face is unattached so as to be available to form the lining of a duct or the external face of tissue; this unattached face is the **apical** surface. The plasma membrane of each of these faces has unique architectural features that play a role in cellular and tissue functions.

Apical Surface: Specialization & Modifications

Specialized membrane regions are found on the apical face of a polarized cell. All surfaces of an organism are covered by a layer of cells known as the epithelium. Epithelial layers differ depending on the body location. The differences are due mostly to variations in the apical surface and *reflect a specialized function carried out by the apical surface.* Careful microscopic and functional analyses of the linings of the human body have revealed four major types of epithelial coverings:

1. Simple squamous
2. Simple columnar
3. Transitional
4. Stratified squamous.

Often these coverings are referred to as epithelial membranes, but they constitute a thin layer of cells. Some contain two layers of cells and others have 8–10 layers. Keep in mind, too, that the term epithelial membrane refers to a lipid bilayer interspersed with proteins. Epithelial membranes have been further subdivided for more precise characterization. For more on these subdivisions, the student is referred to a standard histology text.

Apical Surfaces: Architectural Variations

Apical surfaces can contain the following structural variations:

Microvilli: Under the microscope, these highly specialized membrane projections look like bristles on a brush. Microvilli increase the absorption of nutrients by greatly expanding the surface area of epithelial cells. The cell is columnar in shape, and the villi protrude into the lumenal space for maximal absorption.

Closer examination of the microvilli reveal that an actin filament inserts at the tip of the villus and extends downward through the villus to about midway in the columnar cell to a specialized plate of transverse actin filaments and other actin-binding proteins. Through this cytoskeletal filament, each villus is maintained in an extended form and moves with the flow of fluids in the lumen. The terminal web is structurally reinforced by a well-defined actin bundle that surrounds the cell. This bundle is known as a **belt desmosome** (see Figure 8–2).

Cilia: In certain epithelial linings—eg, the bronchioles of the airways—the apical surface has pseudostratified columnar epithelial cells called **cilia** that extend into the luminal space. Cilia are specialized structures composed of microtubules in a 9 + 2 arrangement. These apical modifications are especially designed to help the epithelial cell move particulate material out of the air passage (Chapter 8).

MEMBRANE SPECIALIZATION

Basolateral Surface of Epithelial Cells

Epithelial cells perform various critical functions, not the least of which is the formation of sheets of cells that adhere tightly to one another and to their basal surfaces. Epithelial linings provide an impervious barrier between the external environment and the organism's interior. Often the epithelial boundary is subject to great stress, and if the boundary is to maintain its integrity, epithelial cells must remain tightly connected. Examination of the surfaces between epithelial cells reveals the presence of several specialized membrane structures (Figure 8–1):

Tight junction or zona occludens: These are located between cells closest to the apical surface. This junction between two cells closes off any space between the cells and outer leaflets, and the cells can appear to fuse. Tight junctions prevent fluids from leaking through the epithelial barrier.

Zonula adherens: This junction surrounds the cell and appears to link two cells. On the inner surface of these junctions, a number of cytoskeletal proteins appear to form a dense plaque. Proteins that comprise this plaque include myosin, α-actinin, tropomyosin, and vinculin.

Gap junction or nexus: This occurs along the basolateral surface between two cells. A protein complex containing six dumbbell-shaped polypeptide subunits called **connexons**—with a central pore in the middle of the complex—is located on the basolateral face of an epithelial cell. This complex faces up precisely with another hexameric structure, and the two central pores align with each other to form a channel between the two cells. The pore size of the channel is large enough to allow molecules of several hundred daltons to pass through.

Of particular interest is that the pores close in the presence of high concentrations of **calcium.** It also has been shown that cyclic adenosine monophosphate (cAMP) and important second messenger molecules can pass from one cell to another through gap junctions. Gap junctions are of particular importance in muscle tissue, where many cells must function in a highly coordinated fashion to effect muscle contraction. Gap junctions allow for the passage between cells of chemical signals that aid in muscle contraction (Chapter 8).

CELL MEMBRANE SURFACE RECEPTORS

All cells have specialized transmembrane proteins that are able to specifically bind **information molecules** and, after this binding, transmit information into the cell. These membrane proteins are known as **receptors.** Within the past decade, an array of receptors have been identified on the surface of cells. Indeed much of what is known about how cells communicate with one another has been learned through research on surface receptors. We will discuss intracellular events of information signaling in detail in Chapters 9 and 10; here it is instructive to examine the types and characteristics of surface receptors.

The quantity of specific surface receptors for any given cell is probably in the hundreds, if not thousands. It has been shown that receptors are grouped into families, and some have a surprisingly large number of members. Each is characterized in part by its binding specificity. For example, the number of proteins in the olfactory receptor family is thought to be in the thousands. The human can detect as many as 10,000 different odorant molecules, and not surprisingly the number of odorant molecule receptors is in the same range. Consider also the family of growth factor receptors; their number is quite large, since the 8–10 types of growth factors have many isoforms. Table 2–10 lists major types of growth factors.

Of course not all cells have the same complement of surface receptors. Yet even with the huge number of different receptors on the surfaces of cells, most receptors share certain features, eg, domain characteristics. Surface receptors have three domains:

1. An extracellular domain or ectodomain.
2. A transmembrane region, which can be either single-pass or multipass.
3. A cytoplasmic domain that contains the site for effector activation.

Table 2–10. Growth factors: Major categories and families.[1]

Major categories
  Endocrine
    The systemic hormones, eg, pituitary hormones, steroid hormones, thyroid hormones, insulin
  Paracrine
    Locally acting hormones, eg, the neuroendocrine system of the gastrointestinal tract
  Autocrine
    Same cell produces growth factor and corresponding receptor (autocrine loop)
Families
  Epidermal growth factor (EGF)
  Platelet-derived growth factor (PDGF)
  Transforming growth factor (TGF)
  Interleukin
  Insulin-like growth factors
  Fibroblast growth factors
  The interferons

[1]Reproduced, with permission, from Chandrasoma P, Taylor CR: *Concise Pathology,* Appleton & Lange, 1995, p. 246.

Surface Receptor Extracellular Domain

The **extracellular domain (ectodomain)** contains the binding site for the signal molecule or **ligand.** This domain is usually the largest part of the protein receptor. It is usually glycosylated and possesses amino acid sequences that are common to other receptor families. The ectodomain often has a conserved intramolecular disulfide bridge, as well as enriched regions for certain types of amino acids, eg, leucine-rich or proline-rich regions. The binding affinity of the ligand to the binding site in the ectodomain is often quite high, on the order of 10^{-9}–10^{-11} M.

Transmembrane Domains

The **transmembrane domains** of receptors are grouped into two types. One very large family of signaling receptors are *threaded* through the membrane seven times. So characteristic is this feature for this family, they are often referred to as the *seven-membrane–spanning receptors—or serpentine* receptors. One notable characteristic of these multipass receptors is that they use a family of intracellular trimeric **guanosine triphosphatases (GTPases) (G proteins)** as their initial effector-activating substrate (Chapter 9).

The β_2 adrenergic receptor and rhodopsin, with their seven-membrane–spanning regions, are shown in Figure 2–18.

Although the overall structure is similar for each member of the family of seven-membrane–spanning receptors, numerous variations account for the ability of different forms of this receptor to bind to different classes of ligands.

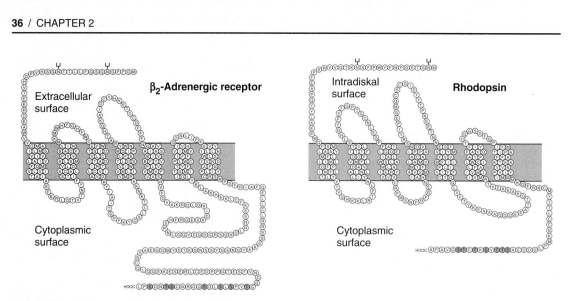

Figure 2–18. Structures of the β₂-adrenergic receptor and rhodopsin, two serpentine receptors. Each protein shows the characteristic seven membrane-spanning–domains. Individual amino acids are identified by single-letter codes. The Y-shaped symbols on N residues identify glycosylated sites on the external surfaces of the cell membranes. For each protein, the amino terminal is extracellular and the carboxyl terminal intracellular. (Modified and reproduced, with permission, from Benovic JL et al: Light-dependent phosphorylation of rhodopsin by β-adrenergic receptor kinase. Reprinted by permission from Nature 1986;321:869. Copyright © 1986. Macmillan Journals limited.)

Single-Pass Transmembrane Domain

An equally large number of surface receptors have a single transmembrane domain. These receptors do not use the G protein; instead some have an enzymatic—ie, kinase—domain as a part of their cytoplasmic region. Other single-pass receptors do not have a kinase region in their cytoplasmic regions. Instead the cytoplasmic regions are a substrate for a kinase that resides in close proximity to the cytoplasmic domain. After ligand binding, the receptor becomes phosphorylated by a cytoplasmic protein kinase, and this activates this type of single-pass receptor.

Cytoplasmic Domain

The **cytoplasmic domain** is where activation occurs. A main feature is that this region of the protein has a catalytic structure that is built into the sequence. Also, all signaling events involve **phosphorylation** of substrate molecules on a serine, threonine, or tyrosine residue.

MECHANISM OF TRANSMEMBRANE SIGNALING

How information is transmitted across the membrane after a ligand binds to its receptor remains a key area of research. **Binding of the ligand** to its receptor is the first step in information transfer. For this to occur, at least four events must transpire:

1. The ligand must be synthesized.
2. The ligand must be in the correct conformation to fit into the binding domain of the receptor.
3. The receptor must be present on the cell surface.
4. The receptor must possess the correct conformation to receive the ligand.

Serious alterations in any of these steps can lead to deleterious effects with potential clinical implications.

The second step of information transfer involves **transducing the ligand signal** into the cell. How this occurs is not entirely clear. In an attempt to elucidate the molecular steps involved, the following four models have been proposed:

1. The ligand binds two subunits and induces their cytoplasmic associations, which generates a new site for the signaling molecule.
2. The ligand induces a conformational change in the receptor, and this is transmitted from the extracellular domain through the transmembrane regions to the intracellular portion of the receptor. The receptor can be either a monomer or a dimer.
3. A combination of events takes place. The ligand induces a conformational change in both the ectodomain and in the cytoplasmic domain. These associations generate new reactive sites in the cytoplasmic domains of the receptor.
4. Ligand binding to the receptor causes it to transphosphorylate another subunit—either a ligand-binding subunit or a nonligand-binding

subunit, which, in turn, leads to the formation of new reactive sites in the receptor.

These model systems and other variations provide some understanding of the process of information exchange that is essential for cellular function in tissues. Not all cells have the same complement of re-

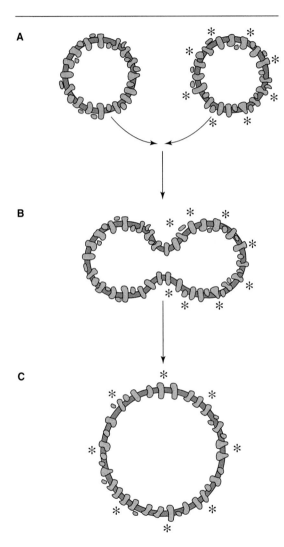

Figure 2–19. Demonstration of the fluid nature of protein movement within membranes. The lipid bilayer of the cell membrane is shown as two parallel lines in which proteins are embedded. Some plasma membrane proteins of the cell at the top right are identified by asterisks. In the experiment, two types of cells (one with a fluorescent marker, right, and one without, left) were fused (A). Minutes after the cell membranes fused (B), the fluorescent marker of the labeled cell spread over the surface of the fused cell, eventually covering the surface uniformly (C). (Modified and reproduced, with permission, from Junqueira LC, Carneiro J, Kelley RO: *Basic Histology,* 7th ed. Appleton & Lange, 1992, p. 30.)

ceptors, and when sufficient receptors are lacking, cells cannot respond to the ligand. Like all proteins on the cell surface, receptors have the potential to turnover and be replaced. Such an outcome depends on the function of the cell.

It is important to reiterate that proteins move within the plane of the membrane, as suggested by the experiment depicted in Figure 2–19. To form dimers, protein molecules within the cytoplasm are tucked close to the inner surface, where activation can occur. Although certain cells have a preponderance of one type of receptor, the cell can synthesize and insert receptors into the membrane during various times of the cell's life. Some incoming signals tell the cell to make and expose a particular type of receptor so it, in turn, can respond to new messages to which the cell, tissue, organ, and organism respond to remain viable. More about these critical downstream signaling pathways is presented in Chapters 9 and 10.

SUMMARY

This chapter discussed the types of lipids and proteins that comprise the plasma membrane and addressed the physical and chemical properties that allow lipids and proteins to carry out the functions of a membrane. Selected clinical correlates were noted, eg, certain glycolipids and glycoproteins are involved in the identification of cells that constitute self versus nonself and thus play a role in successful graft transplantations and blood transfusions.

The general functional properties and arrangement of major membrane lipids and proteins were discussed and examples of how they are assembled were provided. Of special note: all components of biological membranes are assembled in the endoplasmic reticulum and, once intact, are transported as vesicles through the cell to the plasma membrane.

The functional role of peripheral proteins and how they give structure to the lipid bilayer were discussed. The concept of a membrane skeleton was introduced. Proteins in the membrane form a strong association with cytoskeletal proteins and, through this association, help to form and maintain the phenotypic character of a cell.

Also introduced were cell surface receptors, their functional domains, how those receptors transmit a signal across the bilayer, and how they begin an intracellular signaling cascade. The plasma membrane is constantly undergoing change, and it is through this dynamic process that cells can (1) hone in to specific locations, (2) differentiate and specialize to respond to foreign invaders, and (3) repair and rebuild wounded tissue. These bioclinical themes are elaborated on in remaining chapters (Table 2–11).

Additional insights into the architecture of the cell membrane are expected as more is learned about membrane structure in the coming years.

Table 2–11. Some human and animal diseases related to altered cellular components.[1]

Cell Component Involved	Disease	Molecular Defect	Morphologic Change	Clinical Consequence
Mitochondrion	Mitochondrial cytopathy	Defect of oxidative phosphorylation	Increase in size and number of muscle mitochondria	High basal metabolism without hyperthyroidism
Microtubule	Kartagener's syndrome	Lack of dynein in cilia and flagella	Lack of arms of the doublet microtubules	Immotile cilia and flagella with male sterility and chronic respiratory infection
	Mouse (*Acomys*) diabetes	Reduction of tubulin in pancreatic β cells	Reduction of microtubules in β cells	High blood sugar content (diabetes)
Lysosome	Metachromatic leukodystrophy	Lack of lysosomal sulfatase	Accumulation of lipid (cerebroside) in tissues	Motor and mental impairment
	Hurler's disease	Lack of lysosomal α-L-iduronidase	Accumulation of dermatan sulfate in tissues	Growth and mental retardation
Secretory granule	Proinsulin diabetes	Defect of proinsulin-cleaving enzyme	None	High blood proinsulin content (diabetes)
Golgi complex	I-cell disease	Phosphotransferase deficiency	Inclusion-particle storage in fibroblasts	Psychomotor retardation, bone abnormalities

[1]Reproduced, with permission, from Junqueira LC et al: *Basic Histology,* Appleton & Lange, 1995, p. 47.

REFERENCES

Alberts B et al: *Molecular Biology of the Cell.* Garland Publishing, 1994.

Barbacid M: Neurotrophic factors and their receptors. Curr Opin Cell Biol 1995;7:150.

Bennett V, Gilligan DM: The spectrin-based membrane skeleton and micron-scale organization of the plasma membrane. Ann Rev Cell Biol 1993;9:27.

Coughlin SR: Expanding horizons for receptors coupled to G proteins: Diversity and disease. Curr Opin Cell Biol 1994;6:191.

Ganong WF: *Review of Medical Physiology.* Appleton & Lange, 1995.

Houslay MD, Stanley KK: *Dynamics of Biological Membranes.* John Wiley & Sons, 1982.

Hunter T et al: *The Cell Surface.* Vol. 57. Cold Spring Harbor Laboratory Press, 1992.

Lodish H et al: *Molecular Cell Biology.* Scientific American Books, 1995.

Murray RK et al: *Harper's Biochemistry.* Appleton & Lange, 1990.

Simon MI: Summary: The cell surface regulates information flow, material transport, and cell identity. Pages 673–688 in: *The Cell Surface: Symposia on Quantitative Biology.* Vol. 57. Cold Spring Harbor Laboratory Press, 1992.

Stoddard BL, Biemann HP, Koshland JDE: Receptors and transmembrane signaling. Pages 1–15 in: *The Cell Surface: Symposia on Quantitative Biology.* Vol. 57. Cold Spring Harbor Laboratory Press, 1992.

Vance DE, Vance JE: *Biochemistry of Lipids and Membranes.* The Benjamin/Cummings Publishing Co, 1985.

Voet D, Voet JG: *Biochemistry.* John Wiley & Sons, 1990.

Zubay G: *Biochemistry.* Macmillan, 1983.

SUGGESTED READING

Bretscher MS, Munro S: Cholesterol and the Golgi apparatus. Science 1993;261:1280.

Englander SW: In pursuit of protein folding. Science 1993;262:848.

Fish EM, Molitoris BA: Alterations in epithelial polarity and the pathogenesis of disease states. N Engl J Med 1994;330:1580.

Mark J: Forging a path to the nucleus. Science 1993;260:1588.

Marx J: Two major signal pathways linked. Science 1993;262:988.

Murray RK et al: *Harper's Biochemistry.* 24th ed. Appleton & Lange, 1996.

Sell S: *Immunology, Immunopathology & Immunity.* Appleton & Lange, 1996.

Sudhof TC: The synaptic vesicle cycle: A cascade of protein-protein interactions. Nature 1995;375:645.

Structure & Function of Intracellular Organelles

3

KEY TERMS

Organelles
Nuclear envelope
Nuclear pore complex
Nuclear import, disassembly, assembly
Mitochondria
Mitochondrial chaperones
Peroxisomes
Smooth endoplasmic reticulum
Rough endoplasmic reticulum
Protein translocation
Ribosomes
Signal recognition particle
Secretory protein
Core glycosylation

All cells of the human body have the same basic set of intracellular compartments in which major functions of the cell occur. This chapter focuses on the structure and function of the following intracellular components:

- nucleus
- mitochondria
- peroxisomes
- smooth endoplasmic reticulum
- rough endoplasmic reticulum.

Special attention is given to how these compartments deliver their cellular products to adjacent organelles. As discussed in Chapter 2, all intracellular organelles are surrounded by a membrane consisting of lipoprotein bimolecular leaflets. Highly specific variations in membrane lipids and proteins characterize each compartment. Such variations in membrane composition help to determine the functions of organelles, as well as interactions among compartments (Figure 3–1, Tables 3–1 and 3–2).

INTRACELLULAR MOVEMENT

Protein Flow: Vesicle Flow

The major types of movement within a cell involve **protein flow** and **vesicle flow.** One of the major tasks of the cell is to deliver molecules to different locations within the cell's boundaries and to the extracellular space. Defined routes or pathways exist for the intracellular and intercellular movement of material. Although some variations may occur in highly differentiated cells that display specialized phenotypes, cellular flow usually follows similar pathways in eukaryotic cells. For example, although bidirectional flow sometimes occurs between organelles, protein and vesicle flow is for the most part one-way—the flow of membrane proteins from the endoplasmic reticulum (ER) to the cell surface (Figure 3–2, see page 42).

Delivery of material from one compartment to the next involves specific proteins. Specific polypeptide sequences within the protein are employed as an **address label.** One major discovery in medicine in the last two decades has been the recognition that a defect in any of these transport routes can lead to human disease. A defect in the address label or in the site that recognizes the label can greatly affect the health of the cell and the organism. An awareness of the details of these pathways is essential to understanding the molecular basis of many human diseases.

CELL NUCLEUS

The **nucleus** of the eukaryotic cell usually appears as a prominent rounded structure near the center of the cell (Figure 3–3). The nuclear material, referred to as **chromatin,** consists of deoxyribonucleic acid (DNA), histones, and various nuclear proteins that participate in one or more of the following:

- Formation of scaffolding complexes for DNA
- Binding to specific DNA sequences and participating in DNA transcription
- DNA replication.

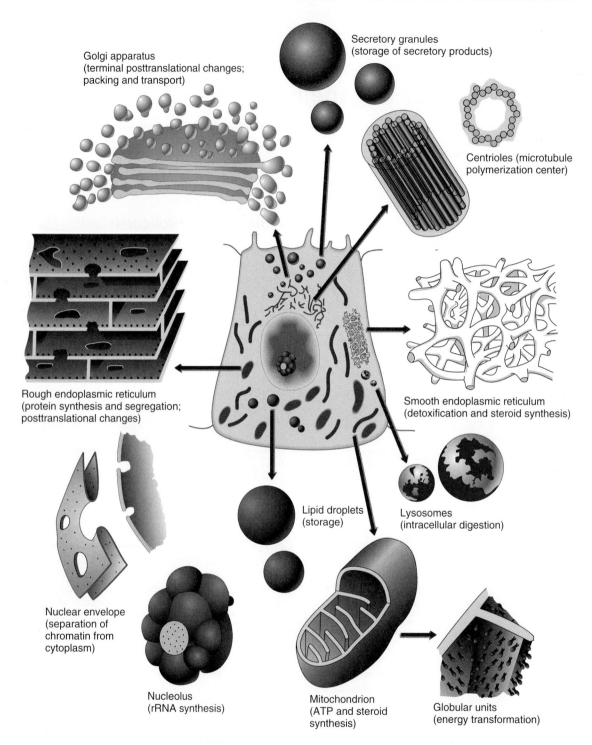

Figure 3–1. Eukaryotic organelles. The organelles found in a typical eukaryotic cell are shown as visualized using an electron microscope. Nucleoli are within the boundaries of the nuclear envelope. (Redrawn and reproduced, with permission, from Bloom W, Fawcett DW: *A Textbook of Histology,* 9th ed. Saunders, 1968.)

Table 3–1. General features of eucaryotic cells.

Feature	Principle
Membranes	All the compartments or organelles are surrounded by the same type of basic unit membrane, a **lipoprotein bimolecular leaflet.** Specific variations in lipid and protein composition characterize compartments and help to determine the directional pathways to and from respective organelles.
Intracellular movement	Movement of materials from one compartment to another occurs in an orderly and directed manner, but material flow—the transport or migration of proteins—occurs by different mechanisms, in particular, **protein flow** or **vesicle flow.**
Formation of intracellular compartments	Intracellular compartments are dynamic and can increase and decrease in size, but no compartment can form de novo; this requires information in the form of a remnant or template from an existing compartment.
Relative position within the cell	The relative position or placement of each cellular component is not random; rather, each component is positioned to best carry out its specialized function.

Located within the nucleus is a structural body known as the nucleolus. Within this structure are chromosomes containing loops of DNA and large clusters of ribosomal ribonucleic acid (rRNA) genes. Each gene cluster is known as a **nucleolar organizer** region. Within the nucleolus, the following processes occur:

1. **Transcription** of ribosomal DNA by RNA polymerase I

Table 3–2. Major intracellular organelles and their functions. Only the major functions associated with each organelle are listed. In a number of instances, many other pathways, processes, or reactions occur in the organelle.[1]

Organelle or Fraction[2]	Marker	Major Functions
Nucleus	DNA	Site of chromosomes Site of DNA-directed RNA synthesis (**transcription**)
Mitochondrion	Glutamic dehydrogenase	Citric acid cycle, oxidative phosphorylation
Ribosome[2]	High content of RNA	Site of protein synthesis (**translation** of mRNA into protein)
Endoplasmic reticulum	Glucose-6-phosphatase	Membrane-bound ribosomes are a major site of protein synthesis Synthesis of various lipids Oxidation of many xenobiotics (cytochrome P450)
Lysosome	Acid phosphatase	Site of many hydrolases (enzymes catalyzing degradative reactions)
Plasma membrane	Na^+ - K^+ ATPase 5′-Nucleotidase	Transport of molecules in and out of cells Intercellular adhesion and communication
Golgi apparatus	Galactosyl transferase	Intracellular sorting of proteins Glycosylation reactions Sulfation reactions
Peroxisome	Catalase Uric acid oxidase	Degradation of certain fatty acids and amino acids Production and degradation of hydrogen peroxide
Cytoskeleton[2]	No specific enzyme markers[3]	Microfilaments, microtubules, intermediate filaments
Cytosol[2]	Lactate dehydrogenase	Enzymes of glycolysis, fatty acid synthesis

[1]Reproduced, with permission, from Murray RK et al: *Harper's Biochemistry*, 24th ed., Appleton & Lange, 1996, p. 9.
[2]An organelle can be defined as a subcellular entity that is membrane-limited and is isolated by centrifugation at high speeds. According to this definition, ribosomes, the cytoskeleton, and the cytosol are not organelles. However, they are considered in this table along with the organelles because they also are usually isolated by centrifugation. They can be considered subcellular entities or fractions. An organelle as isolated by one cycle of differential centrifugation is rarely pure; to obtain a pure fraction usually requires at least several cycles.
[3]The cytoskeletal fractions can be recognized by electron microscopy or by analysis by electrophoresis of the characteristic proteins that they contain.

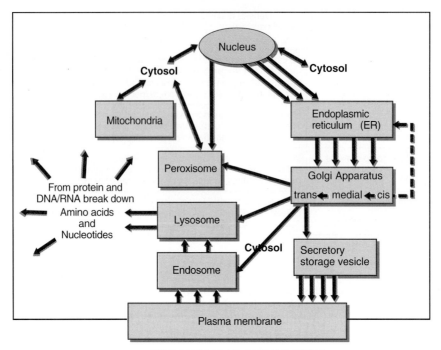

Figure 3–2. Flow of membrane proteins. Note that while bidirectional flow of proteins commonly occurs among some cytoplasmic organelles (eg, ER to Golgi and Golgi to ER), surface membrane proteins are transported from the ER to plasma membrane.

2. **Packaging of rRNA** into ribonucleoprotein complexes that eventually become the two major subunits of the ribosome (the 40S and 60S subunits).

The size of the nucleolus is a reflection of the protein-synthesizing activity of the cell. The more active the cell, the larger the nucleolus.

Synthesis of Ribosomes in the Nucleolus

The nucleolus is not surrounded by a membrane; rather it is a collection of ribosomal particles in the process of assembly. Synthesis of **ribosomes** is a major activity that occurs in the nucleus. In fact, most active eucaryotic cells use about 10 million ribosomes during one round of the cell cycle. As part of this process, a number of very specific proteins are prescribed around the rRNA of each subunit. The small subunit—a 40S particle—has 30 unique proteins assembled around an 18S RNA molecule. The larger unit—a 60S particle—has 51 proteins around its major 28S RNA molecule. The large subunit also has a 5.8S RNA as part of its complex.

A more in-depth review of the mechanics of protein synthesis appears later in the chapter (Figure 3–4).

NUCLEAR ENVELOPE (NE)

The **nuclear envelope** is a double membrane structure that encloses the chromatin and is contiguous with the endoplasmic reticulum (ER). The inner membrane has a different complement of proteins from that of the outer membrane. The inner leaflet of this membrane has a fibrous network of proteins called **lamins** that plays a key role in maintaining the membrane's structural integrity. The outer envelope is continuous with the ER membrane and has docking proteins required for the ribosome to bind to its outer leaflet (Figure 3–5).

NUCLEAR PORE & NUCLEAR PORE COMPLEX

Nuclear pores are huge macromolecular complexes that mediate the active exchange of proteins and ribonucleoproteins between the nucleus and the cytoplasm. The **nuclear pore complex (NPC)** forms a cylinder that is approximately 1200 Å in diameter and 500 Å in thickness and has an eightfold symmetry. An estimated 100–200 proteins comprise the NPC. It has a mass of 124×10^6 daltons, which is about 30 times the size of a ribosome.

This complex is the major gateway for movement of substances in and out of the nucleus. Molecules pass in and out of the nucleus continuously. For example, messenger ribonucleic acid (mRNA) molecules, ribosomal subunits, histones, ribosomal proteins, transcription factors, ions, and smaller molecules are rapidly exchanged between the nuclear compartment and either the lumen of the endoplasmic reticulum or the cytosol (Figure 3–6).

Mechanisms of Nuclear Import & Export

Passage of molecules in and out of the nucleus occurs by active transport, passive diffusion, or by special nuclear localization that occurs via signal sequences on certain proteins. Passive diffusion and active transport into and out of the nucleus occur through the nuclear pore complex. Small molecules and ions (< 9 kDa) undergo passive diffusion through the NPC's aqueous channel, which is about 10 nm in diameter. Larger molecules (> 9 kDa) undergo active transport by a process that involves a nuclear signal (Chapter 9 and 10), as well as by energy-dependent mechanisms.

The main steps of active nuclear import are:

1. A soluble receptor in the cytosol recognizes the molecule to be imported, and the receptor and molecule form a linked complex.
2. The receptor complex associates with the cytoplasmic face of the NPC.
3. The receptor-ligand complex moves close to the central channel of the NPC. GTP hydrolysis by guanosine triphosphatase (GTPase) molecules provides energy to activate the gating mechanism of the central pore, and translocation of the complex into the nucleoplasm follows. Once inside the nucleus, the translocation complex dissociates, and transport factors—including the soluble receptor—are recycled to the cytoplasm (Figure 3–7).

NUCLEAR LOCALIZATION SIGNAL

Role of Importin

Proteins imported into the nucleus have a nuclear localization signal (NLS) that contains a highly enriched stretch of five or six basic amino acids. An example is proline-proline-lysine-lysine-lysine-lysine-alanine-lysine-valine (P-P-K-K-K-K-A-K-V).

Contiguous basic amino acids in the NLS can be located anywhere in the protein. Moreover, the nuclear localization signal is not altered by translocation events. Of particular note is the fact that during nuclear import, the 60 kDa protein **importin** binds to the NLS to initiate and facilitate the import of proteins. Cytoplasmic factors also participate in nuclear import.

Nuclear Dissolution & Reassembly

The interphase nuclei are completely assembled with pore complexes. The nuclear lamina, a lattice of specialized intermediate filaments (Chapter 7), forms a hair net–like structure that connects with the lipoprotein complex of the inner nuclear membrane.

When the cell enters early prophase, cytosolic kinases phosphorylate the subunits of the nuclear lamins. Following phosphorylation, the net-like structure disassembles. The lipoprotein component of the inner nuclear envelope then disassociates into small vesicles—as does the outer nuclear envelope, which is contiguous with the ER compartment. The contents of the nucleus then disperse into the cytosol.

Reassembly of the nuclear envelope begins in late anaphase, when cytoplasmic phosphatases begin to remove the phosphate residues on the nuclear lamins. The nuclear lamins start to repolymerize on the surface of the condensed chromosome. At the same time, vesicles from the inner nuclear membrane (INM) begin to fuse, and an envelope forms around chromosomes. By the end of late telophase, total fusion of INM membranes occurs. These fused membranes, together with dephosphorylated lamins, form the net-like structure on the inner surface of the NE.

Not all integral proteins of the inner nuclear envelope have been fully characterized. Like the lamins, these proteins undoubtedly participate in the nuclear envelope's reassembly process (Chapter 6).

MITOCHONDRIA

Overall Structure & Function

Mitochondria are double membrane–bound organelles that function as the metabolic center of the cell. Mitochondria are the site of adenosine triphosphate (ATP) production. This process requires a large number of enzymes, most of which must be imported from the cytosol (Figure 3–8).

This import process is complex and involves several steps, described below. Mitochondria are thought to be evolutionary remnants of an organism that invaded a primitive prokaryotic cell and became symbiotic with its host. General principles of mitochondria are listed in Table 3–3.

Mitochondrial DNA

Unlike other organelles in the cell, mitochondria possess unique DNA that differs from nuclear DNA and encodes mitochondrial-specific genes. Mitochondrial DNA is

- Small and contains about 16.5 kb, ie, about 10^5 less than that located in the nucleus
- Circular and encodes for two ribosomal RNAs, 22 transfer RNAs (tRNAs), and 13 proteins.

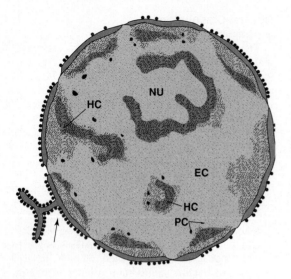

Figure 3–3. Structure of the nucleus. The arrow indicates the junction of the nuclear envelope with the endoplasmic reticulum. Within the nucleus are regions of euchromatin (EC) and heterochromatin (HC) and granules of perichromatin (PC). The nucleolus (NU) is visualized as a distinct body surrounded by heterochromatin and with scattered spots of euchromatin within it. Nucleolar euchromatin contains the genes that encode rRNAs. (Modified and reproduced, with permission, from Junqueira LC, Carneiro J, Kelley RO: *Basic Histology.* Appleton & Lange. 1995, p. 48.)

The mitochondrial genetic code that designates specific amino acids differs slightly from that of nuclear DNA. The mitochondrial code, for example, has altered stop codon signals.

This organelle has functional ribosomes that translate mitochondrial DNA into proteins used in the organelle. The amount of translated protein made by mitochondrial mRNA is limited and forms subunits of larger enzyme complexes. Mitochondria can and do exhibit many morphological forms. A mitochondrion typically undergoes division at least once per cell cycle after replication of its DNA, which occurs during interphase. This replication is not linked to the S phase of the cell. Division occurs by *pinching* in two, which begins when a cleavage furrow develops at the inner mitochondrial membrane.

Mitochondrial Outer Membrane & Inner Membrane

The double-membrane mitochondrion has two lumenal spaces and four membrane faces. The **outer membrane** is composed of a high copy number of the protein **porin.** This protein forms pores that have a diameter that allows molecules of about 5000 daltons or less to pass freely into the first compartment. Thus ions, amino acids, sugars, and other cytosolic components pass unrestricted into the first mitochondrial space, the **intermembrane space.** A family of enzymes located in this space function in the phosphorylation of nucleotides and nucleotide sugars.

The **inner membrane** of the mitochondria forms a much tighter barrier, which is significantly larger

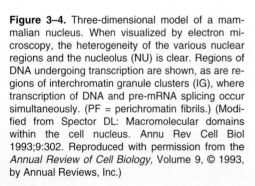

Figure 3–4. Three-dimensional model of a mammalian nucleus. When visualized by electron microscopy, the heterogeneity of the various nuclear regions and the nucleolus (NU) is clear. Regions of DNA undergoing transcription are shown, as are regions of interchromatin granule clusters (IG), where transcription of DNA and pre-mRNA splicing occur simultaneously. (PF = perichromatin fibrils.) (Modified from Spector DL: Macromolecular domains within the cell nucleus. Annu Rev Cell Biol 1993;9:302. Reproduced with permission from the *Annual Review of Cell Biology,* Volume 9, © 1993, by Annual Reviews, Inc.)

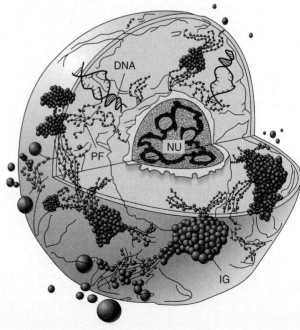

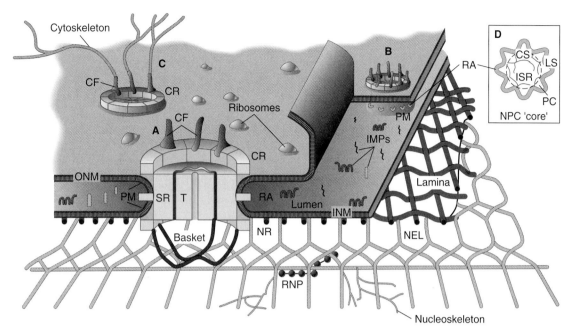

Figure 3–5. Cut-away view of nuclear envelope showing details of nuclear pore complex (NPC). One NPC is depicted in longitudinal section (**A**). Part of the outer nuclear membrane is peeled back in another NPC to give a proposed lumenal view (**B**). A third is depicted as seen from the cytoplasm (**C**). Note that the cytoskeletal and nucleoskeletal attachments are hypothetical. (CF = cytoplasmic filaments; CR = cytoplasmic ring; IMPs = integral membrane proteins; INM = inner nuclear membrane; NEL = nuclear envelope lattice; NR = nucleoplasmic ring; PM = pore membrane; RA = radial arms; RNP = ribnucleoproteins, attached to NEL; SR = spoke ring; T = transporter.) The inset (**D**) depicts a cross-section through the core of the nuclear pore complex. (CS = central spoke domain; ISR = inner spoke ring; LS = lumenal spoke domain; PC = peripheral channel.) The dashed line indicates the possible position of the pore membrane. (Modified and reproduced, with permission, from Goldberg MW et al: Structural and functional organization of the nuclear envelope. Curr Opin Cell Biol 1995;7:302.)

than the outer membrane and is folded into a series of contiguous partitions called **cristae.** These foldings greatly increase the surface area of the mitochondria. Many enzymatic reactions are performed more efficiently if the enzyme can associate with a mitochondrial surface; the cristae facilitate this (see Figure 5–1).

Mitochondrial Matrix

The mitochondrial matrix is a busy place. The matrix face of the inner membrane is studded with a protein complex involved in the production of ATP. A large number of **metabolic enzymes** reside in the **mitochondrial matrix,** including enzymes involved in lipid oxidation, in carbohydrate oxidation, and in the tricarboxylic acid (TCA) cycle or Krebs cycle. In addition, the mitochondrial genome is located in the matrix, together with ribosomes, tRNA, and enzymes required to transcribe mitochondrial DNA and express the corresponding genes. These genes are relatively small in number compared to genes found in the nucleus.

Mechanism of Mitochondrial Protein Import

Mitochondria function as the metabolic center of the cell; these organelles are the site of ATP production, a process that requires many enzymes, most of which are imported from the cytosol (Figure 3–8). Almost all proteins destined to be imported into the mitochondria are made on polyribosomes located in the cytosol.

Proteins targeted for the mitochondria have a **signal peptide** located at the amino terminal end. This signal peptide varies in length from as few as 12 residues to as many as 80. In addition, this region of the protein forms an **amphipathic helix:** the charged residues are clustered on one side of an alpha helix, and the apolar residues are located on the other side. The amphipathic helix fits into a binding domain on a **mitochondrial recognition receptor** located on the outer membrane.

The import process is complex and involves several elements (Table 3–4).

Nucleus

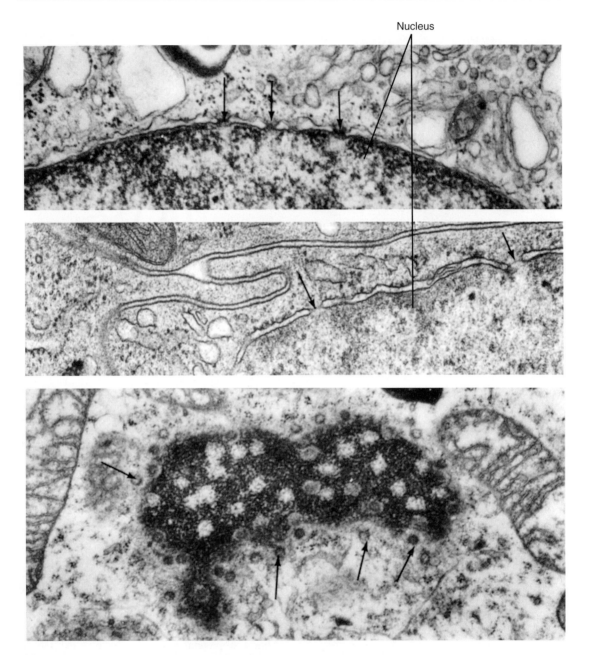

Figure 3–6. Structure of the nuclear envelope as visualized using electron microscopy. The envelope is composed of two membranes (the outer membrane is contiguous with the ER) with nuclear pores (arrows). The two upper micrographs show transverse sections, while the bottom shows a tangential section. The chromatin that is frequently condensed below the nuclear envelope is not usually seen in pore regions. × 80,000. (From Junqueira LC, Carneiro J, Kelley RO: *Basic Histology.* Appleton & Lange. 1995, p. 50, with permission.)

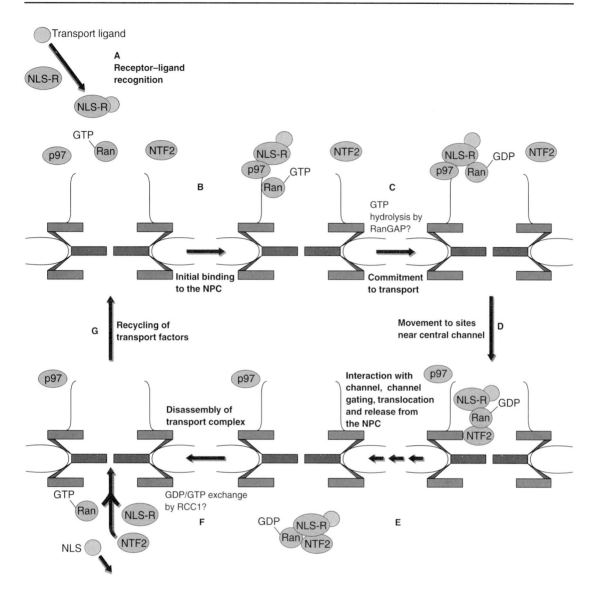

Figure 3–7. Model for protein import through the nuclear pore complex. This diagram integrates data on the NLS receptor/importin (NLS-R), p97; Ran/TC4 (presented as Ran·GTP and Ran·GDP, respectively); and NTF/B-2. The NLS receptor binds its transport ligand (containing an NLS) (A) before it interacts with p97 at the pore complex (B). Subsequent hydrolysis of Ran·GTP at the initial binding site permits commitment to the distal steps of the pathway (C). Ran·GDP becomes part of the complex, while p97 dissociates. NTF2 mediates interaction with sites near the central channel (D) and is cotransported into the nucleus (E). In the nucleus the transport complex is disassembled (F), and transport factors are recycled back into the cytoplasm (G). Note that data on transport intermediates are insufficient to rule out other possibilities for a transport mechanism. The proposed involvement of RanGAP in (C) and the RCC1-catalyzed nucleotide exchange in (F) are not based on direct experimental evidence. (From Melchior F et al: Mechanisms of nuclear protein import. Curr Opin Cell Biol 1995;7:311, with permission.)

Motor neuron in spinal cord

Dorsal root ganglion cell (sensory neuron)

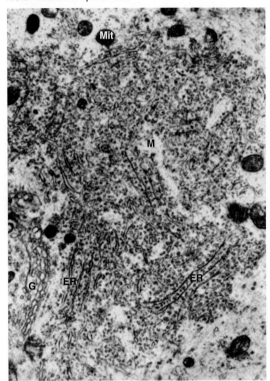
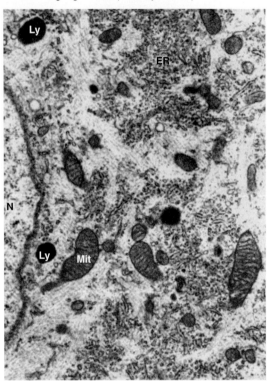

Figure 3–8. Protein synthesis and processing. After leaving the nucleus (N), mRNA enters the cytoplasm and forms polyribosomes for protein synthesis. While many proteins remain in the cytoplasm, some are transported into mitochondria (Mit). Other organelles involved with protein synthesis and processing include the endoplasmic reticulum (ER) and the Golgi apparatus (G). (Ly = lysosome.) (Modified and reproduced, with permission, from Kandel ER et al: *Essentials of Neural Science and Behavior.* Appleton & Lange, 1995, p. 61. Courtesy of Peters et al 1991).

MITOCHONDRIAL CHAPERONES

Newly synthesized proteins bound for the mitochondria associate with another class of cytosolic proteins in preparation for import. Several types of these latter proteins called **chaperones** have been identified. They are found in almost all cellular organelles and in the cytoplasm. Among other things, chaperones help to determine the correct folding pattern and final conformation for other proteins and thus are essential to the health of the cell and the organism.

Chaperones are found in organisms ranging from bacteria to mammals. In some cases, these proteins have other names. One family of chaperones is called **heat shock proteins (hsps)** (Figure 3–9). Their identification occurred unexpectedly: Researchers discovered that these distinctive proteins are produced when cells of the fruit fly are exposed to temperatures increased by only a few degrees. Heat shock proteins

are highly conserved among species and are expressed at rather significant levels in all cells, even under normal growth conditions. Their transcription and translation is significantly increased during environmental stress. It is believed additional chaperones are needed to aid in protein folding as a response to heat stress.

Protein Folding: hsp60 & hsp70 Chaperones

Members of the **hsp60** (also known as GroEL) and **hsp70** (or DnaK) families are involved in protein folding, protein translocation, and the formation of higher orders of protein assembly.

Within the inner mitochondrial space, hsp60 and hsp70 bind to unfolded protein and aid in an orderly conformational assembly. This folding step is energy-dependent and requires the utilization of ATP.

To this end, the **hsp90** family of chaperones are involved in regulating certain transcription factors and

Table 3–3. General principles of mitochondria.

Feature	Principle
Origin	Mitochondria are believed to be evolutionary remnants of an organism that invaded a primitive prokaryotic cell and became symbiotic.
Shape	These organelles exhibit many morphological forms. Some are shaped as spheres while others appear as elongated ribbons.
Mitochondrial DNA	Mitochondrial DNA is replicated during interphase, and this process is not synchronized with DNA replication of the cell. Mitochondrial DNA differs from nuclear DNA and encodes mitochondrial-specific genes.
Protein formation	The amount of translated protein made by mitochondrial mRNA is limited and forms subunits of larger enzyme complexes. Mitochondria have functional **ribosomes** that translate mitochondrial DNA into proteins used in the organelle.
Cell division	Mitochondria undergo division once per cell cycle by a process of pinching in two. A type of cleavage furrow develops beginning with the inner mitochondrial membrane.

Table 3–4. Main elements of protein import into mitochondria.

Element	Role
Ribosomes	Almost all imported proteins are made on polyribosomes in the cytosol.
Signal peptide	Proteins targeted for the mitochondria have a signal peptide located at the amino terminal end.
Amphipathic helix	The signal peptide forms an amphipathic helix. The charged residues are clustered on one side of an alpha helix, and the apolar residues are located on the other side.
Mitochondrial recognition receptor	The amphipathic helix fits into a binding domain on a mitochondrial recognition receptor located on the outer membrane.
Chaperones	Newly synthesized proteins bound for the mitochondria associate with chaperone proteins that help to determine the correct folding pattern and the function of imported proteins.

dria and release of a folded protein requires ATP hydrolysis (Tables 3–5 and 3–6).

PEROXISOMES

Structure & Function: Clinical Correlates

Found in all major eukaryotic cells, **peroxisomes** are single membrane–bound organelles. They are a major site of oxygen utilization, and in this way perform a function similar to that of mitochondria. Peroxisomes appear circular in cross-section, but serial sectioning reveals a reticular form. The name "peroxisomes" is derived from the organelle's high content of oxidases that generate toxic hydrogen peroxide (H_2O_2). The reaction is

$$RH_2 + O_2 \rightarrow R + H_2O_2,$$

where R is an organic substrate.

Fortunately, the enzyme catalase is found in high concentrations in peroxisomes and degrades hydrogen peroxide (H_2O_2) to oxygen and water. This type of oxidation reaction is particularly important in liver and kidney cells that carry out a large number of the body's detoxification reactions. For example, the peroxisomes in hepatocytes detoxify ingested alcohol by converting it to acetaldehyde.

Peroxisomes are also involved in **β-oxidation.** This oxidation involves the breakdown of fatty acids into 2-carbon fragments that are (1) converted to acetyl coenzyme A (CoA), (2) exported from the per-

various protein kinases. With relatively low protein concentrations, a protein likely folds properly because there is little opportunity for the protein's reactive groups to associate with those of other proteins. With large protein concentrations, however, the probability that a protein will fold properly decreases considerably. Typically, the protein concentration in the organelles of the eukaryotic cell is high.

How Chaperones Act

As stated previously, chaperones are found in nearly all organelles and in the cytoplasm. Chaperone proteins act primarily by binding to the reactive surfaces of polypeptides, eg, the hydrophilic surfaces. In so doing, the chaperones sequester these reactive surfaces and effectively prevent aggregation, thus favoring a proper folding pathway.

Chaperones do not covalently modify their polypeptide substrate. Often a protein must be unfolded to be imported and then refolded after it has passed through the membrane of the organelle, and this is accomplished in part by a chaperone.

For example, heat shock proteins bind to elongating polypeptides as the latter are extruded from the ribosome. These chaperones hold the nascent molecule in a conformation that prevents premature random folding and aid in its translocation into the mitochondrial space. Transport of proteins into the mitochon-

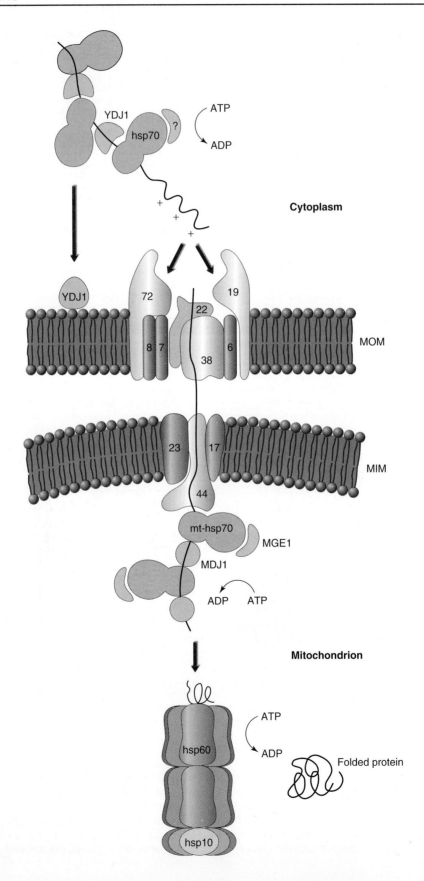

Table 3–5. Some properties of chaperone proteins.[1]

- Present in a wide range of species from bacteria to humans.
- Many are so-called heat shock proteins (hsp).
- Some are inducible by conditions that cause unfolding of newly synthesized proteins (eg, elevated temperature and various chemicals).
- They bind unfolded and aggregated proteins.
- Most chaperones show associated ATPase activity, with ATP or ADP being involved in the protein-chaperone interaction.
- Found in various cellular compartments such as cytosol, mitochondria, and the lumen of the endoplasmic reticulum.

[1]Reproduced, with permission, from Murray RK et al: *Harper's Biochemistry,* 24th ed., Appleton & Lange, 1996, p. 497.

Table 3–6. Some chaperones and enzymes involved in folding that are located in the rough endoplasmic reticulum.[1]

- BiP (immunoglobulin heavy chain binding protein)
- GRP94 (glucose-regulated protein)
- Calnexin
- PDI (protein disulfide isomerase)
- PPI (peptidyl prolyl *cis-trans* isomerase)

[1]Reproduced, with permission, from Murray RK et al: *Harper's Biochemistry,* 24th ed., Appleton & Lange, 1996, p. 497.

oxisome, and (3) used as building blocks for other compounds of the cell.

Peroxisomes contain approximately 50 enzymes that are involved in various metabolic pathways. The peroxisome contains the first two enzymes involved in the synthesis of **plasmalogens,** which account for 19% of the total phospholipid content of the body. Plasmalogens are found in high concentrations in the brain and heart.

Biogenesis of Peroxisomes

Peroxisomal proliferation appears to be an adaptive response to environmental stimuli that require peroxisomal enzymes for growth and survival. Induction consists of two phases:

1. Proliferation of the organelle by budding from preexisting peroxisomes
2. Growth of the organelle by the import of peroxisomal matrix proteins.

Proliferation starts in response to environmental or developmental signals. In mammalian cells, for example, many types of **hypolipemic drugs** can initiate peroxisomal expansion, although the precise mechanism is not fully understood. These drugs appear to mimic an unknown cytoplasmic factor or factors that up-regulate latent transcription factors called **peroxisomal-proliferation-activation-receptors (PPARs).** On activation, these receptors translocate to the nu-

cleus and bind to promoters of genes that encode for cytoplasmic receptors for steroid hormones, thyroid hormone, or retinoic acid.

PPARs bind to DNA elements in the promoters of the genes that encode many peroxisomal enzymes, leading to an increased synthesis of these proteins. The newly made proteins translocate by targeting signals into existing peroxisomes. The resulting increase in protein within the organelle likely initiates its budding, eventually leading to formation of new peroxisomal vesicles. Budding is generally regarded as the major mechanism for increasing the number of peroxisomes; however, a small **peroxisomal precursor compartment** also exists. This compartment seems to incorporate newly synthesized peroxisomal matrix proteins to a greater extent than do mature peroxisomes. This precursor may be another site where peroxisomes originate, thus facilitating expansion of this organelle.

Import of Proteins Into Peroxisomes

Proteins destined for the peroxisome have two types of import signals. By far the most prevalent is a **carboxyl-terminal tripeptide** that contains the amino acids Ser-Lys-Leu-COOH (S-K-L-). Some variation in each of these residues can occur, but for the most part the same type of residue must be present.

The most critical part of the **peroxisomal targeting signal** (PTS) is the status of its location. That is to say, these residues must reside at the **C-terminal** of the protein. Most enzymes located in the peroxisome have their targeting signal peptides located at the C-terminus. However, a few peroxisomal en-

Figure 3–9. Translocation and folding of proteins into the mitochondrial matrix. After synthesis, mitochondrial proteins are maintained in an unfolded conformation by the cytoplasmic proteins hsp70 and YDJ1. The unfolded protein binds to receptor proteins on the mitochondrial outer membrane (MOM) and is transported across the two mitochondrial membranes (MIM = mitochondrial inner membrane). In the matrix, mt-hsp70 works with homologs of the *E coli* stress proteins DnaJ and GrpE, MDJ1 and MGE1, respectively. Folding of the newly imported protein is mediated by the hsp60/hsp10 chaperone complex, a homolog of *E coli* GroEL/GroES. (Numbering on MOM and MIM proteins reflects molecular mass.) (From Hohfeld J, Hartl U: Post-translational protein import and folding. Curr Opin Cell Biol 1994;6:503, with permission.)

zymes have an import sequence located near the amino terminal. The importance of these targeting signals is underscored by the fact that various human metabolic disorders are caused by an inability to import peroxisomal proteins into the organelle or by the mistargeting of the peroxisomal enzyme to the wrong subcellular compartment.

Various disorders of peroxisomes are listed in Table 3–7, and salient characteristics of some of those disorders are provided in Table 3–8.

Major Human Peroxisomal Disorders

Certain inherited disorders are due to nonfunctional peroxisomes. For example, Zellweger syndrome (ZS) is due to an almost complete loss of peroxisomal function and is classified as a group I peroxisomal disorder—the most severe of this type of inherited abnormality. In ZS, a large number of critical enzymes are missing from the peroxisome. Patients with group I disorders die early in life. In group II peroxisomal disorders—eg, Zellweger-like syndrome—cellular organelles have a greater complement of peroxisomal enzymes; therefore, less severe disease results. In group III peroxisomal disease—eg, adrenoleukodystrophy (ALD)—only one dysfunctional peroxisomal enzyme exists. Thus, this form of disease tends to be less severe than group I or group II.

Table 3–7. Disorders of peroxisomes.[1]

Name	MIM Number	Chromosomal Location
Zellweger syndrome	214100	7q11.23
Neonatal adrenoleukodystrophy	202370	
Infantile Refsum disease	266510	
Hyperpipecolic acidemia	239400	
Rhizomelic chondrodysplasia punctata	215100	
Adrenoleukodystrophy	300100	Xq28
Pseudo-neonatal adrenoleukodystrophy	264470	
Pseudo-Zellweger syndrome	261510	3p23-p22
Hyperoxaluria type I	259900	2q36-q37
Acatalasemia	115500	11p13
Glutaryl-CoA oxidase deficiency	231690	

[1]Reproduced, with permission, from Seashore MR, Wappner RS: *Genetics in Primary Care & Clinical Medicine,* Appleton & Lange, 1996, p. 296.
(MIM number = Mendelian Inheritance in Man. The number refers to a reference to additional information.)

ENDOPLASMIC RETICULUM

The endoplasmic reticulum (ER) consists of branching tubules and flattened sacs that extend through a large area of the cytoplasm of all eucaryotic cells. This labyrinthine membrane structure lies close to the nucleus. The ER lumen appears to be interconnected, like passageways in an underground cave.

A very large number of biosynthetic events occur in the ER. The ER membrane contributes to the formation of the cell's plasma membrane, Golgi apparatus, lysosomal membrane, secretory vesicles, and endosomes.

The ER lumen has special characteristics and components. It contains two main structures that differ operationally: the smooth endoplasmic reticulum (SER) and the rough endoplasmic reticulum (RER). The SER is the site of lipid biosynthesis and a major compartment for intracellular calcium sequestration. The SER is also where the family of detoxifying P450 enzymes originate. In the SER, enzymes are rapidly synthesized and degraded, depending on environmental signals, eg, p-450 proteins.

Rough Endoplasmic Reticulum

The term rough endoplasmic reticulum describes a membrane compartment to which many ribosomes are bound. Findings from studies in protein synthesis and cellular compartmentalization suggest that biosynthesis of all membranes occurs in and through the RER. *This membrane network is the origin of the proteins and lipids that comprise almost all other membranes of the cell.* Precisely how the components of the membrane are made and distributed remains a key area of investigation in cell biology. Although not all the details are known, there is sufficient information to account for most of the mechanisms involved (Figures 3–10 and 3–11).

THE ER LUMEN

Physiochemical Environment

The lumen of the endoplasmic reticulum provides an environment in which major successive events of newly synthesized proteins occur, notably, **core glycosylation, disulfide bond formation, polypeptide folding,** and **subunit assembly.** If these steps do not occur accurately, a protein does not exit the lumen of the ER.

For proteins to form disulfide bridges, they must reside in an oxidizing environment. The reduction-oxidation or **redox potential** of the ER lumen has been measured and is shifted toward oxidizing conditions. For example, the ratio of glutathione (GSH) to the oxidized glutathione (GSSG) is about 1-3:1, whereas in the cytosol, the ratio is nearer to 30-100:1.

Table 3–8. Characteristics of peroxisomal disorders.[1]

	Enzymatic Deficiency or Biochemical Defect	Elevated VLCFA	Faulty Plasmalogen Synthesis	Abnormal Bile Acid Synthesis	Abnormal Phytanic Acid Oxidation	Elevated Pipecolic Acid	Other
Group 1: Generalized peroxisomal dysfunction due to faulty peroxisome biosynthesis							
Zellweger syndrome	Multiple	+	+	+	+/–	+	–
Neonatal ALD	Multiple	+	+	+	+/–	+	–
Infantile Refsum disease	Multiple	+	+	+	+	+	–
Hyperpipecolic acdemia	Multiple	+	+	+	+/–	+	–
Group 2: Defects in more than one peroxisomal enzyme, intact peroxisomes							
Zellweger-like syndrome	Multiple	+	+	+	–	–	–
Rhizomelic chondrodysplasia punctata	Acyl-CoA:DHAPAT, phytanic acid α-oxidation	–	+	–	+	–	–
Group 3: Defect in a single peroxisomal enzyme, intact peroxisomes							
ALD/AMN	Lignoceroyl-CoA ligase	+	–	–	–	–	–
Pseudo-neonatal ALD	Acyl-CoA oxidase	+	–	–	–	–	–
Bifunctional enzyme deficiency	Bifunctional enzyme	+	–	+	–	–	–
Pseudo-Zellweger syndrome	3-Oxoacyl-CoA thiolase	+	–	+	–	–	+/–
Hyperoxaluria type I	Alanine:glyoxylate aminotransferase	–	–	–	–	–	+
Acatalasemia	Catalase	–	–	–	–	–	+
Glutaryl-CoA oxidase deficiency	Glutaryl-CoA oxidase	–	–	–	–	–	+

[1]Reproduced, with permission, from Seashore MR, Wappner RS: *Genetics in Primary Care & Clinical Medicine*, Appleton & Lange, 1996, p. 218.
ALD = Adrenoleukodystrophy; AMN = Adrenomyeloneuropathy; CoA = coenzyme A; DHAPAT = dihydroxyacetone phosphate acyltransferase; VLCFA = Very long chain fatty acids;
+ = abnormal; – = normal.

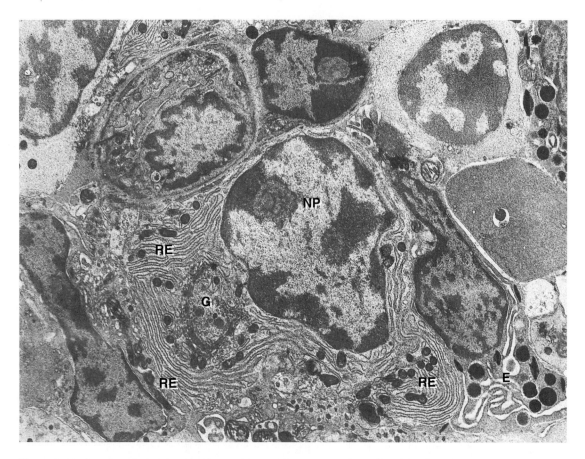

Figure 3–10. Rough endoplasmic reticulum. A plasma cell shows a well-developed rough endoplasmic reticulum (RE), which is characteristic of cells that secrete high levels of protein. An eosinophil (E) is also depicted. (NP = nucleus of plasma cell; G = Golgi.) Rat; × 5010. (From Berman I: *Color Atlas of Basic Histology,* 2nd ed. Appleton & Lange, 1997, p. 23, with permission.)

Thus, the lumen provides a favorable environment for the formation of disulfide bridges.

Researchers have used isolated ER vesicles in an attempt to identify the necessary components for correct protein folding. These studies have demonstrated that ATP is essential to the formation of functional molecules in these ER vesicles. There are several potential steps in the process that could require an energy source. For example, ATP is required to release the hsp60 chaperone in the matrix of the mitochondria. It is also likely that an energy step is needed for the release of chaperones in this compartment (Tables 3–9 and 3–10).

Components of the ER Lumen

The ER lumen contains the following components:

A. Protein disulfide isomerase (PDI). This protein has two thioredox domains. PDI is located primarily in the lumen and is especially abundant in the ER of cells that produce disulfide-bonded secretory or membrane proteins. As the nascent chain threads its way through the ER membrane—and as the molecule enters the lumen where conditions for disulfide bond formation are favorable—any two cysteine residues are likely to bond by a disulfide link. This bond may or may not lead to the correct folding of the protein.

It is thought that PDI associates with the elongating polypeptide and retards the formation of incorrect disulfide bonds. Precisely how PDI surveys a protein to ensure proper -S-S- bridging is not fully understood. One proposed mechanism is that PDI forms a disulfide bond with the cysteine on the nascent protein, but this bond is more labile than that formed from two cysteines in the new protein. Thus, PDI is transiently bound to the new polypeptide during folding actions dictated by other forces (hydrophobic interactions, hydrogen bonding events, and ionic associations with the aqueous solvent within the ER).

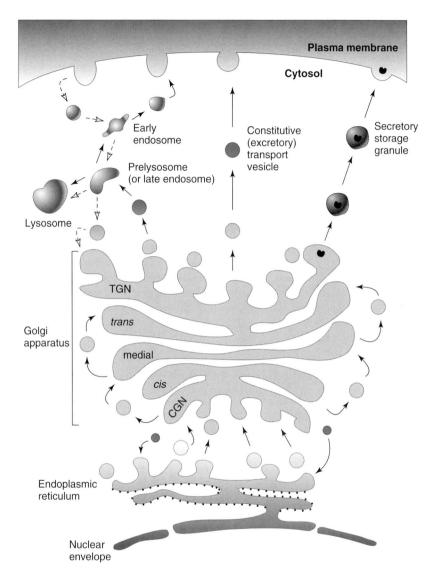

Figure 3–11. Protein sorting. Nascent polypeptides are inserted into either the membrane or lumen of the endoplasmic reticulum (ER) during synthesis on membrane-bound polyribosomes (small black circles studding the cytoplasmic face of the ER). Proteins that will be transported out of the ER (solid black arrows) are moved through ribosome-free transitional elements. These proteins may then pass through regions of the Golgi until they reach the *trans* Golgi network (TGN), the exit face of the Golgi. In the TGN, proteins are sorted. Secretory proteins accumulate in secretory storage granules from which they may be released by exocytosis (upper right of figure). Proteins destined for the plasma membrane and those secreted in a constitutive fashion are carried to the cell surface in small (50- to 100-nm) transport vesicles (upper middle of figure). Other proteins are transferred to lysosomes. Small shaded circles and arrows from the *cis* Golgi network (CGN) indicate retrograde vesicle trafficking to the ER. (Modified and reproduced from Murray RK et al: *Harper's Biochemistry.* Appleton & Lange. 1996, p. 492.)

Table 3–9. Sequences or compounds that direct proteins to specific organelles.[1]

Targeting Sequence or Compound	Organelle Targeted
Signal peptide sequence	Membrane of ER
C-terminal KDEL sequence (Lys·Asp·Glu·Leu)	Luminal surface of ER
N-terminal sequence (70-residue positive region)	Mitochondrion
Short, basic amino acid sequences	Nucleus
Mannose 6-phosphate	Lysosome

[1]Reproduced, with permission, from Murray RK: *Harper's Biochemistry,* 24th ed., Appleton & Lange, 1996, p. 497.

When the nearly correct three-dimensional structure is reached, PDI reduces its linkage to the new protein, thereby allowing two cysteines that are now in close proximity (due to other forces) to form the correct disulfide linkage.

B. Calcium. The ER lumen contains a relatively high concentration of Ca^{2+} (approximately 5 mmol). This ability to store calcium ions suggests that the ER lumen is an important site of Ca^{2+} storage for various metabolic needs. PDI and other lumenal proteins act as low-affinity, high-capacity binders of calcium ions.

C. ER Chaperones. These molecules include

Table 3–10. Mechanisms by which antibiotics and related drugs inhibit protein synthesis.[1]

Agent	Effect
Chloramphenicol	Prevents normal association of mRNA with ribosomes.
Streptomycin, neomycin, kanamycin	Cause misreading of genetic code.
Cycloheximide, tetracycline	Inhibit transfer of tRNA-amino acid complex to polypeptide.
Puromycin	Puromycin-amino acid complex substitutes for tRNA-amino acid complex and prevents addition of further amino acids to polypeptide.
Mithramycin, mitomycin C, dactinomycin (actinomycin D)	Bind to DNA, preventing polymerization of RNA on DNA.
Chloroquine, colchicine, novobiocin	Inhibit DNA polymerase.
Nitrogen mustards, eg, mechlorethamine (Mustargen)	Bind to guanine in base pairs.
Diphtheria toxin	Prevents ribosome from moving on mRNA.

[1]Reproduced, with permission, from Ganong WF: *Review of Medical Physiology,* 17th ed., Appleton & Lange, 1995, p. 19.

members of the hsp70 and hsp90 families, the binding protein (BiP), Grp-94, and peptidylpropyl isomerase. Evidence suggests that the chaperones function primarily to prevent premature folding and to prevent the aggregation of intermediates, thus leading to more productive folding events. Proteins that do not fold properly or that are delayed in acquiring a native structure remain associated with the chaperone for a longer time. The prolonged presence of these proteins in the lumen of the ER is thought to be an important signal for their subsequent degradation by resident proteases in this compartment.

D. Calnexin. Calnexin is an 88-kDa protein that resides in the ER. The protein is not a member of the hsp60, hsp70, or hsp90 families. Unlike the other components of the ER, calnexin is an **integral ER protein** with a catalytic domain that faces the lumenal space. One of its functions is to bind incorrectly folded proteins and retain them in the ER. Calnexin is therefore thought to function as a quality control molecule that prevents release of inappropriately folded proteins.

E. Calreticulin. This 46-kDa molecule was first identified as a Ca^{2+}-binding protein in the sarcoplasmic reticulum of muscle cells. Also an ubiquitous resident in the lumen of the ER, calreticulin has two types of Ca^{2+}-binding domains:

1. A high-affinity site, thus indicating that calreticulin binds calcium at very low concentrations of calcium
2. A high-capacity site for binding several molecules of calcium at the same time.

In the ER, calreticulin has retention signals for amino acids and for carboxyl groups—further indication that the protein plays a strategic metabolic role in this cellular compartment. In addition, calreticulin has a nuclear localization signal, and the protein has been shown to play a modulating role in the binding of the steroid receptor to its DNA site. This observation indicates that calreticulin must escape from the retrieval pathway in order to arrive in the cytoplasm. Precisely how this occurs is not known. Of interest is the fact that calreticulin also has been implicated in several other functions. It appears, for example, to act as an integrin-binding protein, a plasma anticoagulant, and as a "memory molecule" (a molecule that appears to facilitate long-term potentiation) in the sea snail *Aplysia.* It is possible that other roles for calreticulin will be discovered as the full range of this protein's biological activity is elucidated.

RETENTION OF PROTEINS IN THE ER

Movement of material out of the ER occurs by formation of transport vesicles that possess a specific proteinaceous coat, designated COP II. Thus, soluble proteins that are translocated into the lumen are delivered to other cellular locations by vesicles that bud from the ER. Some proteins need to remain in the ER as part of the function of this compartment, ie, for protein folding and core glycosylation.

Several mechanisms act to retain proteins in the ER (Figure 3–12). It appears that certain proteins are excluded from transport vesicles by their characteristic shape, or they misfold and become permanently associated with ER proteins, such as BiP or ER chaperones, and are later degraded within the lumen of the ER.

In addition, amino acid sequences called **retention sequences** appear in proteins that remain in the ER membrane.

The retention system in the ER is imperfect, and some important lumenal proteins are transported inadvertently out of the ER to the next compartment, the Golgi complex. Fortunately, proteins critical to the ER have a **retrieval-retention sequence** composed of four amino acids (KDEL) located near the carboxyl terminal. Proteins containing the KDEL sequence are slower to move toward transport vesicles, and this suggests that exclusion from the vesicles may contribute to the retention of those proteins. Findings from in vitro experiments suggest that

KDEL ligand binding to retrieval receptors is pH-dependent. Maximum binding occurs between pH 5 and pH 6, which is the pH range within the Golgi complex. (Figure 3–12)

ER proteins that contain the KDEL sequence and are inadvertently transported to the Golgi complex bind to the retrieval receptor, which is located in a region of the Golgi where vesicles bud and then move back toward the ER. These are called **retrograde vesicles.** The pH of the ER is nearer neutrality, and proteins with KDEL quickly dissociate from the receptor on returning to the ER environment.

It should be emphasized that retrograde vesicles can form at any site in the Golgi complex and are not limited to the Golgi stack closest to the ER membrane.

PROTEIN TRANSLOCATION

Review of Protein Synthesis: Ribosomes, mRNA, & Signal Peptides

Before considering the mechanisms involved in formation of lipids and proteins that comprise mem-

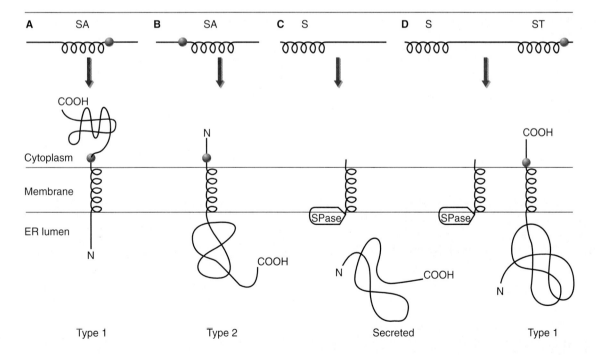

Figure 3–12. Membrane protein orientation in the endoplasmic reticulum. Insertion into the membrane in opposite orientations is mediated by type 1 and type 2 signal-anchor sequences (SA) (A, B respectively). The interaction of the enzyme signal peptidase (SPase) and cleavable signal sequences (S) within the protein (C) results in membrane translocation of secretory proteins. The interaction of SPase and a stop-transfer (ST) sequence in the protein (D) results in membrane insertion in type I orientation. (Sphere = clusters of charged amino acid residues that often flank SA and ST sequences on the cytoplasmic side of the membrane-spanning domain.) (From High S et al: Mechanisms that determine the transmembrane disposition of proteins. Curr Opin Cell Biol 1995;7:582, with permission.)

branes, a brief review of the mechanics of protein synthesis is warranted.

All protein synthesis begins in the cytosol. Ribosomal subunits leave the nucleus fully assembled as 40S and 60S complexes. These subunits are disassembled into a functional ribosome until they form a complex with an mRNA. The small subunit (40S) associates with the 5′ region of an mRNA, together with other components of the protein translation complexes. After the association of the mRNA with the initiation complex, the 60S subunit binds and forms the mature 80S ribosome. Translation of the mRNA commences immediately when a functional ribosome forms. A well-defined channel exists in the 60S subunit; this channel is long enough to contain approximately 30 amino acid residues of the polypeptide. The elongating polypeptide passes into this channel.

After the initial ribosome forms and moves the mRNA by six nucleotides—and a second translational complex develops following its reading of six nucleotides—a third complex forms. This ribosomal loading process continues until the mRNA is saturated with ribosomal complexes.

A typical mRNA contains 10–12 ribosomes, thus forming a polyribosome complex or a **polysome.** When an individual ribosome reaches the **translational end** of the mRNA—**the termination codon**—the ribosome leaves the mRNA. The two subunits then separate and form pools in the cytosol from which new ribosomes can be derived. These ribosomes are able to reassemble on the same or other mRNA molecules. Ribosomal subunits can be used repeatedly and will faithfully translate any competent mRNA.

Messenger RNAs undergoing translation fall into two functional categories:

1. mRNAs that encode for proteins that undergo secretion or form an integral membrane protein. These molecules are directed to the surface of the endoplasmic reticulum.
2. mRNAs that encode for proteins that remain in the cell. Their synthesizing complexes remain in the cytosol, unattached to membranes.

It should be emphasized that newly made proteins in this group constitute the bulk of proteins made by the cell. As we have already seen, some of these proteins have **address signals** as part of their amino acid sequence. These signals help direct the proteins to their correct cellular location.

Membranes and secreted proteins are biosynthesized in the RER. This cellular organelle is where all membrane biosynthesis occurs and also where the initial steps of post-translational glycosylation take place. Moreover, protein folding and subunit assembly occur in the lumen of the RER.

SIGNAL RECOGNITION PARTICLE

The delivery of secretory proteins or membrane proteins into the ER begins when the growing polypeptide first emerges from the channel of the large ribosomal subunit as described above. These types of proteins have a **signal peptide** located near the amino-terminal end of the polypeptide. The signal peptide contains a high proportion of hydrophobic amino acids. The type and length of the signal peptide can vary, but its overall composition must be predominantly hydrophobic.

When this sequence of the growing chain emerges from the protection of the ribosome, several events occur. First a **signal recognition particle (SRP)** recognizes the peptide and immediately binds to it (Figure 3–13).

As a result of this binding, elongation of the peptide ceases temporarily. The newly formed complex (the translation complex plus the SRP) associates with an integral membrane protein receptor located within the membrane of the endoplasmic reticulum. The signal recognition particle receptor (SRP-R)—also called the docking protein—is a heterodimer with two subunits, SRα and SRβ. After attachment of the SRP, the translational complex is guided to another membrane junctional complex called the **translocon.**

Before describing in detail the events of translocation of the polypeptide, additional information concerning the SRP and the SRP-R is instructive. The SRP is composed of a single 7S RNA molecule with six polypeptides associated with it (9, 14, 19, 54, 68, 70 kDa, respectively). Each polypeptide has an abundance of basic amino acids.

The overall area of the SRP complex is 240×60 Å. It is thought that formation of the SRP is analogous to the association of the ribosomal proteins with the ribosomal RNA (rRNA)—that the binding of one molecule of protein begins a cooperative association with the other five.

SRP-54 is the protein to which the newly exposed signal peptide associates. SRP-54 has a large domain containing a high concentration of methionine residues, and this is called the M-domain. This region of the protein folds to provide an elongated hydrophobic binding groove studded with methionine residues that extend into the apolar environment, somewhat analogous to bristles of a brush.

Another important feature of SRP-54 is its recently discovered GTPase domain, which is located in a portion of the protein that resides outside the M-domain. The SRP-R is a heterodimer that consists of an alpha chain and a beta chain. Both subunits have a GTPase domain, thus increasing to three the number of GTPases involved in protein targeting.

Ribosomal Targeting

Ribosomal targeting involves three steps:

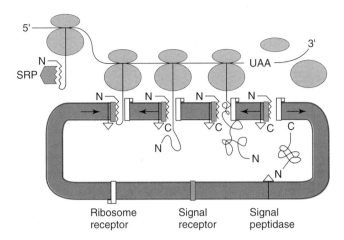

Figure 3–13. Translocation of proteins into the endoplasmic reticulum. Ribosomes synthesizing proteins move along the mRNA from the 5′ to 3′ end. When the signal peptide of a protein destined for secretion, the cell membrane, or lysosomes comes out of the large unit of the ribosome, it binds to a signal recognition particle (SRP). This arrests further translation until the ribosome–nascent chain–SRP complex binds to the SRP receptor on the cytoplasmic face of the endoplasmic reticulum (ER). In a reaction that requires GTP hydrolysis, SRP is recycled in the cytoplasm, and protein synthesis (elongation) continues. Upon translocation, the nascent chain causes the opening of a proteinaceous tunnel so that the growing protein chain enters the ER. The signal peptide is then cleaved by signal peptidase. After protein synthesis ends, the two subunits of the ribosome dissociate, the carboxyl terminus of the protein enters the ER, and the tunnel units disassemble. (N = amino terminus of protein; C = carboxyl terminus of protein.) (Modified and reproduced, with permission, from Perara E, Linappa VR: Transport of proteins into and across the endoplasmic reticulum membrane. In: *Protein Transfer and Organelle Biogenesis.* Das RC, Robbins RW [editors]. Academic Press, 1988.)

1. Signal sequence recognition
2. Elongation arrest
3. Targeting to the ER membrane.

The SRP complex (SRP + ribosome) targets to the ER membrane and binds to the SRP-R (SRα and SRβ). This binding causes the GTPase of SRP-54 and the GTPases of the two receptor subunits to activate. This in turn releases the SRP from the ribosome and causes the receptors to attach the ribosome to a translocon, a protein complex in the ER membrane.

Passage of the nascent chain through the membrane occurs through an enlarged channel. The precise way the channel is formed is not completely understood. Using unique types of fluorescent dyes attached to an artificial signal sequence, researchers have shown that an aqueous channel is formed by the translocon proteins and the ribosome. Nearly all proteins made for secretion or for membrane insertion are translated and translocated by the ribosomes attached to the ER membrane. A model for GTP utilization of SRP-54 is depicted below.

Immediately following the transfer of the translational complex to the translocon and the release of the signal peptide from the SRP-54 and SRP-9\14, translational events resume. The signal peptide remains associated with the lipid bilayer, perhaps embedded in the hydrophobic regions of the membrane.

As the polypeptide elongates, it remains tethered to the inner surface of the membrane via the signal peptide. When the translational termination codon is reached, the ribosome falls off the mRNA, and the final residues of the protein are transferred across the ER membrane. The final exit translocation of the new peptide activates a protease that is bound to the inner surface of the ER membrane, and this action cleaves the signal peptide from the newly made protein. The signal peptide is released from the membrane and degraded by other resident proteases in the lumen.

MECHANISMS OF TRANSLOCATING SECRETORY PROTEINS & MONOTYPIC MEMBRANE PROTEINS

Variations of the polypeptide translocation process occur for proteins that remain located in the membrane. Recall that there are two basic types of integral membrane proteins: those with a single transmembrane domain (**monotypic**) and those with multiple loops that traverse the membrane bilayer (**multipass, polytopic**).

We consider first the monotopic membrane protein. Keep in mind that the functional and locational destiny of any protein is encoded in its gene. Just as there is an amino-terminal signal sequence (as described earlier) that programs the secretory protein for translocation across the ER membrane, so also an internal signal sequence is recognized by the SRP that attaches to it and causes a destabilization of the ribosomal-translocon complex. This in turn *prevents* the translocation of the peptide *but does not prevent* continued translation. Thus the **stop transfer sequence** anchors the elongating protein in the membrane and becomes the transmembrane domain of this single-pass membrane protein.

Two variations of this process warrant attention. The simple version described above allows the single pass protein to orient with the amino terminal (NH_2) located in the lumen of the ER and the carboxyl terminal (COOH) located on the cytosolic side. Various membrane proteins have the opposite orientation—ie, they have a **signal sequence** (also called a **start transfer sequence**) located many residues past the NH_2 end of the protein. When this sequence emerges from the ribosomal channel, the SRP recognizes it and brings the ribosomal complex to the ER membrane. The internal start transfer sig-

nal functions precisely as the **signal peptide** and associates with components of the translocon, which hold it fast within the translocating channel. Unlike the amino-terminal signal sequence of secreted proteins, this sequence is not recognized by the signal peptidase and is not cleaved. Presumably, the membrane channel can increase in size to accommodate both the growing chain and the tethered signal peptide.

The types of amino acids on either side of the hydrophobic transmembrane sequence provide a key to understanding how binding occurs to the M-domain of the SRP-54 protein. There are clusters of positively charged amino acids on both sides of the hydrophobic signal sequence, and these charges help to lock this protein into the bilayer. Key to understanding how the signal peptide is oriented is the number of positively charged residues on each side. The greater the charge, the more likely the peptide will be oriented on the cytosolic side of the membrane, as illustrated by the type I membrane protein shown in Figure 3–14.

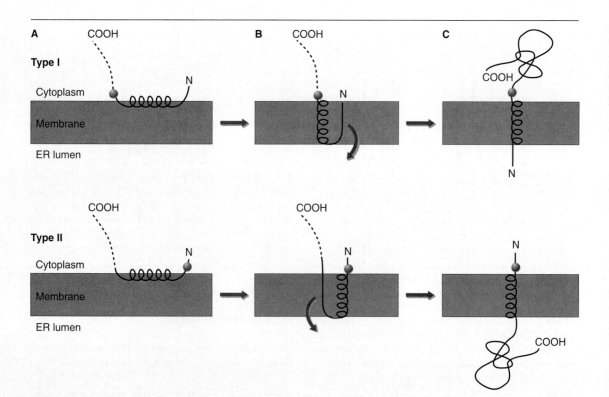

Figure 3–14. Intermediate steps during membrane insertion of signal anchor–containing proteins. The hydrophobic core of the signal-anchor sequence (A) interacts with the endoplasmic reticulum (ER) membrane and (B) inserts into the membrane to form a loop with either the amino-terminal (type I) or carboxyl-terminal (type II) flanking region of the protein. Next (C), the appropriate terminus of the protein is translocated into the ER lumen. (Sphere = clusters of charged amino acid residues that often flank signal-anchor sequences on the cytoplasmic side of the membrane-spanning domain.) (Modified and reproduced, with permission, from High S et al: Mechanisms that determine the transmembrane disposition of proteins. Curr Opin Cell Biol 1995;7:583.)

MECHANISMS THAT DETERMINE POLYTOPIC PROTEINS

Various membrane proteins are "stitched" through the lipid bilayer. These *polytopic* membrane proteins are formed when **start transfer** and **stop transfer** sequences are encoded at appropriate sites within the polypeptide chain. When a start transfer sequence emerges from the ribosomal channel, SRP interacts with it, and the complex binds to the SRP-R for attachment to the translocon. As a stop transfer sequence is encountered, translocation through the membrane ceases, but translation does not.

When a second start transfer sequence is recognized by SRP, it binds and brings the complex to the ER via SRP-R, for transfer across the membrane. Thus by possessing a series of start transfer and stop transfer sequences, polytopic proteins are threaded through the bilayer. Whether a given hydrophobic sequence is a *start* or *stop* depends on the extent and distribution of clustered positively charged amino acids flanking it. The larger cluster of charges usually remains on the cytosolic side of the ER, the orientation of the NH_2.

CORE GLYCOSYLATION OF PROTEINS & LIPIDS OCCURS IN THE ER

Most proteins made on membrane-bound ribosomes are glycosylated as they undergo translocation into the lumen of the ER. This results from the transfer of a large oligosaccharide that has been synthesized on a special membrane-bound lipid, the **dolichol,** which is embedded in the lumenal leaflet of the ER. Dolichols are long-chain polyisoprenols (n = 14–24), with the last isoprene unit saturated. At this site, phosphate linkages form, and glycosyl transferase enzymes add carbohydrate residues. Formation of the oligosaccharides to the dolichol begins by phosphorylation of the saturated residue, thereby making a reactive site (Figure 3–15).

Following this reaction, five mannose residues are quickly added sequentially by five mannoside transferases. These three reactions occur while the dolichol complex is oriented toward the cytosol. This complex "flips" through the membrane and faces the lumenal surface, at which point four mannose residues are added, followed by three glucose residues. A com-

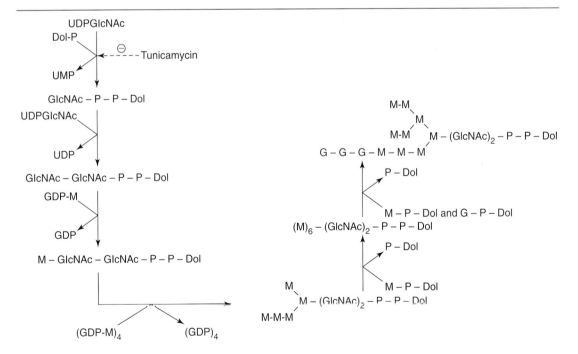

Figure 3–15. Biosynthesis of oligosaccharide-P-P-dolichol. Note that GDP-mannose donates the internal mannose residues, whereas dolichol-P-mannose and dolichol-P-glucose provide the more external mannose residues and the glucose residues. (UDP = uridine diphosphate; Dol = dolichol; P = phosphate; UMP = uridine monophosphate; GDP = guanosine diphosphate; M = mannose; G = glucose.) (Modified and reproduced, with permission, from High S et al: Mechanisms that determine the transmembrane disposition of proteins. Curr Opin Cell Biol 1995;7:583.)

pleted dolichol-phosphate-oligosaccharide contains two *N*-acetylglucosamine residues, nine mannose residues, and three glucose residues. This entire carbohydrate complex is transferred to an asparagine residue that is part of a site containing Asn-X-Ser\Thr.

This tripeptide sequence has the potential to receive the large group of sugars en mass; the result is N-glycosylation (N designating the asparagine residue). Not all Asn-X-Ser\Thr found in a protein are eligible for glycosylation. Rather, glycosylation appears to favor the asparagine residue of the tripeptide that is part of a β-turn or loop, in which the Asn peptide N-H group is hydrogen that *bonds* to the Ser or Thr hydroxyl-O atom.

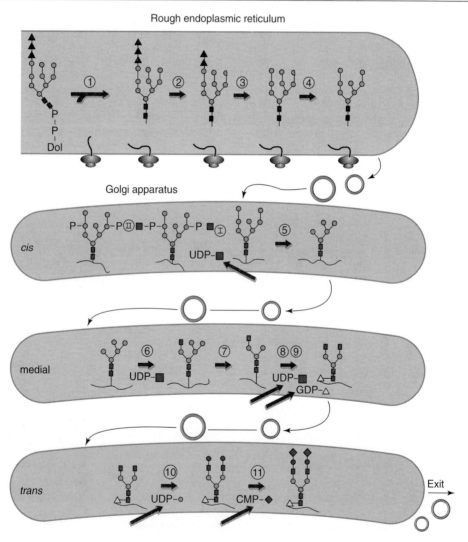

Figure 3–16. Oligosaccharide processing. Reactions are catalyzed by the following enzymes: ① = oligosaccharyltransferase; ② = α-glucosidase I; ③ = α-glucosidase II; ④ = endoplasmic reticulum α1,2 mannosidase; Ⓘ = *N*-acetylglucosaminylphosphotransferase; Ⓘ = *N*-acetylglucosamine-1-phosphodiester α-*N*-acetylglucosaminidase; ⑤ = Golgi apparatus α-mannosidase I; ⑥ = *N*-acetylglucosaminyltransferase I; ⑦ = Golgi apparatus α-mannosidase II; ⑧ = *N*-acetylglucosaminyltransferase II; ⑨ = fucosyltransferase; ⑩ = galactosyltransferase; ⑪ = sialtransferase; ■ = *N*-acetylglucosamine; O = mannose; ▲ = glucose; △ = fucose; ● = galactose; ◆ = sialic acid. (Modified from Kornfeld R, Kornfeld S: Assembly of asparagine-linked oligosaccharides. Annu Rev Biochem 1985;54:631. Reproduced with permission from the *Annual Review of Biochemistry*, Volume 54, © 1985, by Annual Reviews, Inc.).

Table 3–11. Key tasks[1] the cell must accomplish in the synthesis of membrane lipids in the ER.

Task	Requirement
Lipid manufacture	Determine ER location for—and biomolecular pathways of—lipid manufacture
Lipid sorting and transfer	Determine sorting and transport mechanisms for lipids to be distributed from the site of synthesis to their appropriate location in the bilayer; most cells have polarity and lipid composition is not the same at different sites (eg, apical vs basolateral sites).
Lipid distribution	Determine the assymetrical distribution of lipids in the bilayer.

[1]These tasks are also the subject of ongoing biological research and elucidation.

Figure 3–16 presents a schematic model of oligosaccharide processing.

MEMBRANE LIPID BIOSYNTHESIS

Biosynthesis of membrane lipids occurs mostly in the ER. Key tasks the cell must address in the synthesis of membrane lipids are listed in Table 3–11.

The three major varieties of membrane lipids are

1. Glycerolphospholipids: eg, phosphatidylcholine (PC), phosphatidylethanolamine (PE), phosphatidylserine (PS), and phosphatidylinositol(PI).
2. Sphingophospholipids: eg, sphingomyelin (SM) and ceramide (CER).
3. Cholesterol: very low density lipoprotein (VLDL) cholesterol, low density lipoprotein (LDL) cholesterol, and high density lipoprotein (HDL) cholesterol.

Enzymes involved in the synthetic pathway for these lipids are positioned as **integral membrane proteins** in the ER, and their catalytic domains face the cytosol. How the cell synthesizes and transports these lipids poses a special problem because aliphatic hydrocarbon chains are insoluble in the aqueous milieu of the cytosol. Fatty acids are esterified to special proteins called **acyl carrier proteins (ACP),** thereby keeping them in a soluble form.

An early step in the formation of the membrane lipid is a transfer reaction that leads to the formation of phosphatidic acid by replacing the acyl-CoA derivative of two fatty acids with glycerol-3-phosphate, thereby forming diacylglycerolphosphatidic acid. This transfer reaction also involves the release of the fatty acids from the ACP and inserts them into the cytosolic leaflet of the ER bilayer.

A second reaction involves removal of the phosphate by a phosphatase reaction leading to the formation of diacylglycerol, which forms the substrate for the formation of CTP-choline by utilizing the third enzyme of the reaction, choline phosphotransferase. The formation of ceramide occurs in four reactions from the precursors palmityl-CoA and serine. Once ceramide is made, it is transported to the Golgi for conversion to sphingomyelin and glycosphingolipids. The enzyme, sphingomyelin synthase, transfers a phosphocholine head group from phosphatidylcholine (PC) to ceramide, thereby forming sphingomyelin. The other members of this family of membrane lipids are made in the *cis* Golgi (Chapter 4) (Tables 3–12 and 3–13).

Mechanisms of Lipid Sorting and Transport

All synthesis of glycerolphospholipids occurs on the cytosolic face of the ER, and this involves several enzymatic pathways. New lipids freely diffuse within

Table 3–12. Composition of the major lipoprotein complexes.[1]

Complex	Source	Density (g/mL)	% Protein	% TG[2]	% PL[3]	% CE[4]	% C[5]	% FFA[6]
Chylomicron	Intestine	< 0.95	1–2	85–88	8	3	1	0
VLDL	Liver	0.95–1.006	7–10	50–55	18–20	12–15	8–10	1
IDL	VLDL	1.006–1.019	10–12	25–30	25–27	32–35	8–10	1
LDL	VLDL	1.019–1.063	20–22	10–15	20–28	37–48	8–10	1
*HDL$_2$	Intestine, liver (chylomicrons and VLDLs)	1.063–1.125	33–35	5–15	32–43	20–30	5–10	0
*HDL$_3$	Intestine, liver (chylomicrons and VLDLs)	1.125–1.21	55–57	3–13	26–46	15–30	2–6	6
Albumin-FFA	Adipose tissue	> 1.281	99	0	0	0	0	100

[1]Reproduced, with permission, from Balcavage WX, King MW: *Biochemistry: Examination & Board Review,* Appleton & Lange, 1995, p. 212.
[2]Triacylglycerols; [3]Phospholipids; [4]Cholesterol esters; [5]Free cholesterol; [6]Free fatty acids.
*HDL$_2$ and HDL$_3$ derived from nascent HDL as a result of the acquisition of cholesteryl esters.

the plane of this bilayer, and hence quickly equilibrate with existing lipids in this membrane leaflet. Moreover, nonspecific **flippases** in the ER membrane also move the newly made lipids to the lumenal leaflet. Thus, rapid equilibration of all glycerolphospholipids occurs within the ER.

This is not the entire story, however. Recall that a hallmark of the membrane is the asymmetric distribution of the various lipids. How does such distribution occur? In the plasma membrane and Golgi complex, an ATP-dependent translocase—**aminophospholipid translocase**—pumps phosphotidylserine (PS) and to a lesser extent phosphatidylcholine (PC) toward the cytoplasmic side of the membrane. As a result, the cytosolic leaflet contains all the PS and most of the PE and PI. Note that this enzyme does not pump ceramide or sphingosine. This differential movement of lipids is a key factor in the establishment of lipid asymmetry in the membrane (Tables 3–14 and 3–15).

MEMBRANE LIPID TRAFFICKING PATHWAYS

Vesicular Pathway & Monomeric Exchange

There are two major trafficking pathways for membrane lipids:

1. The **vesicular pathway** transports lipids to the plasma membrane, Golgi complex, and lysosomes. This pathway involves **budding of the ER membrane** to form a vesicle that fuses with the Golgi complex then moves to other organelles along this pathway.
2. **Monomeric exchange** is the pathway in which organelles such as mitochondria and peroxisomes undergo direct transfer from the ER surface via **lipid exchange proteins.** Phosphatidylcholine (PC) is involved in both types of movement. PC is made on the cytosolic surface. Some PC mole-

Table 3–13. Apoprotein classification.[1]

Apoprotein-MW(Da)	Lipoprotein Association	Function and Comments
apo-A-I–29,016	Chylomicrons, HDL	Major protein of HDL, activates LCAT
apo-A-II–17,400	Chylomicrons, HDL	Primarily in HDL, enhances hepatic lipase activity
apo-A-IV–46,000	Chylomicrons and HDL	Present in triacylglycerol-rich lipoproteins
apo-B-48–241,000	Chylomicrons	Exclusively found in chylomicrons; derived from apo-B-100 gene by RNA editing in intestinal epithelium; lacks the LDL receptor-binding domain of apo-B-100
apo-B-100–513,000	VLDL, IDL, and LDL	Major protein of LDL; binds to LDL receptor; one of the longest known proteins in humans
apo-C-I–7,600	Chylomicrons, VLDL, IDL, and HDL	May also activate LCAT
apo-C-II–8,916	Chylomicrons, VLDL, IDL, and HDL	Activates lipoprotein lipase
apo-C-III–8,750	Chylomicrons, VLDL, IDL, and HDL	Inhibits lipoprotein lipase
apo-D–20,000; also called cholesterol ester transfer protein, CETP	HDL	Exclusively associated with HDL, cholesteryl ester transfer
apo-E–34,000 (at least 3 alleles [E2, E3, E4] each of which may have multiple isoforms)	Chylomicron remnants, VLDL, IDL, and HDL	Binds to LDL receptor, apo-E-ε4 allele amplification associated with late-onset Alzheimer's disease
apo-H–50,000 (also known as β-2-glyco-protein I)	Chylomicrons	Triacylglycerol metabolism
apo(a)–at least 19 different alleles; protein ranges in size from 300,000–800,000	LDL	Disulfide bonded to apo-B-100, forms a complex with LDL identified as lipoprotein(a), Lp(a); strongly resembles plasminogen; may deliver cholesterol to sites of vascular injury; high-risk association with premature coronary artery disease and stroke

[1]Reproduced, with permission, from Balcavage WX, King MW: *Biochemistry: Examination & Board Review,* Appleton & Lange, 1995, p. 213.

Table 3–14. Hyperlipoproteinemias.[1]

Disorder	Defect	Comments
Type I (familial LPL deficiency, familial hyperchylomicronemia)	(a) deficiency of LPL; (b) production of abnormal LPL; (c) apo-C-II deficiency	Slow chylomicron clearance, reduced LDL and HDL levels; treated by low fat/complex carbohydrate diet; no increased risk of coronary artery disease
Type II (FH)	Four classes of LDL receptor defect (see text above)	Reduced LDL clearance leads to hypercholesterolemia, resulting in atherscleosis and coronary artery disease
Type III (familial dysbetalipoproteinemia, remnant removal disease, broad beta disease)	Hepatic remnant clearance impaired due to apo-E abnormality; patients only express the apo-E2 isoform that interacts poorly with the apo-E receptor	Causes xanthomas, hypercholesterolemia and atherscleosis in peripheral and coronary arteries due to elevated levels of chylomicrons and VLDLs
Type IV (familial hypertriacylglycerolemia)	Elevated production of VLDL associated with glucose intolerance and hyperinsulinemia	Frequently associated with type-II (non-insulin dependent) diabetes mellitus, obesity, alcoholism or administration of progestational hormones; elevated cholesterol as a result of increased VLDLs
Type V familial	Elevated chylomicrons and VLDLs due to unknown cause	Hypertriacylglycerolemia and hypercholesterolemia with decreased LDLs and HDLs
Familial hyperalphalipoproteinemia	Increased level of HDLs	A rare condition that is beneficial for health and longevity
Familial hyperapobetalipoproteinemia	Increased LDL production and delayed clearance of triacylglycerols and fatty acids	Strongly associated with increased risk of coronary artery disease
Familial defective apo-B-100	Gln for Arg mutation in exon 26 of apo-B gene (amino acid 3500); leads to reduced affinity of LDL for LDL receptor	Dramatic increase in LDL levels; no affect on HDL, VLDL or plasma triglyceride levels; significant cause of hypercholesterolemia and premature coronary artery disease
Familial LCAT deficiency	Absence of LCAT leads to inability of HDLs to take up cholesterol (reverse cholesterol transport)	Decreased levels of plasma cholesteryl esters and lysolecithin; abnormal LDLs (Lp-X) and VLDLs; symptoms also found associated with cholestasis
Wolman's disease (cholesteryl ester storage disease)	Defect in lysosomal cholesteryl ester hydrolase, affects metabolism of LDLs	Reduced LDL clearance leads to hypercholesterolemia resulting in atherscleosis and coronary artery disease
Hormone-releasable hepatic lipase deficiency	Deficiency of the lipase leads to accumulation of triacylglycerol-rich HDLs and VLDL remnants (IDLs)	Causes xanthomas and coronary artery disease

[1]Reproduced, with permission, from Balcavage WX, King MW: *Biochemistry: Examination & Board Review,* Appleton & Lange, 1995, p. 216.

cules are translocated across the membrane to the lumenal surface, then follow the endocytic pathway through the Golgi complex to the plasma membrane—and to their final destination on the exterior of the cell. Alternately, some PC remains on the cytosolic surface and can be extracted and translocated directly to the mitochondria when that organelle contacts the cytosol.

Vesicle budding and **vesicle fusion** are the major pathways that move lumenal contents and membranes, including lipids and integral proteins. It is believed that, in some instances, the rapid synthesis of lipids in the cytosolic leaflet causes a membrane cur-

vature that initiates the budding process of the ER (Chapter 4). It is also important to note that the membrane lipids phosphoinositol (PI) and ceramide are critical participants in **signal transduction** (Chapter 9). Note also that PI is the precursor for the GPI-anchored proteins PI, PIP, PIP_2 and PIP_3, which are synthesized in the ER.

Most cells of the body exhibit polarity, ie, one surface of the cell differs from the other. This is particularly true of epithelial cells. Techniques have been developed to examine the lipid and protein composition of the basolateral and apical surfaces.

For more information, readers are referred to a standard text on the physiology of cellular structure and function.

Table 3–15. Hypolipoproteinemias.[1]

Disorder	Defect	Comments
Abetalipoproteinemia (acanthocytosis, Bassen-Kornzweig syndrome)	No chylomicrons, VLDLs or LDLs, due to defect in apo-B expression	Rare defect; intestine and liver accumulate, malabsorption of fat, retinitis pigmentosa, ataxic neuropathic disease; erythrocytes have "thorny" appearance
Familial hypobetalipoproteinemia	At least 20 different apoB gene mutations identified; LDL concentrations 10–20% of normal; VLDL slightly lower, HDL normal	Mild or no pathological changes
Familial alpha-lipoprotein deficiency (Tangier disease, Fish-eye disease, apo-A-1 and -C-III deficiencies)	All of these related syndromes have reduced HDL concentrations, no effect on chylomicron or VLDL production	Tendency to hypertriacylglycerolemia; some elevation in VLDLs; Fish-eye disease characterized by severe corneal opacity

[1]Reproduced, with permission, from Balcavage WX, King MW: *Biochemistry: Examination & Board Review,* Appleton & Lange, 1995, p. 218.

REFERENCES

Bergeron JJM et al: Calnexin: A membrane-bound chaperone of the endoplasmic reticulum. Trends in Biochem Sci 1994;19:124.

Burns K et al: Calreticulin: From Ca^{2+} to control of gene expression. Trends in Cell Biol 1994;4:152.

Crowley K, Reinhart G, Johnson A: The signal sequence moves through a ribosomal tunnel into a noncytoplasmic aqueous environment at the ER membrane early in translocation. Cell 1993;73:1101.

Dobson C, Evans P, Radford S: Understanding how proteins fold: The lysozyme story so far. Trends in Biochem Sci 1994;19:31.

Freeman RB, Hirst TR, Tuite MF: Protein disulfide isomerase: Building bridges in protein folding. Trends in Biochem Sci 1994;19:331.

Gaut JR, Hendershot LM: The modification and assembly of proteins in the endoplasmic reticulum. Curr Opin Cell Biol 1993;5:589.

Georgopoulos C, Welch W: Role of the major heat shock proteins as molecular chaperones. Annu Rev Cell Biol 1993;9:610.

Goldberg MW, Allen TD: Structural and functional organization of the nuclear envelope. Curr Opin Cell Biol 1995;7:301.

Hartl F, Hlodan R, Langer T: Molecular chaperones in protein folding: The art of avoiding sticky situations. Trends in Biochem Sci 1994;19:20.

Hartl FU: Molecular chaperones in cellular protein folding. Nature 1996;381:571.

High S, Dobberstein B: Mechanisms that determine the transmembrane disposition of proteins. Curr Opin Cell Biol 1992;4:581.

Kobe B, Deisenhofer J: The leucine-rich repeat: A versatile binding motif. Trends in Biochem Sci 1994;19:415.

Melchior F, Gerace L: Mechanisms of nuclear protein import. Curr Opin Cell Biol 1995;7:310.

Ng D, Walter P: Protein translocation across the endoplasmic reticulum. Curr Opin Cell Biol 1994;6:510.

Peters JM: Proteosomes: Protein degradation machines of the cell. Trends in Biochem Sci 1994;19:377.

Pfanner N, Craig E, Meijer M: The protein import machinery of the mitochondrial inner membrane. Trends in Biochem Sci 1994;19:368.

Sander L et al: Sec61p and BiP directly facilitate polypeptide translocation into the ER. Cell 1992;69:353.

Seashore MR, Wappner RS: *Genetics in Primary Care.* Appleton & Lange, 1995.

van Meer G: Transport and sorting of membrane lipids. Curr Opin Cell Biol 1993;5:661.

Walter P, Johnson AJ: Signal sequence recognition and protein targeting to the endoplasmic reticulum membrane. Annu Rev Cell Biol 1994;10:87.

SUGGESTED READING

Birge RR: Protein-based computers. Sci Am (March) 1995;90.

Craig EA: Chaperones: Helpers along the pathways to protein folding. Science 1993;260:1902.

Goto K, Warner TD: Endothelin versatility. Nature 1995;375:539.

Lei K et al: Mutations in the glucose-6-phosphatase gene that cause glycogen storage disease Type 1a. Science 1993;262:580.

Marx J: Forging a path to the nucleus. Science 1993;260:1588.

Morimoto RI: Cells in stress: Transcriptional activation of heat shock genes. Science 1993;259:1409.

Richards FM: Obituary: Christian B. Anfinsen (1916–95). Nature 1995;376:19.

Ungewickell E et al: Role of auxilin in uncoating clathrin-coated vesicles. Nature 1995;378:632.

Organelles & Vesicle Traffic

4

In this chapter we consider several fundamental principles of cell biology, with special attention to the key biomolecular mechanisms that enable proteins and lipids to travel to various *intracellular* locations.

Carrier vesicles are the major means by which proteins and lipids are transported between organelles. During this transport process, the cell benefits from an elegant and marvelous economy: the proteins and lipids that are transported constitute the membrane of the carrier vesicle, and within the lumen of this membrane, **cargo molecules** can be concentrated and delivered to other organelles (Figure 4–1).

Many human diseases result from defects in the intracellular delivery system (Table 4–1). Consequently, to understand the molecular basis of these diseases and to devise therapeutic modalities, we must understand how vesicle trafficking and delivery occur. Toward this end, the chapter addresses several important issues, including:

- initiation of vesicle formation (Table 4–2)
- formation of vesicles at selective sites on the membrane surface

- vectorial pathways for vesicle migration
- proteins required for vesicle formation and vesicle fusion with a target membrane
- energy requirements for vesicular transport.

For a review of the bioenergetics of cellular metabolism—including the biochemistry underlying oxidation, phosphorylation, and other processes involved in the metabolism of proteins and lipids—readers are referred to a standard biochemistry text.

SECRETORY PATHWAY

The cellular mechanisms of protein trafficking and membrane fusion in the secretory pathway are conserved across species, from yeast to mammalian cells. Much of the current understanding of intracellular vesicular trafficking, in fact, has emerged from studies on the secretory pathway in yeast cells. In that model system, advanced techniques in genetics, molecular biology, biochemistry, and microscopy are being used to identify and characterize many components that mediate intracellular protein sorting and vesicular trafficking.

The classic studies on the secretory pathway in the exocrine pancreas led to the concept of **vectorial trafficking,** in which proteins are transported through the secretory pathway by carriers that consist of small membrane-bound vesicles (Palade, 1975). Many biochemical components of this vesicle carrier system have been characterized. Still to be elucidated, however, are various steps in this pathway and the function of some membrane components (Mellman, 1995). Transport from the endoplasmic reticulum (ER) to the *cis* Golgi, the *trans* Golgi network (TGN), and then to the plasma membrane is vesicle-mediated, as is membrane recycling from the Golgi apparatus back to the ER. Conversely, the mechanism of intra-Golgi transport—whether by vesicle carriers or intercisternal tubular connections between

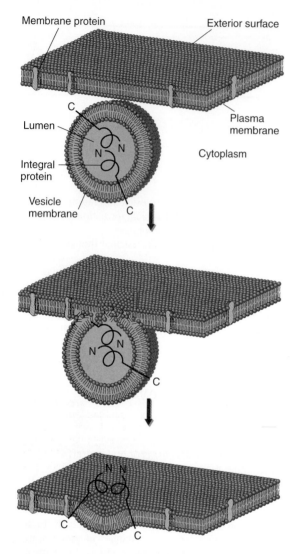

Figure 4–1. Vesicle fusion and integral membrane protein orientation. When vesicle membranes fuse with the plasma membrane, the surface of the vesicle membrane that faced the cytoplasm remains on the cytoplasmic face of the plasma membrane. Consequently, integral membrane proteins that had carboxyl terminals on the cytoplasmic face of the vesicle have carboxyl terminals on the cytoplasmic face of the plasma membrane after fusion is complete. (Modified and redrawn, with permission, from Lodish HF, Rothman JE: The assembly of cell membranes. Sci Am 1979;240:43.)

Golgi stacks—is still not clearly understood (Figure 4–2).

Elucidating the Secretory Pathway

Although the basic **secretory pathway** was outlined more than 30 years ago, the molecular details of these processes are still being elucidated. The pio-

Table 4–1. Diseases associated with defective intracellular trafficking signals.

Disease	Proteins Affected	Fate of Protein
Congenital sucrase-isomaltase deficiency	Sucrase-isomaltase	ER,[1] Golgi complexes, or basolateral surface but not apically located
Cystic fibrosis	CFTR[2]	Degraded in ER: fails to reach surface or other sites
Familial hyper-cholestero-lemia	LDL[3] receptor	Class 2 fails to exit ER Class 4 fails to cluster in coated pits Class 5 fails to recycle after endocytosis
Hereditary emphysema	α_1-antitrypsin	Accumulates and degraded in ER; not secreted
I-cell disease	Lysosomal hydrolases	Secreted
Leukocyte adhesion deficiency	CD18	β subunit of receptor is not made or is degraded; a subunit does not mature in absence of β subunit
Zellweger syndrome	Peroxisomal proteins	No peroxisome made because of mutation in peroxisome assembly factor

[1]Endoplasmic reticulum.
[2]Cystic fibrosis transmembrane regulator.
[3]Low-density lipoprotein.

neering work of Palade and colleagues was based on a number of experimental techniques used to dissect the secretory pathway in mammalian cells, for example:

1. Electron microscopy (EM) was used to identify organelles of the secretory pathway in numerous

Table 4–2. Principal events of vesicle formation.

- Material synthesized in the ER is destined to be delivered into a **compartment,** not into the cytosol.
- Substances enter the cell by the physical process of vesicle formation and fusion; this process of cellular entry is called **endocytosis.**
- Material within the lumen of the vesicles is often modified with an **address label** that allows the material to be sorted and concentrated to regions within the lumen that are active in vesicle formation.
- Proteins and lipids within the lumen are modified by **enzymes** that reside in the lumen of each compartment.
- The major site of **glycosylation** of proteins and lipids is the **Golgi** apparatus.
- The **lysosome,** the major hydrolytic compartment of the cell, receives its enzymes from diferent sources.

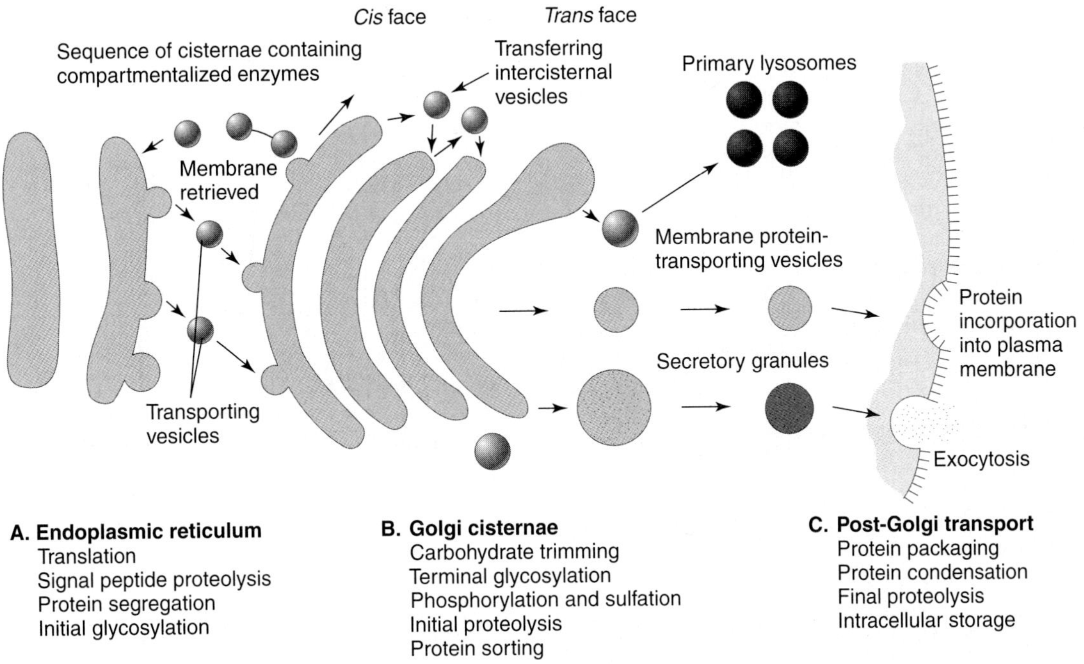

Cis face   Trans face

Sequence of cisternae containing
compartmentalized enzymes

Transferring
intercisternal
vesicles

Primary lysosomes

Membrane
retrieved

Membrane protein-
transporting vesicles

Protein
incorporation
into plasma
membrane

Secretory granules

Transporting
vesicles

Exocytosis

A. Endoplasmic reticulum
  Translation
  Signal peptide proteolysis
  Protein segregation
  Initial glycosylation

B. Golgi cisternae
  Carbohydrate trimming
  Terminal glycosylation
  Phosphorylation and sulfation
  Initial proteolysis
  Protein sorting

C. Post-Golgi transport
  Protein packaging
  Protein condensation
  Final proteolysis
  Intracellular storage

Figure 4–2. Movement of proteins through the Golgi apparatus. Proteins destined for secretion, lysosomes, or the plasma membrane are translocated across the membrane of the endoplasmic reticulum (A), where the initial steps in the glycosylation of glycoproteins occurs. Proteins are sorted into transport vesicles, which carry them to the *cis* face of the Golgi apparatus. Within the Golgi cisternae (B), the carbohydrate moieties of glycoproteins are trimmed before terminal glycosylation in the *trans* Golgi. Phosphorylation and sulfation of certain proteins occurs in the *trans* Golgi and the *trans* Golgi network (TGN), respectively. Proteins are transferred within the cisternae by intracisternal coated vesicles. On the most *trans* face of the Golgi—the TGN—proteins are sorted to different cellular destinations. In the post-Golgi phase (C), proteins are distributed to primary lysosomes, constitutive vesicles, and secretory granules depending on their destination within the cell or cell membrane. (Modified and reproduced, with permission, from Junqueira LC et al: *Basic Histology,* 8th ed. Appleton & Lange, 1995, p. 35.)

cell types during controlled and stimulated secretion.

2. EM autoradiography was used to follow the passage of proteins through the various organelles of the secretory pathway.

3. Data gained by subcellular fractionation techniques in which organelles were isolated and characterized biochemically provided major contributions to the identification of the intracellular pathway.

4. Pulse-chase experiments were conducted in which cells were incubated with radioactive amino acids (or other precursors) and the kinetics and biochemical fate of specific proteins were followed through the secretory pathway. Pulse-chase experiments in concert with cell fractionation and the use of antibodies to specific protein(s), coupled with analytical biochemical techniques to characterize the post-translational modifications, enabled investigators to map very precisely the route that many

proteins take through the secretory pathway. By the mid 1980s it became apparent that soluble proteins, membrane glycoproteins destined for the plasma membrane, and other organelles are transported via the secretory pathway.

5. Novel procedures using simple envelope viruses in which the tracking of one or two well-characterized viral envelope (membrane) proteins could be followed by use of pulse-chase protocols became useful strategies for studying the cell biology of vesicle transport. Expansion of immunoelectron micromicroscopy (using immunogold localization) and of monoclonal antibodies has enabled investigators to further probe the secretory pathway in greater detail and has led to identification of major sites of protein sorting for secretion or for lysosomal targeting as well as to the identification of protein molecules of the plasma membrane (Griffiths & Simons, 1986).

6. Bakers' yeast, *Saccharomyces cerevisiae,* was

used by Scheckman and colleagues to generate scores of mutant cells defective at different steps in the secretory pathway. This pioneering work refined the details of the pathway.

7. The biochemical dissection and *reconstitution* of vesicular movement within mammalian cells from the early to the late Golgi cisternae, the identification of the vesicle fusogenic machinery, and the demonstration of its conservation in synaptic vesicle exocytosis by Rothman and colleagues have had a major impact on our understanding of the secretory process in cells ranging from yeast to those of the human brain.

CONSTITUTIVE SECRETORY PATHWAY

The research strategies just described have provided much evidence regarding the secretory properties of cells. Many cells and tissues, depending on their structure and function, produce peptide hormones, digestive enzymes, antibodies, serum proteins, growth factors, and other secretory molecules. Even fibroblasts secrete components of the basal lamina, including collagen, laminin, and fibronectin (Chapter 8).

In fact, all cells have what has been termed a **constitutive secretory pathway.** In this pathway, proteins are continuously delivered in membrane-bound vesicles from the TGN to the plasma membrane, where they fuse and extrude their contents—by exocytosis—to the external milieu. As far as is known, this is a continuous process that (1) does not require an external signal to be delivered to the cell and (2) is independent of a calcium requirement.

REGULATED SECRETORY PATHWAY

Calcium Required

Endocrine and exocrine cells and neurons possess a **regulated secretory pathway.** In these cells, secretory proteins are stored for hours or even days in large granules (up to 0.5 μm in diameter), which are docked below the plasma membrane. These granules do not fuse with the plasma membrane to release their contents until the cell is activated for exocytosis by an external stimulus—hormonal or neuronal. The signaling stimulus is followed by a transient influx of calcium ions across the plasma membrane, which raises the cytosolic concentration to ~ 1 μm. This transient increase in Ca^{2+} activates other intracellular effector molecules, causing the membrane of the granule to fuse with the plasma membrane, thereby

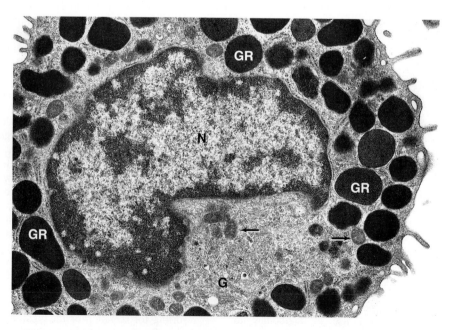

Figure 4–3. Secretory granules. A mast cell has numerous secretory granules containing vasoactive substances such as histamine and serotonin. This electron micrograph of a rat mast cell clearly shows large dense core granules (GR). (N = nucleus; G = Golgi apparatus; arrows = mitochondria.) × 16,086. (Reproduced, with permission, from Berman I: *Color Atlas of Basic Histology.* Appleton & Lange, 1993, p. 27. Courtesy of Dr. Jacques Padawer.)

releasing the granule's contents into the extracellular milieu. Thus, in contrast to constitutive secretion, regulated secretion has an absolute requirement for calcium. Indeed, chelation of extracellular calcium inhibits stimulated secretion in endocrine cells and neurons.

Dense Core Secretory Granules

Concentration of the cargo proteins within the vesicle is initiated in the late Golgi apparatus and in the TGN and is completed in immature secretory granules (Figure 4–3). An approximately 200-fold concentration of content proteins occurs in the secretory granules, compared with the lumen of the ER. The large secretory granules formed by this process are often referred to as **dense core secretory granules** because of their morphological appearance upon electron microscopy. They contain highly concentrated protein that forms a semicrystalline structure that is electron opaque—hence their appearance in the electron microscope.

Cells that possess a regulated secretory pathway also have a constitutive secretory pathway—eg, islet β cells that secrete insulin, pituitary somatomammotrophs that produce growth hormone, and exocrine pancreatic cells responsible for production of digestive enzymes. This means endocrine cells must have a mechanism for distinguishing proteins destined for the regulated pathway from proteins targeted to the constitutive pathway. The nature of these signals remains elusive, and how the cell discriminates between different classes of proteins to ensure their correct packaging into the appropriate vesicles remains an area of intense investigation.

Many components of the vesicle trafficking machinery are functionally conserved—from yeast cells that secrete only constitutively to mammalian cells that have a regulated secretory pathway, eg, neurons. This suggests that regulated secretion may require only subtle differences in the secretory apparatus to generate a dense core secretory granule, rather than a constitutively released vesicle. The nature of the components that confer a regulated secretory phenotype on cells remains unknown, however (Figure 4–4).

DEFAULT SECRETION

Clinical Correlate: Cystic Fibrosis

Complementary deoxyribonucleic acids (cDNAs) encoding the transcript for native and mutated secretory or membrane proteins have been introduced into mammalian tissue culture cells. Findings from this research suggest that proteins are secreted from cells constitutively in the absence of a targeting signal, or a **topogenic signal,** to direct a protein to a particular cellular destination. By analogy to computer programming, this became known as **default secretion.**

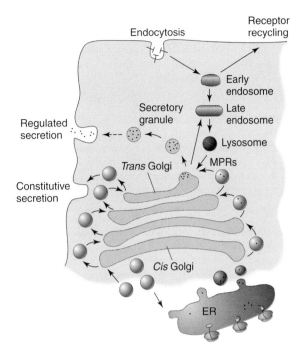

Figure 4–4. Constitutive and regulated secretion. Neuroendocrine cells are capable both of constitutive, or nonregulated, secretion of proteins, whereby proteins are delivered constantly to the plasma membrane in secretory vesicles, and regulated secretion of peptide hormones or neuropeptides. In the latter case, the polypeptides are stored intracellularly in dense core secretory granules, often for prolonged periods. In this model, all polypeptides flow from the endoplasmic reticulum (ER) to the Golgi apparatus. Exit from the *trans* Golgi is different in the constitutive and regulated pathways, as is final protein packaging into constitutive vesicles or secretory granules. Note recycling of membrane and receptors through endocytosis. MPRs = mannose-6-phosphate receptors. (Modified and reproduced, with permission, from Ganong WF: *Review of Medical Physiology,* 17th ed. Appleton & Lange, 1995, p. 20.)

When recombinant DNA techniques are used to add a topogenic signal to a normally secreted protein, the chimeric protein is sorted to the appropriate organelle. For example, if an ER retention signal like KDEL (Lys-Asp-Glu-Leu; see Chapter 3) is added to the C-terminus of a protein, that protein is retained in the ER rather than secreted.

Findings from experiments performed in the mid 1980s suggest that the transport of soluble cargo proteins through the secretory pathway could occur by **bulk flow,** ie, at the proteins' prevailing concentration in the ER lumen. In the absence of targeting or retention sequences—called **topogenic domains—**

proteins are thought to traverse the secretory pathway very rapidly. Most likely this model is not entirely complete. It is known, for instance, that all proteins must undergo a quality control check in the ER lumen to determine whether:

1. the protein is folded correctly,
2. disulfide bonds are formed correctly,
3. the polypeptide is part of an oligomeric protein (eg, the T-cell receptor, which consists of seven subunits),
4. all subunit interactions have occurred to form a stable protein.

To ensure that folding and assembly events have occurred properly, a variety of chaperone molecules exist in the lumen of the ER. If correct intramolecular interactions do not occur or if a protein remains misfolded, degrading enzymes in the lumen of the ER destroy the defective protein.

Cystic fibrosis results from a single amino acid change that causes misfolded cystic fibrosis transmembrane conductance regulator (CTFR) polypeptides to accumulate in the ER instead of being transported to the plasma membrane. These misfolded CTFR polypeptides are also degraded in the ER.

All proteins that traverse the secretory pathway are subject to these chaperone interactions and are concentrated within the vesicle approximately fivefold. There is evidence suggesting a sorting transfer mechanism governs protein transport rather than simple bulk flow. The details of this mechanism, however, remain poorly understood. Figure 4–4 shows some of the main events occurring during trafficking and sorting of proteins through the Golgi complex.

The transport of material into the cell—endocytosis—is also a complex task, and as in the secretory pathway, variations exist in the cellular control of the endocytotic process.

MOLECULAR EVENTS OF VESICLE FORMATION & MOVEMENT

VESICLE BUDDING

In this section we consider the conditions and components involved in the formation, targeting, and fusion of vesicles. These are the components and mechanisms that ensure each membrane of intracellular compartments maintains its molecular composition after intercompartmental transfer. Targeting a vesicle to the correct membrane is essential for individual cell activity and is also critical in its development and its maintenance of tissues.

The major mechanism by which proteins and lipids move within the cell is called **vesicle budding.** Vesicles form from the membrane of one compartment—called the **donor** compartment—and then move to another membrane compartment—called the **acceptor.** This leads to fusion of donor membranes with acceptor membranes and to the delivery of the vesicle contents into the lumenal space of the acceptor compartment. This process remakes cell compartments, reforms cell surfaces, and maintains or alters cell-to-cell contacts.

One might think that the contents and components of the donor compartment would eventually be lost during fusion, and the size of the donor compartment would diminish and that of the acceptor would therefore increase. If this were the case, the ER would disappear while the Golgi would substantially increase in size. This does not occur because cells possess homeostatic mechanisms that regulate and maintain the composition of each organelle membrane. This is achieved, in part, by membrane recycling (Figure 4–4).

Thus, when ER transport vesicles fuse with acceptor membranes of the *cis* Golgi, certain organelle receptor proteins—eg, those responsible for maintaining soluble proteins in the ER—and lipids are recycled from the early Golgi apparatus back to the ER. This is known as **retrograde transport.** In contrast, soluble cargo proteins continue along the secretory pathway, a process known as **anterograde transport.** The differential trafficking of anterograde cargo proteins and the retrieval and recycling—or retrograde trafficking—of components are achieved by at least two classes of proteins with specific protein **coats** that bind to transport vesicles. These protein complexes are called **coatomers,** or **COPs** (Figure 4–5).

COP-I

Using cell-free systems to follow the transport of membrane glycoproteins through the Golgi apparatus, Rothman and colleagues characterized a set of cytosolic proteins that form a proteinaceous coat after being recruited onto Golgi membranes. These proteins form a complex of eight subunits and are designated coatomer, or **COP-I.** The coatomer complex has a small guanosine triphosphate (GTP)–binding protein called ARF, or adenosine diphosphate (ADP)–ribosylation factor. Genetic evidence mainly from yeast cells suggests that mutations that inactivate coatomer subunits or isoforms of ARF also block intracellular vesicular transport and secretion. This evidence established the role for COP-I vesicles in mediating intracellular vesicular transport. Additional evidence came from observations in which microinjection of antibodies directed against one of the

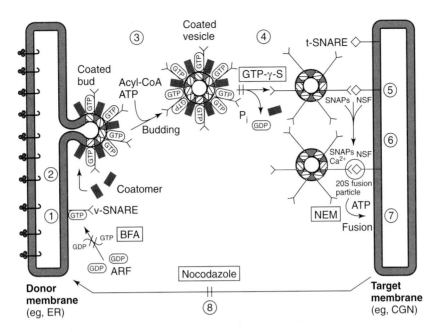

Figure 4–5. Anterograde and retrograde transport. Anterograde transport of cargo proteins from the endoplasmic reticulum (ER) to the Golgi (CGN) involves transport vesicles and coat proteins called coatomers or COPs. To date, at least two types of COPs have been described: Those implicated in anterograde vesicle transport are designated COP-II, whereas those with coats that mediate retrograde transport from the Golgi to the ER (see below) are referred to as COP-I coated vesicles. Note that although the coats of COP-I and COP-II vesicles are similar morphologically, their biochemical composition is different. A budding vesicle associates with a coatomer before release from the ER and travels to the Golgi. The dissociation of the coatomer from the "donor" vesicle is necessary for the vesicle to fuse with the acceptor, or target, membrane and release its protein cargo. (Adapted from Rothman JE: Mechanisms of intracellular protein transport. Nature 1994;372:55. Courtesy of E Degen.)

coatomer subunits, β-COP, into mammalian cells inhibited ER to Golgi transport.

Genetic evidence from yeast cells also has demonstrated that COP-I, rather than functioning in anterograde protein trafficking, most likely plays a role in the recycling and retrieval of membrane components from the Golgi apparatus to the ER during retrograde transport (Figure 4–6).

COP-II

A second set of vesicle coat proteins, with five subunits, has been characterized biochemically and genetically from yeast cells. This protein complex, designated COP-II, appears to function in anterograde transport and mediates vesicle trafficking from the ER to the Golgi apparatus. Mammalian equivalents of some COP-II subunits have been detected by virtue of their cross-reactivity to antibodies raised against the yeast proteins. Consistent with their proposed role in anterograde vesicle transport, these proteins are concentrated in transitional elements of the

ER of pancreatic acinar cells and insulin-secreting β-cells of the islets of Langerhans. The transitional elements, originally described by Palade (1975), are derived from the ribosome-free part of the ER and contain cargo proteins en route to the Golgi apparatus.

VESICLE RECYCLING

On the basis of the biochemical characterization of COP-I and COP-II and their interactions with membranes, a straightforward model for COP action in mediating vesicular transport was formulated. It is believed that the major cargo proteins—soluble or membrane bound—are transported in the anterograde direction by COP-II–coated vesicles. A restricted set of proteins and lipids, on the other hand, is believed to return from the *cis* Golgi to the ER. Among these retrograde-trafficked proteins are receptor molecules responsible for maintaining soluble resident proteins in the ER.

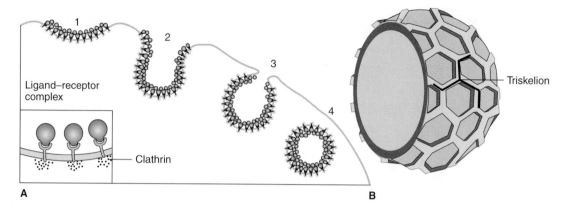

Figure 4–6. Formation of a coated vesicle. A coated pit (A) folds inward progressively to form a coated vesicle, which is released in step 4. As shown in the inset, the coat proteins clathrin and adaptor complex AP-2 are present on the opposite side of the membrane from the receptor. At the time of vesicle release, the coat proteins are present in a lattice pattern on the external surface of the vesicle (B), whereas bound ligand is carried in a ligand-receptor complex on the internal face of the vesicle. (Modified and reproduced from Cormack, DH: *Essential Histology.* JB Lippincott, 1993, p. 71, with permission.)

Molecular Switches

Within the cell are several families of molecules called **molecular switches** that play a pivotal role in activating downstream biochemical events. Biochemically the switch is a hydrolytic enzyme that removes the terminal phosphate from a guanine or adenosine triphosphate (GTP or ATP). Mostly the switches involve the guanine nucleotides. The way the switch works is that in the "off" condition the bound nucleotide is in the diphosphate form (GDP). When the GDP is replaced with a GTP (by another protein), the conformation of the switch protein is altered and it will then bind to a target molecule and activate it. Soon after the molecule in the "on" condition activates its target, the hydrolytic portion of the protein cleaves off the terminal phosphate of the bound nucleotide triphosphate, and the protein reverts back to the GDP-bound, or "off," conformation. We will encounter many different forms of this basic mechanism in the discussions to follow.

ARF is a protein of ~ 20 kDa that is myristoylated at its N-terminus. The possession of fatty acyl myristate enhances ARF's interaction with membranes. On exchanging GTP for guanosine diphosphate (GDP), the ARF-GTP complex binds to membranes. This is mediated by a conformational change that causes the N-terminal domain to interact with its target membrane by insertion into the membrane lipid bilayer. This activated form of ARF—or its yeast functional equivalent Sar1p—then recruits COP-I or COP-II coats, respectively, to the membrane.

In contrast to membrane-bound ARF-GTP, ARF-GDP is cytosolic and is unable to recruit COPs to membranes. This has led to the hypothesis that ARF-GTP promotes vesicle coat recruitment and that on

GTP hydrolysis, ARF-GDP dissociates from membranes, leading to disassembly of the coat complex.

Exactly how ARF recruits COP-I to membranes is still being elucidated. Originally, it was postulated that ARF was present in stoichiometric amounts with coatomer. However, it is now believed that ARF may activate a lipid-modifying enzyme present in the Golgi apparatus—phospholipase D (PLD). It has been suggested that the products of PLD, phosphatidic acid, rather than ARF, may recruit coatomer subunits to Golgi membranes. The study of how ARF facilitates coat recruitment is an area of active research.

SNARES & VESICLE TARGETING

Findings from in vitro experiments suggest that coatomer-coated vesicles cannot fuse with an acceptor membrane unless the proteinaceous coat is removed. Uncoated transport vesicles can fuse with target vesicles, but this requires a cytosolic factor—N-ethylmaleimide sensitive factor (NSF)—because of sensitivity (ie, inactivation) to the sulfhydryl alkylating reagent, N-ethylmaleimide (Figure 4–5). Not surprisingly, NSF has a counterpart in yeast: the product of the *sec18* gene. Yeast with mutations in the Sec18 protein have defective secretion because transport vesicles that bud from the ER accumulate to high levels since they are unable to fuse with Golgi acceptor membranes.

Conservation Across Species: NSF

NSF is a trimer containing three identical 76-kDa subunits that also requires a set of soluble attachment proteins, designated **SNAPs** (**s**oluble **N**SF **a**ttachment **p**roteins), to mediate its binding to Golgi membranes. The NSF-SNAPs complex binds to membranes by a membrane-bound receptor—a SNAP receptor designated **SNARE.**

The first mammalian SNAREs to be characterized, **synatobrevin** and **syntaxin,** are two major proteins in the membranes of neuronal synaptic vesicles. Remarkably, functional homologues of synatobrevin, syntaxin, and a third soluble synaptic vesicle–associated membrane protein, SNAP-25, are also present in yeast cells. Mutation of any of the three yeast proteins inhibits late stages in the yeast cell secretory pathway. We now recognize that the same basic molecules or families of related polypeptides are conserved (1) in the mammalian secretory pathway, (2) in synaptic vesicle docking and fusion during neurotransmitter release, and (3) in the yeast cell secretory pathway (Figure 4–5).

CLATHRIN-COATED VESICLES

Interestingly, the paradigm for coated vesicle formation was derived not from the exocytotic secretory pathway but from endocytosis. Internalization of receptor-ligand complexes from the plasma membrane is known to occur by coated pits that mature into coated vesicles (Figure 4–6). This particular protein complex is assembled from a protein known as **clathrin.** Clathrin forms a basket-like cage that helps pull the membrane bilayer into the basket as it is being formed. This invagination of the membrane also concentrates material located on the lipids and proteins that reside on the surface. In the case of the plasma membrane, extracellular substances are bound at the site of the invaginating vesicle. Conversely, material from the lumen of the TGN is pulled into the vesicle being formed on this intracellular membrane.

The **clathrin-coated vesicle** is involved in the movement of material from the plasma membrane to endosomes, and from the TGN to the plasma membrane.

Components of the Clathrin Coat

Clathrin is a hexamer composed of three large polypeptides linked with three smaller ones. EM shadowing techniques reveal that this hexameric structure—called a **triskelion**—forms a cage-like structure when joined with five or six other clathrin units.

The structure can have either a pentagonal or hexagonal configuration. It is not clear what initiates the formation of the clathrin basket. Electron microscopic analysis of the plasma membrane of cells undergoing endocytosis reveals regions of membrane thickening where clathrin forms a cage-like structure. The membrane invaginates into the cage, thus forming a **membrane pit.** The continued assembly of clathrin results in a pinching off of the plasma membrane, thus forming a fully coated vesicle.

Once the vesicle pinches off, the clathrin basket promptly disassembles by a process that requires adenosine triphosphate (ATP). It has also been suggested that Ca^{2+} binding is involved in the disassembly process. In the formation of much larger membrane invaginations, as in the case of phagocytosis (see below), **clathrin patches** form but do not cover the entire structure being endocytosed. Whether these patches are functionally significant is not clearly established. Clathrin-coated vesicles also form from the *trans* Golgi network and transport secreted proteins to the plasma membrane, to which they fuse and then can deliver their contents to the extracellular space (Figure 4–6).

Adaptins

The cytoplasmic portion of a transmembrane protein often bears sequences that initiate biomolecular cascades within the cytoplasm (Chapter 9). When receptors bind to their ligand, the binding exposes an internalization signal domain that flags the receptor ligand complex for removal from the cell surface. In this case, a protein complex called **adaptin,** located just beneath the membrane, recognizes the internalization signal and helps to initiate internalization by activating clathrin coat formation. Various adaptins have been identified, and it is believed that they help to establish specificity for transport of a number of receptors.

VESICLE TARGETING

A newly formed vesicle can fuse with a number of possible target membranes. To ensure accurate targeting of the vesicle, each vesicle has a special receptor molecule called the SNARE-v (for vesicle). The acceptor or target membrane also has a receptor that binds with the SNARE-v, and it is called the SNARE-t (for target membrane). SNAREs ensure proper localization as vesicles bud from the donor compartment (Figure 4–5).

Formation of the Fusion Complex

The actual fusion of two membranes (ie, a vesicle membrane to a target membrane) requires a special **fusion protein.** This protein destabilizes hydrophilic forces at the interface of the two membranes. It is thought that as the two faces of each bilayer approach each other, a hydrophobic domain of the fusion protein drives the water molecules from the site and the outer lipid leaflets flow together. This same event occurs with the inner leaflets.

A mammalian **fusigen** protein has been identified, but the precise physiochemical details of how the two membranes flow together have not been established.

GTPases: DOCKING & FUSION

Two types of guanosine triphosphatases (GTPases) exist in the cell, and both are involved in controlling molecular switching processes. Trimers comprise one type, and they have three important subunits (α, β, and γ). Monomers, having only one polypeptide, comprise the other type of GTPases.

G-proteins

The trimeric GTPases are a major family of proteins commonly called the **G-proteins.** They are involved in transducing signals from outside the cell to inside. Each trimer subunit appears to be involved in relaying different signals to target molecules in the cell. The G-protein family of trimers is discussed in more detail in Chapter 9.

Monomeric GTPases

The second major class of GTPases are monomeric. To date, five subfamilies have been identified, and they are listed in Table 4–3. Each GTPase subfamily contains many members, and some of the most notable are Ran and ARF; these molecules are found in different subcellular situations. The monomeric GTPases also function as molecular switches; they change their conformation when they are in either the GDP-bound or GTP-bound state. Two auxiliary proteins also function as a part of the switch: a GTP-activating protein (GAP) and a GTP-releasing protein (GRP).

Rab Proteins

Rab proteins function in vesicle transport in the following way. The vesicle formed from the donor membrane has both the v-SNARE and Rab in its GTP configuration. When the vesicle docks at the correct SNARE-t, Rab-GTP hydrolyzes. This action appears to initiate vesicle fusion with the acceptor membrane. Rab, in its GDP configuration, dissociates from the membrane and then cycles back to a donor membrane, where the GAP resets Rab by catalyzing GTP-binding. This event causes Rab to bind to the membrane through its lipid moiety and to participate in

another targeting event. Of interest, specific Rabs exist for each subcellular membrane, and this feature helps to ensure targeting specificity.

VESICLE TRANSPORT IN SUM

We have pointed out the key experimental techniques and the investigators who used them to study vesicle movement in order to emphasize the importance of understanding some of the details of the secretory pathway. These processes are essential for cell function and are involved in every aspect of bodily function. For example, the transmission of electrical impulses by nerve cells, secretion of hormones, production of blood components, cellular defense, embryonic development and organ formation, cell nourishment, and excretion all rely on the movement of vesicles. Thus is it essential that the student understand the basic molecular schemes of vesicle trafficking, recognize how vesicles are targeted to specific compartments, and appreciate the large number of molecules involved in this process.

GOLGI COMPLEX

The Golgi complex (or apparatus) is composed of a set of flattened cisternae with dilated rims arranged in a stack. The cisternae are also associated with a vast array of small vesicles—in effect, a network of tubules emanating from both sides of the stacks. The Golgi complex resides near the ER.

The Golgi apparatus exists in all cells and serves several crucial functions, yet it is diverse in structure depending on the cell type. For example, in secretory cells like hepatocytes or pancreatic cells, the Golgi complex has many layers known as **flattened cisternae** or **saccules.** In fibroblasts, conversely, the Golgi has only a few saccules. A number of biochemical events occur on molecules that pass through the Golgi stack; most of them involve attaching carbohydrate complexes onto proteins and lipids. The Golgi is often referred to as the carbohydrate factory of the cell (Figure 4–7).

POLARITY IN THE GOLGI COMPLEX

cis–medial–trans Golgi Stacks

Morphologically and functionally, the Golgi complex exhibits polarity. The polarity of the Golgi is expressed in the following terminology: the side of the flattened membrane where vesicles fuse is called the

Table 4–3. Monomeric GTPases.

GTPase	Function
Ras	Involved in growth and differentiation
Rho	Associated with integrin activity and formation of the actin cytoskeleton
Rab	Involved in vesicle transport within the cell
ARF	Associated with vesicle formation
Ran	Involved in nuclear protein transport

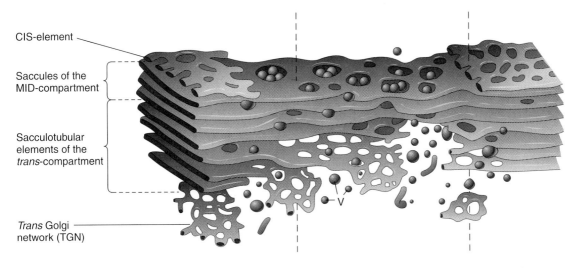

CIS-element

Saccules of the
MID-compartment

Sacculotubular
elements of the
trans-compartment

Trans Golgi
network (TGN)

V

Figure 4–7. Three-dimensional reconstruction of a Golgi complex derived from several electron micrographs of a rat epithelial cell. The various compartments and morphologies of the Golgi stacks are shown. The reconstruction depicts the complexity and arrangements of *cis, medial,* and *trans* Golgi compartments. V = vesicles. (Adapted from Rambourg and Clemont [1990], with permission. Modified and reproduced from Mellman I, Simons K: The Golgi complex: In vitro veritas? Cell 1992;68:832, with permission.)

cis **face,** and the side where vesicles bud is called the ***trans* face.**

The stack of Golgi that resides closest to the ER is operationally called the *cis* Golgi network; the membrane stacks located somewhat in the middle are called the *medial* Golgi network; and the stack that appears most distal to the ER is the *trans* Golgi network (TGN).

An individual flattened membrane is called a cisterna (pl. *cisternae*); any given cisterna has a *cis* and a *trans* face. The regions at the ends of the stack contain a series of tubular structures that may or may not be connected to the cisterna. These vesicles and tubular structures are the Golgi networks—*cis* near the ER and *trans* distal to the ER.

A series of sequential biochemical reactions occurs within separate compartments through which glycoproteins pass by in assembly-line fashion. Newly synthesized membrane and secretory proteins, as well as membrane lipids that are glycosylated, coming from the ER enter the Golgi through the *cis* face. They move through the Golgi stack and leave the complex by the *trans* face, where vesicles and tubules form the TGN, a reticular mesh.

As proteins or lipids traverse the Golgi stacks, they undergo a series of post-translational modifications that involve remodeling of the N-linked oligosaccharides. As the protein passes through the Golgi stacks, these modifications occur sequentially:

- *cis* Golgi: high mannose chains trimmed to M-5 by mannosidase I

- *medial* Golgi: *N*-acetylglucosamine (GlcNAc) transferred by GlcNAc transferase I
- *trans* Golgi: terminal sugars (galactosyl residues) and sialic acid added.

BIOCHEMICAL EVENTS IN THE GOLGI

The following biochemical events occur in the Golgi. Interruption or alteration of these important events can have clinical implications.

A. Glycosylation of proteins and lipids: This involves **glycosidases,** a series of carbohydrate-processing enzymes that remove sugar moieties, and **glycosyltransferases,** which place sugars back onto the core carbohydrate chain.

B. Glycosylation and assembly of proteoglycans in the Golgi: Most sugars added to the proteoglycans' core protein are sulfated. This enzymatic event also takes place in the Golgi stacks.

C. Addition of mannose-6-phosphate (M-6-P): M-6-P is added as a targeting signal to enzymes that are destined for the lysosome.

D. Sorting for transport: Sorting of material for transport to the downstream organelles—the plasma membrane, endosomes, and secretory vesicles—occurs in the TGN (Figure 4–4).

GLYCOSYLATION EVENTS IN THE GOLGI

Recall that the Golgi is the "carbohydrate factory." In the ER, the dolichol phosphate adds a large carbohydrate complex containing 2-GlcNAc-9-mannoses-3-glucoses to an appropriate asparagine residue on a newly growing polypeptide chain. Once the complex is completed, a step-wise trimming of the sugars begins. (See Figure 3–16.)

The terminal glucose is cleaved in two steps. First, the terminal glucose is removed by glucosidase-I. This is followed by the removal of the other two glucoses by glucosidase II. Then one mannose is cleaved, thus completing the early steps of carbohydrate processing in the ER. Next, the proteins bearing this complex are transported to the Golgi.

In the early Golgi stack, processing continues with the removal of three additional mannoses from the core complex. At this stage, the core complex has five mannose residues. N-acetylglucosamine transferase I adds one GlcNAc, which forms a complex that allows for the removal of three more mannose residues. This complex, which now consists of two molecules of GlcNAc-3-mannose-1-GlcNAc, is a core structure to which other carbohydrates are added, each by a special glycosyltransferase that recognizes the evolving carbohydrate structure and adds its own saccharide to the chain.

Complex sugar residues on proteins and lipids are assembled, and they are fundamentally different from those of DNA, RNA, and proteins. In this instance, the sugar complex of one step constitutes the binding domain for the next glycosyl enzyme to place its substrate onto the polysaccharide structure. Thus, the template is formed during biosynthesis. DNA, RNA and proteins use preexisting templates to determine their sequence.

Proteoglycans have complex sugars attached to the core polypeptide through an OH linkage of serine or threonine with a xylose sugar residue. Many of the core peptides of proteoglycans have repeating sequences of Ser or Thr residues to which the carbohydrate chains are attached. The carbohydrates protrude from the core protein, like bristles on a test-tube brush.

TRAFFIC DESTINATIONS FROM THE GOLGI

Because the Golgi complex is a major processing organelle of the cell, proteins, lipids, and membrane components whose final destination is a lysosome, peroxisome, plasma membrane, or secretory vesicle must pass through this complex. When proteins for the various organelles reach the TGN, specialized vesicles bud, carrying their content to the designated sites using SNAPs (as described above). Interest-ingly, passage of some vesicles to their targets occurs by moving along such cytoskeletal components as microtubules, which serve as guiding tracks (Chapter 7).

LYSOSOME

STRUCTURE & FUNCTION

Lysosomes (Figure 4–8) are the major "digestive" organelles of the cell involved in receptor-ligand degradation, cholesterol metabolism via the LDL receptor, and organelle turnover. As such, they contain a large number of specific enzymes (hydrolases) involved in the degradation of proteins, lipids, carbohydrates, and nucleic acids. These organelles are surrounded by a single bilayer that has unique characteristics discussed below. One of the hallmark features of the lysosome is the low pH of its lumen. This

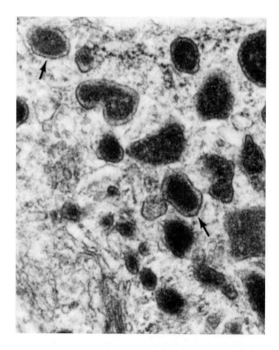

Figure 4–8. Lysosomes. This electron micrograph of a macrophage shows numerous primary lysosomes in the cytoplasm. Lysosomes are characterized visually by uniform content and a clearly defined limiting membrane. Functionally, each lysosome is an organelle filled with hydrolytic enzymes. × 45,000. (Reproduced, with permission, from Junqueira LC et al: *Basic Histology*, 8th ed. Appleton & Lange, 1995, p. 37.)

feature is acquired by a membrane bound ATP-driven proton pump (which exchanges Na^+ for H^+). For the enzymes located in the lysosome to carry out their hydrolytic function, an acidic environment is required. The pH optimum for most of these hydrolases is approximately 5, and thus their activity is quite limited if lysosomes are inadvertently disrupted and the enzymes are released into the cytosol, where the pH is 7.2–7.3. Thus having a specialized compartment for digestion of materials allows for optimum hydrolytic conditions. Amino acids derived from protein hydrolysis are used in biosynthetic pathways as are other components such as nucleotides (Table 4–4).

Membrane Components of the Lysosome Are Unique

The lumen of the lysosome is a site of protein degradation, yet its own membrane structure seems resistant to digestion. This resistance to hydrolytic digestion has prompted a more detailed examination of the molecules that make up the membrane. Using a variety of techniques (lysosomal isolation, membrane isolation, antibodies developed to the various components), investigators have shown that among the various membrane components (which range in size from 20 to greater than 150 kDa) the most abundant are two groups of proteins in the 100–120 kDa range. These proteins have been dubbed **lgpA** and **lgpB.**

Examination of the structure and arrangement of these proteins has shown that they are single pass integral proteins with a large proportion of their structure lumenally directed. Moreover, they are extensively glycosylated. Although glycosylation per se may not be a "protective" feature, it has been shown that the greater the proportion of carbohydrates in a protein, the slower its degradation. Thus it appears that most lysosomal membrane proteins that are involved in the lysosome's function (transport of the newly digested molecules out of lysosome) are heavily glycosylated.

Lysosomal membrane proteins are synthesized in the ER and transported to the Golgi for their extensive glycosylation (Figure 4–9). These proteins also must be targeted to the lysosome, but so far it is unclear how this occurs. They do not have an obvious lysosomal targeting signal (M-6-P, to be discussed below). It is thought that the lysosomal membrane proteins cluster in the trans Golgi and form specific transport vesicles (sorting endosomes) that fuse and help form lysosomes.

Pathways for Import of Material into the Lysosome

Import of material into the lysosome can be roughly divided into two types.

Biosynthetic pathway. The first involves delivery of the soluble hydrolytic enzymes and the specialized lysosomal membrane proteins and as such can be considered the "biosynthetic pathway." Material passing along this route includes that originating in the ER, passing through the Golgi network, and emerging from the TGN. This pathway has several special features discussed below.

Endocytic pathway. The second type of entry into the lysosome involves more of the "hydrolytic function" of the lysosome, that is, material imported for "digestion." This occurs by four different routes.

1. The formation of endocytic vesicles, the major route into the lysosome, involves clathrin coated pits and vesicles and endosomes formed without clathrin coats (see below).
2. **Autophagy** consists of the engulfment and digestion of other organelles, eg dysfunctional mitochondria, within the cell. Precisely how the engulfment occurs is not clear, although it is thought that ER membranes surround the organelle to be digested, which then fuses with the lysosome. This structure is called an autophagosome before fusion with the lysosome.
3. **Phagocytosis** is the engulfment of larger particles such as bacteria or other external cellular debris (Figure 4–10). Although similar to endocytosis, this complex process involves large particles from outside the cell (see below). Nearly all cells can carry out phagocytosis, but two classes of cells are especially designed for this purpose and as such have been designated **professional phagocytes.** The three most prominent members of this club are neutrophils, monocytes, and macrophages.
4. Some cytosolic proteins that carry a lysosomal targeting signal (KFERQ, Lys Phe Glu Arg Gln) are delivered to the lysosome.

The Odyssey of Lysosomal Hydrolases

If the lysosome is to serve as a major degradative compartment of the cell, then obviously the enzymes required to carry out these processes must be selectively delivered to this organelle. The cell has de-

Table 4–4. Some of the enzymes found in lysosomes and the cell components that are their substrates.[1]

Enzyme	Substrate
Ribonuclease	RNA
Deoxyribonuclease	DNA
Phosphatase	Phosphate esters
Glycosidases	Complex carbohydrates; glycosides and polysaccharides
Arylsulfatases	Sulfate esters
Collagenase	Proteins
Cathepsins	Proteins

[1]Reproduced, with permission, from Ganong WF: *Review of Medical Physiology,* 17th ed., Appleton & Lange, 1995, p. 7.

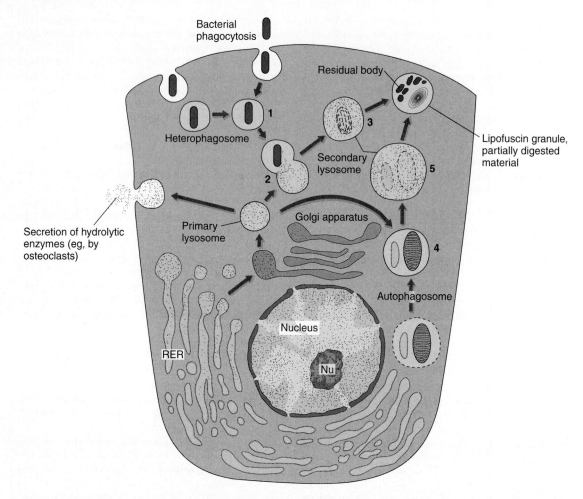

Figure 4–9. Lysosome formation and function. Lysosomal membrane proteins are synthesized on and translocated into the rough endoplasmic reticulum (RER) and glycosylated cotranslationally in the Golgi apparatus. Lysosomes are involved in intracellular digestion of phagocytosed material (1–3) as well as of intracellular material (4, 5), including peptide-receptor complexes. (Modified and reproduced, with permission, from Junqueira LC et al: *Basic Histology,* 8th ed. Appleton & Lange, 1995, p. 39.)

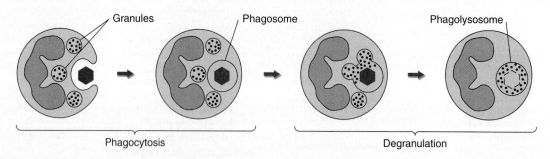

Figure 4–10. Degranulation in a neutrophil. After a neutrophil phagocytoses an extracellular particle such as a bacterium, the phagosome containing the particle fuses with cytoplasmic lysosomes. Degradation of the particle occurs in the resultant phagolysosome. The fusion of lysosomes and phagosome is visualized under the microscope as degranulation. (Modified and reproduced, with permission, from Stites DP et al: *Basic & Clinical Immunology,* 8th ed. Appleton & Lange, 1994, p. 15.)

vised a selective system to ensure that this pathway is maintained.

Creation of the signal patch. The hydrolases bound for lysosomes are synthesized in the ER and, like most proteins made there, receive their N-linked "core" glycosylation. Protein folding also occurs in the ER, and hydrolase proteins fold so that a **signal patch** is created. (A signal patch is a recognition domain composed of amino acids in a nonlinear sequence; it arises when requisite amino acids for a recognition domain are brought into close proximity by the folding of the polypeptide chain.) When the hydrolase is transported to the Golgi, this domain will be recognized and utilized by a Golgi enzyme to alter the N-linked oligosaccharide, thereby providing a special "lysosomal targeting address."

Targeting of the M-6-P receptor. The signal patch of the hydrolase binds to a site on a GlcNAc-phosphotransferase. This enzyme utilizes UDP-glucose as a donor and transfers phospho-GlcNAc to a terminal mannose residue of the N-linked oligosaccharide. A second enzyme, GlcNAc-glycosidase, removes the GlcNAc, leaving a mannose-6-phosphate (M-6-P) available for targeting to a specific protein that has a binding site for M-6-P, the **M-6-P receptor.** The phosphotransferase and glycosidase involved in targeting are located in the *cis* saccules of the Golgi.

There are two types of M-6-P receptors; both are integral membrane proteins with a binding domain facing the lumen and the carboxyl ends protruding into the cytosol. Amino acid sequence comparisons reveal that the two receptors are likely derived from a common ancestor protein. The sizes of the receptors are quite different as are their requirements for binding hydrolases. The most prominent M-6-P receptor has a mass of 215 kDa, whereas the other form is only 46 kDa. Both are involved in Golgi sorting events, but only the larger receptor is able to retrieve secreted hydrolases. These receptors appear to cluster in the TGN.

Early and late endosomes. Binding of a sufficient number of hydrolases to the receptors triggers the formation of a clathrin assembly on the cytosolic surface of the Golgi, causing vesicle formation as described above. These vesicles are transported to another vesicle called the **late endosome.** As will be described in more detail below, the process of endocytosis begins with the formation of another vesicle, called the **early endosome,** that contains material from outside the cell. The ionic concentration and pH of the early endosome are the same as that of the exterior of the cell. In mammalian tissues, the pH is 7.3–7.4. The early endosome will fuse with other vesicles that are deeper in the cell and have, as a part of their membrane structure, the ATP-driven vacuolar-type proton pump. The pH of these vesicles is approximately 6.0. When the early endosomes fuse with these vesicles, they are called late endosomes,

and the pH environment is now decreased to about 6. Vesicles carrying the newly made hydrolases also fuse with the late endosome, and at the lower pH the hydrolases dissociate from the M-6-P receptor and begin their catalytic digestions of the contents of the endosome.

At the same time the hydrolase is unloaded from the late endosome, additional vesicles form on the endosome surface, and the empty M-6-P receptor is recycled back to the TGN. This recycling may be similar to that described for ER-specific resident proteins as well as other essential ER proteins, which are recycled from the *cis* Golgi back to the ER. *Thus both receptor recycling and retrieval of specific proteins are crucial functions within the cell.* Defects that might arise in this normal process can be devastating.

How efficient is the delivery of components to the correct site? If one considers the enormous amount of vesicle movement in the cell it would appear that the process is amazingly efficient, but not 100%. Some hydrolases are lost in the final steps of binding at the *trans* Golgi, and instead of binding to the M-6-P receptor for delivery to the endosome-lysosome complex, they are delivered to the exterior of the cell. In other words, some of the hydrolases are secreted. The hydrolytic enzymes are benign to the cell and its surroundings because of the pH of the environment. Just as some proportion of hydrolases are inadvertently lost through the secretory pathway, so are some of the M-6-P receptors brought to the cell surface by misdirected movement into a secretory vesicle destined for the cell membrane rather than the late endosomal compartment. This is a fortuitous event because the M-6-P receptor is now an integral protein with its M-6-P binding domain directed to the outside of the cell. Secreted hydrolases expressing the M-6-P tag are bound to the receptor and then endocytosed and delivered to the lysosome-late endosome complex.

DISORDERS OF LYSOSOMAL ENZYME SYNTHESIS AND STORAGE

Mucopolysaccharide Storage Diseases

A number of genetic diseases have been described that involve lysosomal hydrolases. One type, encompassing the **mucopolysaccharide storage diseases,** results from a deficiency of specific lysosomal enzymes involved in the degradation of dermatan sulfate, heparan sulfate, or both. These compounds belong to a group of glycosaminoglycans also known as mucopolysaccharides (see Chapter 8). Incompletely degraded mucopolysaccharides accumulate in tissues and are excreted in the urine. Not all of the glycosaminoglycans can be eliminated; they thus begin to accumulate in cells and surrounding intercellular spaces. These diseases cause progressive deterioration and result in death, usually before the age of 10. Deficiency of 10 specific lysosomal enzymes has been demonstrated. Each of the enzymes catalyzes cleavage at a specific site in the polysaccharide. The degradation of the mucopolysaccharide chains occurs sequentially, and a defect at a given linkage prevents cleavage at subsequent linkages in the chain even though the enzyme catalyzing that event is present. Thus one can readily see that seemingly minor alterations in one of the hydrolases can have profound effects (Table 4–5).

I-Cell Disease

Another class of genetic defects involving lysosomes was instrumental in identifying the trafficking pathway for all the lysosomal hydrolases. This disease involved glycosidases, sulfatases, and cathep-

sins, which are essential components in the lysosomal arsenal of hydrolases. This disease is designated the **I-cell** (inclusion body) **disease** because it manifests itself by the appearance of huge inclusion bodies in cells and exceptionally high levels of hydrolases in the circulation. There are two types—mucolipidosis II and mucolipidosis III—but the basic defect is in the post-translational modification of the acid hydrolases. As described above, lysosomal hydrolases are targeted to the lysosome by the formation of an M-6-P residue on specified N-linked carbohydrate residues. Patients, such as the one shown in Figure 4–11, with I-cell disease are deficient in the phosphotransferase that places a phosphodiester-linked *N*-acetylglucosamine on a mannose residue on the glycoprotein. Consequently, these enzymes are not targeted to the M-6-P receptor and are not directed to the lysosome. They are, however, picked up by secre-

Table 4–5. Lysosomal storage disorders.[1]

Disorders of	Name	MIM Number	Chromosomal Location
Mucopolysaccharides	Hurler syndrome; MPS type IH	252800	4p16.3
	Hurler-Scheie syndrome; MPS type IH/IS	252800	4p16.3
	Hunter syndrome; MPS type II	309900	Xq27–28
	β-Glucuronidase deficiency; MPS type VII	253220	7q21.1–q22
Sphingolipids	Generalized gangliosidosis; GM_1 Gangliosidosis, type 1	230500	3p21.33
	Tay-Sachs disease	272800	15q23–q24
	Fabry disease	301500	Xq22.1
	Gaucher disease, type 1	230800	1q21
	Niemann-Pick disease; sphingomyelinase deficiency, type I	257200	11p15.4–15.1
Glycoproteins (Oligosaccharides)	Fucosidosis	230000	1p34
	Mannosidosis; α-mannosidase deficiency	248500	19p13.2–q12
	β-Neuraminidase deficiency	256550	6p21.3
	Sialolipidosis	252650	10pter–q23
	Galactosialidosis	256540	20q12–q13.1
	Aspartylglucosaminuria	208400	4q32–q33
Lysosomal enzyme transport	Mucolipidosis type II; I-cell disease	252500	4q21–23
	Mucolipidosis type III; Pseudo-Hurler polydystrophy	252600	
Lysosomal membrane transport	Infantile free sialic acid storage disease	269920	
Other disorders of lysosomes	Pompe disease, acid maltase deficiency	232300	17q23
	Wolman disease	278000	10q23.2–q23.3
	Cholesteryl ester storage disease	278000	10q23.2–q23.3

[1]Modified and reproduced, with permission, from Seashore MR, Wappner RS: *Genetics in Primary Care & Clinical Medicine,* Appleton & Lange, 1996, pp. 297–298.

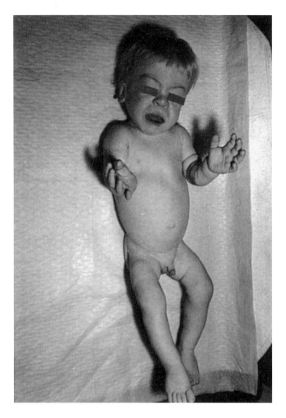

Figure 4–11. Child affected by mucolipidosis II, an I-cell disease. (Reproduced, with permission, from Oski FA et al [editors]: *Principles and Practice of Pediatrics,* 2nd ed. Lippincott, 1994.)

tory vesicles of the TGN and delivered to the outside of the cell. The secretion of these hydrolases accounts for the high levels found in the blood.

Since mucolipidosis primarily affects connective tissue, fibroblasts taken from affected patients have been particularly useful in elucidating the defects and in determining the importance of M-6-P in targeting the protein to the correct intracellular compartment.

ENDOCYTOSIS

Endocytosis is the vesicular uptake of fluids, macromolecules, or small particles into the cell. At least three mechanisms are involved:

1. **Pinocytosis,** which literally means "cell drinking." It is also known as **clathrin-independent endocytosis.**
2. **Receptor-mediated endocytosis** or **clathrin-dependent endocytosis.** This process has received considerable attention because of its involvement in certain human diseases.

3. Phagocytosis, which literally means "cell eating" (Figure 4–12).

Pinocytosis

Pinocytosis is constitutive, ie, it involves a continual dynamic formation of small vesicles at the cell surface. More specifically, small invaginations and vesicles form at the cell surface, then internalize and fuse with other vesicles just below the surface to form primary endosomes. At the cell periphery, these vesicles evaginate and form fusion-vesicles with the surface membrane.

Thus, at the cell surface, vesicles form and act dynamically to bring material into the cell and to recycle the plasma membrane. These vesicles transport small molecules, water, and soluble proteins—material that is part of the fluid phase of the extracellular environment. Although the pinocytic vesicles are small, their massive number accounts for the bulk of the material brought into the cell.

Occasionally the vesicles are larger-forming macropinocytic structures involved in membrane ruffling. Pinocytosis can be extensive; in some cells, as much as 100% of the plasma membrane is internalized and recycled in 1 hour.

After pinocytic vesicles are pinched off in the cytoplasm, many fuse with one another and with larger vesicles to form **early endosomes.** These endosomes eventually move to the interior of the cell and fuse with early-forming lysosomes, where degradation of the lumenal material commences. These latter vesicles, called **late endosomes,** contain the hydrolases brought in by vesicles derived from the TGN.

Receptor-Mediated Endocytosis

As the name implies, **receptor-mediated endocytosis (RME)** uses specific surface-expressed receptors to transport molecules bound to those receptors. RME offers several advantages to the cell.

A. Specificity: Certain cells express surface receptors that are unexpressed by other cells, and this permits selective binding of molecules from the extracellular solution. Expression of certain receptors on one cell type but not another is a common mechanism during development and tissue formation.

B. Capacity to concentrate the ligand at the surface of the cell: The laws of diffusion demonstrate that molecules move from an environment of high concentration to one of low concentration. Thus, if certain cells can selectively remove ligands from the solution surrounding them, they become a "sink" for these molecules. Eventually the ligand will be removed from the surrounding fluid.

C. Refractory: If the specific receptor is not returned to the membrane after binding and internalization, the cell becomes refractory to the ligand. *This is important in the process of signaling and is one way an incoming signal can be turned off* (Chapter 9).

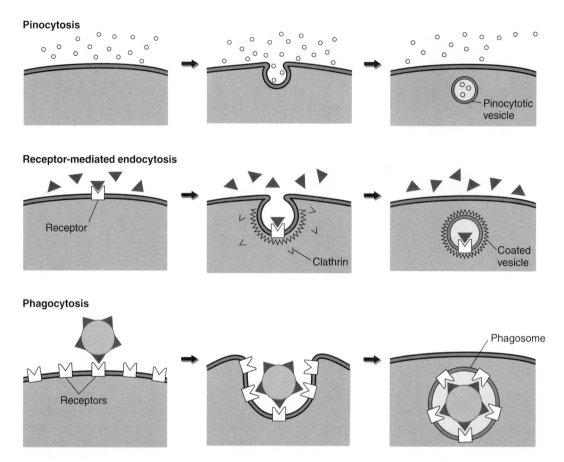

Pinocytosis

Pinocytotic
vesicle

Receptor-mediated endocytosis

Receptor

Clathrin

Coated
vesicle

Phagocytosis

Phagosome

Receptors

Figure 4–12. Mechanisms of endocytosis. Pinocytosis (top) involves the engulfment of fluid phase material via the formation of a vesicle from plasma membrane in order to import extracellular fluid. Receptor-mediated endocytosis (middle) involves ligand-receptor binding on the plasma membrane and subsequent recruitment of clathrin and a family of "adaptor" proteins (AP-2) to the cytoplasmic face of the plasma membrane, leading to formation of a coated pit. The coated pit invaginates to form a coated vesicle, which transports the ligand-receptor complex into the cytoplasm. (See also Figure 4–6.) Phagocytosis (bottom) is initiated by binding of a larger particle to multiple receptors on the plasma membrane. A phagosome is formed by invagination of the plasma membrane involved in the ligand-receptor binding. (Modified and reproduced, with permission, from Stites DP et al: *Basic & Clinical Immunology,* 8th ed. Appleton & Lange, 1994, p. 14.)

ENTRY OF SUBSTANCES INTO THE CELL BY RME

LDL Cholesterol, Transferrin, & Growth Factors

The mechanism of internalization in RME is fundamentally different from the constitutive process of pinocytosis or phagocytosis: ligand-bound receptors appear to accumulate in specific regions called **coated pits,** which exist on the cell surface. These small surface invaginations have an amorphous dense material—clathrin—that resides below them on the cytosolic surface. The number of molecules that enter the cell by this process is extensive and includes transport proteins that deliver nutrients to the cell—notably, **low-density lipoprotein (LDL) cholesterol**—and the iron transport protein **transferrin.**

Another group of molecules that gain entry to the cell by RME are the **growth factors,** including epidermal growth factor (EGF), platelet-derived growth factor (PDGF), insulin, and certain members of the cytokine family (Chapter 10). A key difference for this latter group is that the ligand is not an important part of the endocytic pathway; rather, events that follow receptor-ligand binding are critical for the cellular response. For this class of proteins, RME seems to remove the receptor from the surface and turn down the cell's capacity to respond to the ligand. Certain viruses and toxins can use other receptors and the RME pathway to opportunistically gain entry into the cell.

Unless the ligand is bound to it, some receptors do not move into the coated pit. For example, the EGF receptor remains diffusely distributed on the cell sur-

Table 4–6. Common features of receptor-mediated endocytosis (RME).

After early endosomes fuse with other endosomes that contain the ATPase proton pump and the pH in the lumen decreases, the ligand-receptor complex can follow one of four pathways:
1. The receptor recycles after it has unloaded its cargo.
2. The receptor and the carrier ligand recycle, as occurs with transferrin.
3. The ligand and receptor are degraded in the lysosomal compartment.
4. The receptor and ligand are transported across the cell and delivered to the membrane on the opposite side of the entry surface; this occurs primarily in polarized cells.

face in its unoccupied state. When EGF binds to the receptor, however, the complex moves quickly within the plane of the bilayer to a coated pit and is rapidly internalized. Alternately, many empty receptors move into the coated pit and are internalized without bringing in a bound ligand, eg, receptors for transport molecules like LDL, transferrin, sialoglycoprotein, and α_2-macroglobulin.

The common features of receptor-mediated endocytosis are summarized in Table 4–6 and Figure 4–13.

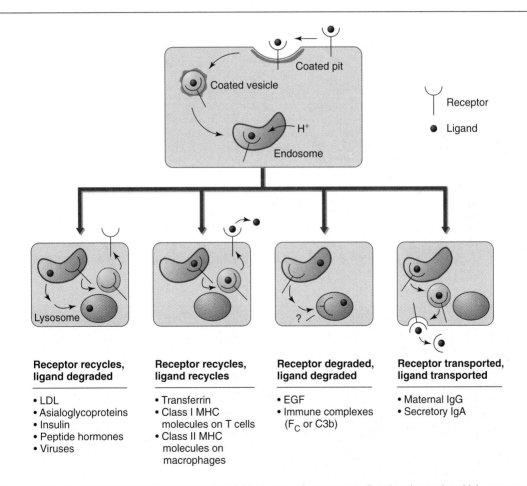

Receptor recycles, ligand degraded	Receptor recycles, ligand recycles	Receptor degraded, ligand degraded	Receptor transported, ligand transported
• LDL • Asialoglycoproteins • Insulin • Peptide hormones • Viruses	• Transferrin • Class I MHC molecules on T cells • Class II MHC molecules on macrophages	• EGF • Immune complexes (F_C or C3b)	• Maternal IgG • Secretory IgA

Figure 4–13. Receptor-mediated endocytosis. The initial events of receptor-mediated endocytosis, which are common to all four types of the process, are shown in the top panel. The first step is ligand-receptor binding (one ligand, one receptor). Binding is followed by formation of a coated pit, which subsequently forms a coated vesicle. The coated vesicle enters the cytoplasm of the cell and fuses with an acidic endosome. The eventual fate of receptor and ligand varies according to the type of endocytosis. (From Goldstein JL et al: Receptor-mediated endocytosis: concepts emerging from the LDL receptor system. Annu Rev Cell Biol 1985;1:5, with permission.)

DEFECTS IN RECEPTOR-MEDIATED ENDOCYTOSIS

Clinical Correlates

A defect in the M-6-P receptor or in the enzyme that places the M-6-P on the lysosomal hydrolases can lead to serious human disease. Greater appreciation of the molecular causes of these diseases has led to a considerable understanding of the mechanisms of vesicle targeting.

Research in the human disease **familial hypercholesterolemia,** for example, has helped to unravel the details of receptor-mediated endocytosis. Familial hypercholesterolemia is characterized by a selective elevation in levels of LDL cholesterol, the major cholesterol transport protein in the plasma. The primary defect in familial hypercholesterolemia results from mutations in the gene for the **LDL receptor,** which is widely distributed on most cells of the body and constitutes a major route for dietary cholesterol to enter cells (Figure 4–14).

Cholesterol is required in the synthesis of cell membranes, in the biosynthesis of steroid hormones, and for the production of bile acids in the liver. If LDL is not taken up by cells, unusually high plasma levels of LDL lead to the formation of atherosclerotic plaques in the coronary vessels and, possibly, myocardial infarction.

In studies using fibroblasts from patients with hypercholesterolemia, Goldstein, Brown, and Anderson discovered the causes of familial hypercholesterolemia (Goldstein & Brown, 1983). In the process, the researchers identified three types of defects in the LDL receptor. In the most prevalent and severe form of hypercholesterolemia, the LDL receptor is incapable of binding LDL, and the respective gene is called **receptor-negative.** A second mutant allele, designated as receptor-defective, binds LDL but at a much reduced capacity. In the third type of defect, the receptor binds LDL normally but is incapable of moving to coated pits for internalization.

PHAGOCYTOSIS

Phagocytosis is the uptake by the cell of relatively large particles (0.5 μm) by a mechanism that is **clathrin-independent but actin-dependent.** Thus, phagocytosis usually requires actin polymerization. The process is triggered by the interaction of molecules on the particle with a surface receptor on the cell. Phagocytosis is a key function in the host defense against invading microorganisms, and the phagocytosis of damaged or senescent cells is essential for tissue remodeling and wound healing. Phagocytosis is critically important in metazoan organisms.

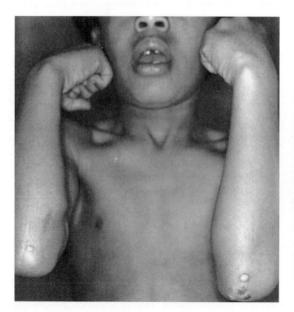
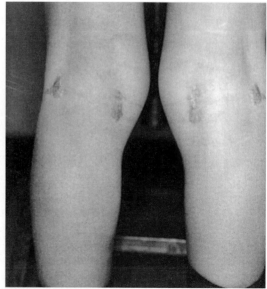

A   B

Figure 4–14. A seven-year-old boy with homozygous hypercholesterolemia. Note the cutaneous xanthomas on the elbows, which first appeared at the age of four years. (Reproduced, with permission, from Oski FA et al [editors]: *Principles and Practice of Pediatrics,* 2nd ed. Lippincott, 1994.)

Also, phagocytosis is a common mechanism used by microorganisms to (1) avoid direct destruction by antibodies and complement proteins and (2) evade cytotoxic cells.

Phagocytosis in mammals is carried out mainly by three types of cells, neutrophils, monocytes, and macrophages. These cells have special surface receptors designed to recognize and carry out the phagocytic process. The receptors recognize the nonantigen-binding domains of immunoglobulins or other immune molecules that comprise the host-defense system. Antibodies and complement proteins in the plasma coat the surface on an invading microorganism, thereby making the microbe accessible to the surface receptor on the phagocyte and initiating the phagocytic event. This process is called opsonization (Figure 4–15).

In addition to their role in phagocytosis, phagocytes also produce other important signaling molecules, including cytotoxic radicals of oxygen and nitrogen (eg, nitric oxide), enzymes that degrade the extracellular matrix, and cytokines and lipid components that mobilize other cells as part of the inflammatory process.

Neutrophils, monocytes, and macrophages are the most voracious phagocytes; however, epithelial cells and fibroblasts are also capable of phagocytosis. Indeed, they are quite active in the ingestion of larger particles, including collagen. In the case of retinal epithelia, discarded portions of the retinal rod following light activation are nibbled up by retinal epithelial cells. Although they lack the surface receptors of professional phagocytes, fibroblasts are also able to engulf microorganisms. Apparently, fibroblasts use receptors for proteins of the extracellular matrix—such as fibronectin, laminin, and certain glycosaminoglycans—that often associate with foreign microorganisms (Chapter 8).

MECHANISMS OF PARTICLE UPTAKE BY PHAGOCYTES

Ingestion of opsonized particles occurs by a zippering mechanism in which the particle is first bound to the surface of the phagocyte through its **Fc receptor.** A sequential recruitment of other cell surface receptors follows. This recruitment results in the formation of a phagosome that conforms to the shape of the ingested particle, so the plasma membrane fits tightly around the particle—analogous to the way Velcro surfaces interact.

Although the basic tenets of the **zipper model** have proved correct, modifications of the process are known to occur. For example, there are similarities between cell spreading on surfaces and phagocytosis, indicating that pseudopod advance over surfaces occurs in many ways (Figure 4–16).

Increased Surface Ruffling

It has recently been shown that the addition of growth factors to phagocytes—such as EGF to fibroblasts or macrophage colony–stimulating factor (M-CSF) to macrophages—results in increased surface ruffling. Ruffles are essentially unguided pseudopodia. **Macropinosomes** are large endocytic vesicles that form as ruffles and fold back against the cell surface, trapping extracellular fluid. Recent findings suggest that certain pathogenic organisms stimulate ruffling of the cell to invade it. Thus, although the

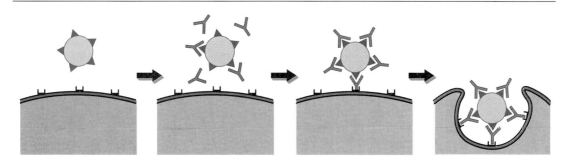

Figure 4–15. Large particles (such as immune complexes) or invading bacteria that have been killed are first coated with proteins (immunoglobins or complement proteins) before they are ingested into the cell. The coating process is called opsonization. The phagocyte has surface receptors that recognize the immunoglobin or complement proteins. Thus the particle to be ingested is first bound to cell surfaces via specific receptors before being engulfed by the cell. (Modified and reproduced, with permission, from Stites DP et al: *Basic & Clinical Immunology,* 8th ed. Appleton & Lange, 1994, p. 15.)

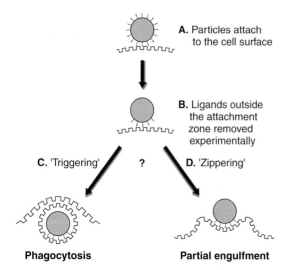

A. Particles attach
to the cell surface

B. Ligands outside
the attachment
zone removed
experimentally

C. 'Triggering'   ?   D. 'Zippering'

Phagocytosis   **Partial engulfment**

Figure 4–16. Model of opsonization. Experiments with macrophages established that the basic points of the zippering model are correct. Particles were allowed to associate with the cell surface (A). After ligand molecules outside the region of association were removed (B), observations were made to see which model more closely represented actual events. The partial engulfment predicted by the zippering model (D) occurred. Later experiments showed that modifications of zippering also occur. Opsonins are represented by spikes protruding from the particle surface, and opsonin receptors are represented by square pits in the cell membrane. (Adapted, with permission, from Swanson JA, Baer SC: Phagocytosis by zippers and triggers. Trends Cell Biol 1995;5:90.)

phagocytic processes are a major means of host defense, some organisms achieve entry into the cell by a variation of phagocytosis.

Transducing the Phagocytic Signal

For a particle to enter the cell by phagocytosis, a reorganization of the **actin-based cytoskeleton** is required. When a particle to be engulfed is bound to the cell's receptor, a signal is generated by the receptor. This signal involves phosphorylation events in molecules that are close to the membrane. These phosphorylation signals are ultimately interpreted by molecules associated with monomeric actin (eg, globular actin, or G-actin), and this in turn causes the actin molecules to polymerize and form a fiber called **F-actin.**

The cell needs this structural element to form the pseudopod that surrounds the particle prior to engulfing. The signal is initiated by a cytoplasmic tyrosine kinase called **src kinase.** On activation, src kinase

phosphorylates tyrosine residues located on the cytoplasmic tail of the Fc receptor. This event, like many other receptor-ligand-binding events, results from the binding process, in this case, binding of the opsonized particle.

Formation of Phagolysosome

After the zippered entrance into the cell of a large particle that includes patches of the plasma membrane, the engulfed particle is called a **phagosome.** The final destination of the phagosome is to fuse with lysosomes bearing the hydrolases, so as to correct the environment for digestion and degradation of the particle. The resulting structure is called a **phagolysosome.** The process is more complex than simple fusion of compartments. Rather, the membrane of the phagosome is remodeled and transported through the cell in a defined pathway.

It is possible to isolate phagosomes from cells at different times after they have been engulfed by the cell. The membranes of the phagosome are then analyzed by gel electrophoresis and antibody staining. In the very early phagosome, such proteins as the M-6-P receptor and the Fc receptor are prominent members of the membrane. Within a short time, however, the number of these proteins in the phagosome membrane decreases. Also decreased at this time are the proton-ATPase pump and certain defined membranes of the lysosomes lgpA and lgpB. In addition, many surface receptor molecules are cycled back to the membrane. Together, these findings indicate that the phagosome membrane remodels and acquires other molecules (eg, SNAREs) that enhance the fusion of the phagosome with other intracellular compartments.

TRANSCYTOSIS

Substances that enter the cell via specific receptors almost always form vesicles, called **early endosomes,** just beneath the plasma membrane. These vesicles act as a sorting station for the endocytosed ligands and receptors. The pH of the lumen of the early endosome is approximately 6.0, which often leads to the dissociation of the ligand from its receptor. If this occurs, both ligand and receptor are usually then sorted to another budding vesicle of the early endosome, which eventually fuses with the lysosome and is digested. However, some of the ligand-receptor complexes do not dissociate at the lower pH. Instead they sort to other regions of the early endosome and form budding vesicles that fuse with other intracellular membranes or at different sites on the plasma membrane. This process is called **transcytosis.** Transcytosis is a way that molecules coming from outside the cell can be delivered to different places within the cell or, in some instances, can be moved entirely across one cell layer to another. One of the best-studied examples of transcytosis is the delivery of certain maternal immunoglobulins across intestinal epithelial cells of the newborn. Maternal antibodies are transported into the milk-secreting cells of the mammary gland and are ingested by the neonate. The maternal antibodies bound to their receptors are sorted in the early endosome of the gut cells and move via other vesicles across the epithelial cell and fuse with the plasma membrane on the basolateral surface of the cell. Here, the pH is nearly neutral and the ligands are released from the receptor. The immunoglobulins are then picked up by the lymphatic vessels and delivered into the general circulation of the newborn. In transcytosis, neither the ligand or its receptor are destroyed; the empty receptor sorts from the basolateral surface back to the apical surface to pick up another cargo molecule.

Exocytosis

Specialized cells that deliver a product on demand—eg, neurotransmitters or digestive enzymes—house these products within storage vesicles near the plasma membrane. When a signal is generated, usually from outside the cell, it rapidly causes the storage vesicle to fuse with the plasma membrane and to release its contents. The process that couples the release of material to a stimulus is called **stimulus-secretion.** Stimulus-secretion occurs in many specialized cells, such as mast cells and pancreatic acinar cells, and especially at junctional complexes where two neurons come into contact.

Examination of specialized secretory cells by electron microscopy reveals that vesicles containing the material to be secreted are **electron dense** and contain high concentrations of the material to be released (Figure 4–6). These compartments are called **secretory vesicles** or **dense-core vesicles.** It is known that hydrolases possess the M-6-P tag and that this aids their selective accumulation into vesicles destined for the lysosome. In addition, it seems that secretory proteins have some type of signal patch within their structure that allows them to aggregate and concentrate into the secretory vesicle. For most secretory proteins, further research is needed to elucidate the biomolecular signal patch.

CONSTITUTIVE VS REGULATED COMPARTMENTS

It appears that vesicles flow continually from the TGN to the plasma membrane. Thus, the TGN is a major compartment for the production of secretory vesicles. The endosomes are another site for vesicle formation. The realization that vesicles bud off large endosomes began with studies of synaptic vesicles that reside in nerve cells. Just below the membrane

surface in the junction between two nerve cells is a population of small secretory vesicles that are poised to fuse with the plasma membrane on activation of the appropriate signal. Synaptic vesicles contain neurotransmitter molecules such as acetylcholine and γ-aminobutyric acid (GABA).

Neurotransmitters & Synaptic Vesicles

When a nerve impulse reaches the synapse, the vesicles fuse with the plasma membrane and release the neurotransmitter. Synaptic receptors pick up the neurotransmitter, thereby initiating the depolarizing electrical current that propagates through the second neuron in the pathway. At the synapse, meanwhile, the membrane of the cell that releases the neurotransmitter quickly forms **endocytic vesicles** that return to a larger endosomal compartment, where they fuse. Vesicles bud from this larger endosome, reload with the neurotransmitter, and return to a position just beneath the membrane at the synapse, where the vesicles await a signal to fuse and release their contents (Figures 4–17 and 4–18).

Studies of exocytotic events involving synaptic vesicles have revealed the presence of proteins quite similar, if not identical, to those involved in vesicle formation, targeting, and fusion within intracellular compartments. For example, an ATP-binding protein called **N-ethylmaleimide-sensitive factor (NSF)** is required for fusion of vesicles to intracellular compartments, and NSF appears to be part of the complex needed for exocytosis.

SORTING TO DIFFERENT SITES ON THE PLASMA MEMBRANE

Address Markers

Most cells in tissue have **polarity.** Because surfaces differ in structure, the lipid and protein compositions of the membrane are not distributed uniformly.

Epithelial cells are a good example of polarized cells. They have an apical surface, which can have any number of specializations. Brush borders, cilia, or microvilli are all modifications that occur at the apical surface (Chapters 2 and 8). Other plasma membrane regions that show specialization are found where the epithelial cells attach to each other and where they attach to the basement membrane. It follows, then, that membrane proteins and lipids must be sorted to different parts of the polarized cell. Products to be sorted that arrive in the TGN must contain some type of **address marker** that allows the membrane component—as well as material to be released—to be directed to the proper site in the polarized cell.

Several mechanisms are employed by the cell.

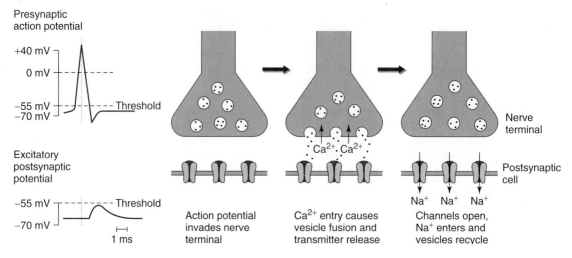

Presynaptic
action potential

Excitatory
postsynaptic
potential

Action potential
invades nerve
terminal

Ca^{2+} entry causes
vesicle fusion and
transmitter release

Channels open,
Na^+ enters and
vesicles recycle

Nerve
terminal

Postsynaptic
cell

Figure 4–17. Chemical transmission in synapses. The events of synaptic transmission are shown in left-to-right order. As the action potential reaches the presynaptic terminal, Ca^{2+} entry into the terminal causes vesicles containing neurotransmitter to fuse with the cell membrane. Neurotransmitter is released into the cleft and taken up by the postsynaptic neuron. While this occurs, endocytic vesicles form in the presynaptic cell to recycle vesicle membrane components. (Modified and reproduced, with permission, from Kandel ER et al: *Essentials of Neural Science and Behavior.* Appleton & Lange, 1995, p. 191.)

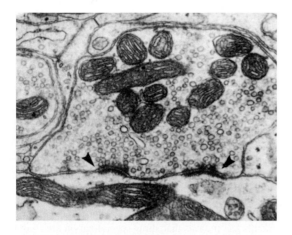

Figure 4–18. A chemical synapse. This electron micrograph shows the structure of the presynaptic terminal of a nerve-muscle synapse. The numerous round forms are vesicles containing the neurotransmitter acetylcholine. The poorly defined dark, thickened areas on the presynaptic side of the cleft (arrows) are thought to be membrane docking sites for vesicles. The large dark forms are mitochondria. (Reproduced, with permission, from Kandel ER et al: *Essentials of Neural Science and Behavior.* Appleton & Lange, 1995, p. 191. Courtesy of JE Heuser & TS Reese.)

Sorting signals on the vesicles preferentially carry cargo to the apical and basolateral surfaces of the cell. For example, vesicles containing proteins that are bound to the lipid bilayer through a **GPI linkage** are sorted to the apical surface of the cell.

Most vesicles that do not have a specific sorting signal go to the apical surface by the default or constitutive pathway. Proteins to be secreted into a lumen lined by epithelial cells thus deliver the protein to the surface through the default pathway.

MEDICAL ASPECTS OF CELL BIOLOGY

Table 4–1 lists principal diseases caused by defects in intracellular vesicle trafficking. In these diseases, proteins are misdirected or are otherwise unable to reach their normal cellular destinations, and cellular dysfunction ensues.

SUMMARY

In this chapter we have focused on the structure, formation, and function of the various organelles in a typical eukaryotic cell, discussing the mechanisms involved in movement of material from one compartment to another. This process is a complicated event that involves many different protein molecules and occurs via the formation of membrane vesicles that bud from the donor compartment and dock on a target compartment. In order for the budding (carrier) vesicle with material in its lumen and new proteins embedded in the membrane to target to a new compartment, an "address label" must be attached. This label can be a single protein or a combination of several proteins. The composition and arrangement of the address molecule gives it specificity to bind to a target membrane that contains on its surface the spe-

cific receptor for the address label. Although there seems to be a general movement of material from the ER to the plasma membrane, there are many sites where retrograde trafficking also occurs.

Several human diseases occur as a result of a defect in various proteins involved in trafficking from compartment to compartment. The processes of moving material from outside the cell to its interior include pinocytosis, phagocytosis, and a special type of endocytosis in which specific molecules are selectively taken into the cell.

REFERENCES

Amara JF, Cheng SH, Smith AE: Intracellular protein trafficking defects in human disease. Trends Cell Biol 1992;2:145.

Austin CD, Shields D: Formation of nascent secretory vesicles from the TGN of endocrine cells is inhibited by tyrosine kinase phosphatase inhibitors. J Cell Biol 1996; 135:000.

Barinaga M: Secrets of secretion revealed. Science 1993; 260:487.

Barlowe CL et al: A membrane coat formed by Sec proteins that drive vesicle budding from the endoplasmic reticulum. Cell 1994;77:895.

Beron W et al: Membrane trafficking along the phagocytic pathway. Trends Cell Biol 1995;5:100.

Boman AL, Kahn RA: Arf proteins: The membrane traffic police. Trends Biochem Sci 1995;20:147.

Chen YG, Shields D: ADP-ribosylation factor-1 stimulates formation of nascent secretory vesicles from the trans Golgi network of endocrine cells. J Biol Chem 1996; 271:5297.

Donaldson JG, Klausner RD: ARF: A key regulatory switch in membrane traffic and organelle structure. Curr Opin Cell Biol 1994;6:527.

Goldstein JL, Brown MS: Familial hypercholesterolemia. In: *The Metabolic Basis of Inherited Disease,* 5th ed. Stanbury JB et al (editors). McGraw-Hill, 1983.

Griffiths G, Simons K: The *trans* Golgi network: Sorting at the exit site of the Golgi complex. Science 1986; 234:438.

Kahn RA, Yucel JK, Malhotra V: ARF signaling: A potential role for phospholipase D in membrane traffic. Cell 1993;75:1045.

Letourneur F et al: Coatomer is essential for retrieval of dilysine-tagged proteins to the endoplasmic reticulum. Cell 1994;79:1199.

Ludwig T, Le Borgne R, Hoflack B: Roles for mannose-6-phosphate receptors in lysosomal enzyme sorting, IGF-II

binding and clathrin-coat assembly. Trends Cell Biol 1995;5:202.

McKusick VA, Neufeld EF: The mucopolysaccharide storage diseases. In: *The Metabolic Basis of Inherited Disease,* 5th ed. Stanbury JB et al (editors). McGraw-Hill, 1983.

Munro S, Pelham HRB: A C-terminal signal prevents secretion of luminal ER proteins. Cell 1987;48:899.

Murray RK et al: *Harper's Biochemistry,* 24th ed. Appleton & Lange, 1996.

Novick P, Field C, Schekman R: Identification of 23 complementation groups required for post-translational events in the yeast secretory pathway. Cell 1980;21:205.

Palade G: Intracellular aspects of the process of protein synthesis (Nobel Lecture). Science 1975;189:347.

Pelham HRB: About turn for the COPs. Cell 1994;79:1125.

Pelham HRB: Heat shock and the sorting of luminal ER proteins. EMBO J 1989;8:3171.

Pryer NK, Wuestehube LJ, Schekman R: Vesicle-mediated protein sorting. Annu Rev Biochem 1992;61:471.

Rabinovitch M: Professional and non-professional phagocytes: An introduction. Trends Cell Biol 1995;5:85.

Rothman JE: Mechanisms of intracellular protein transport. Nature 1994;372:55.

Rothman JE, Orci L: Molecular dissection of the secretory pathway. Nature 1992;355:409.

Rothman JE, Warren G: Implications of the SNARE hypothesis for intracellular membrane topology and dynamics. Curr Biol 1994;4:220.

Sandvig K, van Deurs B: Endocytosis without clathrin. Trends Cell Biol 1994;4:275.

Schwartz-Lippincott J: Membrane dynamic between the endoplasmic reticulum and Golgi apparatus. Trends Cell Biol 1993;3:81.

Schekman R: Protein localization and membrane traffic in yeast. Annu Rev Cell Biol 1985;1:115.

Sudhof TC et al: Membrane fusion machinery: Insights from synaptic proteins. Cell 1993;75:1.

Swanson JA, Baer SC: Phagocytosis by zippers and triggers. Trends Cell Biol 1995;5:89.

Vallee RB, Okamoto PM: The regulation of endocytosis: Identifying dynamin's binding partners. Trends Cell Biol 1995;5:43.

von Mollard GF et al: Rab proteins in regulated exocytosis. Trends Cell Biol 1994;4:164.

Whiteheart SW, Kubalek EW: SNAPS and NSF: General members of the fusion apparatus. Trends Cell Biol 1995;5:64.

SUGGESTED READING

Smith CB, Betz WJ: Simultaneous independent measurement of endocytosis and exocytosis. Nature 1996; 380:531.

Mitochondria & Cellular Energy   **5**

MITOCHONDRIA & ENERGY PRODUCTION

Mitochondria have long been recognized as the "power house" of the cell. These membrane-enclosed organelles are present in all eukaryotic cells, except red blood cells (erythrocytes) and terminal keratinocytes, and are responsible for the production of energy in the form of **adenosine triphosphate (ATP).** Mitochondria are abundant organelles in cells that expend large amounts of energy, such as skeletal and cardiac muscle cells; the exocrine pancreas, where high levels of secretory proteins are synthesized; and motile cells (eg, sperm). Many mitochondrial enzymes are encoded by nuclear deoxyribonucleic acid (DNA) and, after translation of their messenger ribonucleic acids (mRNAs) in the cytoplasm, individual polypeptides are imported into the mitochondrion (see below and Chapter 3). Mitochondria possess their own DNA, which has limited coding capacity, and ribosomes that are similar in size to those of bacteria; consequently, it is thought that these organelles evolved from bacteria that were engulfed by eukaryotic cells some 10^9 years ago.

THE ORGANIZATION OF MITOCHONDRIA

Video microscopy has shown that mitochondria are flexible, mobile organelles that move constantly through the cytoplasm to sites in the cell where energy consumption is high. This image of mitochondria, which range in length from approximately 0.5 to 2 μm, contrasts with the older view that mitochondria are static, elongated cylinders. Mitochondria, unlike organelles of the secretory pathway, possess two membranes. One is a smooth **outer membrane,** which is characterized by the presence of monoamine oxidase, acyl coenzyme A (CoA) synthetase, and phospholipase A_2; the other is a slightly thicker **inner membrane.** The lumen surrounded by the mitochondrial inner membrane is called the **matrix space,** and it contains the soluble enzymes of the citric acid cycle and the enzymes involved in fatty-acid beta-oxidation (β-oxidation). The space between the inner and outer membranes, called the **intermembrane space,** contains the enzymes creatine kinase and adenylate kinase. The inner membrane is arranged into numerous folds called **cristae,** which increase its surface area significantly.

In 1953, Palade and colleagues published the first detailed electron microscopic images of mitochondria and described the cristae. It took another 10 years, however, before these components were analyzed biochemically. By the mid 1960s, investigators had determined the arrangement of the respiratory apparatus on the cristae, and Racker and colleagues had generated "submitochondrial particles." By combining biochemical analysis with electron microscopy, these investigators showed that spherical components on the inner surface of the inner mitochondrial membrane are the sites of the reaction known as **oxidative phosphorylation** and that the respiratory chain components are buried in the membrane (Figures 5–1 and 5–2).

The general characteristics of each mitochondrial subcompartment are summarized below.

Outer membrane. The outer membrane contains multiple copies of porin, an aqueous channel forming

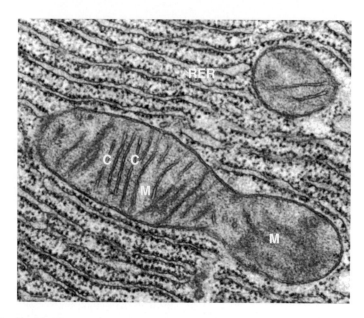

Figure 5–1. The mitochondrion. A complete mitochondrion is visible in this electron micrograph of a rat pancreatic cell. The major parts of the mitochondrion—membranes, cristae (C), and matrix (M)—are clearly seen. On a finer level, note the rough endoplasmic reticulum (RER) with ribosomes on its cytoplasmic surfaces. × 50,000. (From Junqueira LC et al: *Basic Histology,* 8th ed. Appleton & Lange. 1995, p. 28, with permission.)

protein, and is permeable to all molecules with a molecular weight of less than approximately 5000. These molecules, including ions and metabolites, can enter the intermembrane space but cannot penetrate the inner membrane. The outer membrane also possesses receptors for polypeptides that are translocated into the matrix, inner membrane, and intermembrane spaces.

Intermembrane space. This compartment contains a unique set of enzymes, distinct from the matrix, that use the ATP generated in the inner membrane.

Inner membrane. This compartment is a specialized membrane that is rich in the phospholipid cardiolipin, which possesses four fatty acid chains attached to glycerol. Cardiolipin renders the membrane impermeable to ions. The inner membrane is folded into numerous cristae that contain the following: (1) proteins that function in oxidation reactions of the respiratory electron transfer chain, (2) the **ATP synthase** enzyme complex that synthesizes ATP, and (3) transport proteins that regulate metabolic transport into and out of the matrix. The enzymes of the **respiratory chain** are embedded in this membrane and carry out **oxidative phosphorylation,** which generates ATP.

Matrix. The matrix contains enzymes that metabolize pyruvate and fatty acids to produce acetyl CoA and those that oxidize acetyl CoA in the citric acid cycle. The major products of the matrix are carbon dioxide (CO_2) and reduced nicotinamide adenine di-

nucleotide (NADH); the latter is the source of electrons for transport along the respiratory chain. It also contains the mitochondrial DNA, ribosomes, and some transfer RNAs.

Because of this double-membrane structure, enzymes or polypeptide subunits of enzymes (which are synthesized in the cytoplasm) that are destined for the matrix space have to pass through four separate compartments (ie, outer membrane, intermembrane space, inner membrane, and mitochondrial matrix) to reach their cellular destination. The matrix proteins must therefore have specific targeting (topogenic) signals that define their destination and receptor proteins on the outer surface of the inner membrane that recognize these signals. The outer membrane has fewer receptors and allows passage of many polypeptides across its membrane into the intermembrane space. The details of this process, which involves chaperone proteins, are discussed in Chapter 3.

OXIDATION

Protons and Energy Production

All cells use a common mechanism by which energy generated from the oxidation of metabolites in the mitochondrial matrix, in particular carbohydrates and fatty acids, is coupled to drive membrane-bound **proton pumps.** The proton pumps transfer hydrogen ions (H^+) from one side of a membrane to the other. In mitochondria, H^+ are transferred across the inner

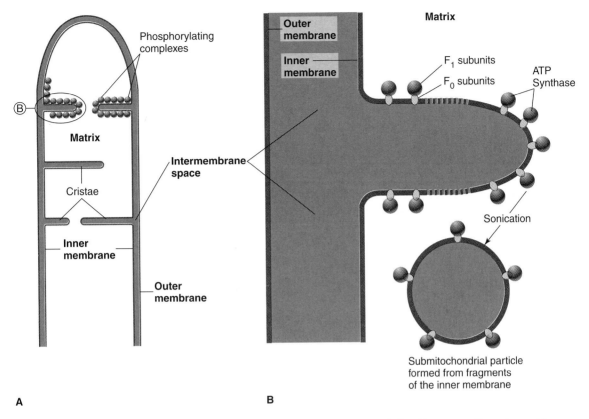

Figure 5–2. Mitochondrial membranes and phosphorylating complexes. The relationships among the outer and inner membranes, the cristae, and the matrix are shown (A). A magnified view (B) shows phosphorylating complexes on the inside surface of the inner membrane and on the cristae. Submitochondrial particles have the complexes on their outer surfaces and are therefore ideal research tools. (Modified and reproduced from Murray RK: *Harper's Biochemistry,* 24th ed. Appleton & Lange, 1996.)

membrane to the intermembrane space; this transfer of protons results in the establishment of an **electrochemical proton gradient** across the inner membrane. This gradient drives reactions that generate energy when the protons flow back "downhill" via integral membrane proteins embedded in the mitochondrial inner membrane. One such protein discussed below is ATP synthase, which synthesizes ATP from adenosine 5′-diphosphate (ADP) and inorganic phosphate (P_i). The proton pumps are themselves driven by the free energy that is released when electrons are sequentially transferred through the electron-transport chain. As electrons flow from a higher to a lower energy state, the released energy drives the translocation of H^+ across the inner mitochondrial membrane. This process occurs in the inner membrane of mitochondria by coupling metabolism to production of ATP via the electron-transport chain.

Oxidative phosphorylation is the process by which the enzymatic oxidation of metabolites is converted into energy in the form of ATP. This process can be separated into three parts:

1. the biochemical reactions that generate electrons with a high level of energy;
2. the membrane-bound electron-transport system, which enables the energy of electron transport to be converted to a proton gradient across the inner mitochondrial membrane;
3. ATP synthase, which uses the proton gradient to generate ATP during the flow of H^+ from the intermembrane space into the mitochondrial matrix.

The source of electrons is the oxidation of carbohydrates, lipids, proteins, or nucleic acids, although the major fuel sources in most cells are carbohydrates and fatty acids. A series of four major protein complexes embedded in the mitochondrial inner membrane, known as the **electron-transport system,** allows the electrons produced by metabolite oxidation to flow sequentially from one electron acceptor to the next. The free energy released (ie, the energy available to perform work) as the electrons pass from one complex to the next is used in the movement of protons into the intermembrane space. This process establishes a proton gradient across the inner mitochondrial membrane, and it is this gradient that drives ATP synthesis. At the end of the transport chain, the electrons combine with the final acceptor, molecular oxygen, to produce water. The protons that accumulate in the intermembrane space then flow down their concentration gradient via the enzyme ATP synthase, which acts like an ATPase running in reverse (ie, instead of hydrolyzing ATP, this enzyme uses the energy of H^+ translocation to generate ATP from ADP and P_i). Both the multiple proteins of the electron-transport complexes and ATP synthase are in the inner mitochondrial membrane and comprise numerous integral membrane proteins that span the inner membrane bilayer. In the early 1960s, Mitchell proposed that the energy of proton translocation across a concentration gradient could be coupled to ATP synthesis. This is the **chemiosmotic theory,** for which Mitchell received the Nobel prize in 1975 (Figure 5–3).The mechanism of electron transfer, which is the result of metabolic oxidation and its coupling to ATP synthesis via the generation of a proton gradient, is the main focus of this chapter.

Carbohydrates and Fats

Carbohydrates and fats are the major fuel sources whose metabolism yields electrons. In the cytoplasm, glucose, a six-carbon sugar, is partially oxidized by a series of 10 separate enzymatic reactions known as **glycolysis** to two three-carbon molecules of pyruvic acid (Figure 5–4). Pyruvate is then transported from the cytosol across the outer and inner mitochondrial membranes into the matrix, where it is completely oxidized. Pyruvate is initially oxidized to acetyl CoA

(see below), and the electrons released during the oxidation of acetyl CoA in the citric acid cycle are then "fed" into and transported along the electron-transport chain to generate ATP. Similarly, fatty acids, derived from the breakdown of insoluble triglycerides in the cytoplasm, are transported into the mitochondrial matrix as fatty acyl CoA. This substance can be completely oxidized by the metabolic cycle β-oxidation, which uses four separate enzymes. The pathway removes two carbons from the fatty acid at each turn of the cycle and generates acetyl CoA, which is metabolized via the citric acid cycle to yield reducing electrons for ATP synthesis.

During glycolysis, each molecule of glucose that enters this metabolic pathway produces two molecules of glyceraldehyde-3-phosphate (the fifth intermediate in the pathway). These molecules are then oxidized to pyruvate, thereby producing a total of four ATP molecules (Figure 5–4). Two ATP molecules, however, are consumed during the glycolytic cycle, one at each of two separate steps in the conversion of glucose into fructose 1,6-diphosphate. The result is a net "profit" of two ATP molecules. The products of glycolysis can be written as:

$$\text{Glucose} + 2\ \text{ADP} + 2\ P_i + 2\ \text{NAD}^+$$
$$\rightarrow 2\ \text{pyruvate} + 2\ \text{NADH} + 2\ \text{ATP}$$

The pyruvate produced by the glycolytic cycle is then oxidized completely in the citric acid cycle. This process provides additional ATP (see below), and the NADH is a source of stored energy that can be used via oxidative phosphorylation in the conversion of ADP to ATP.

During the oxidation of glyceraldehyde 3-phos-

Food

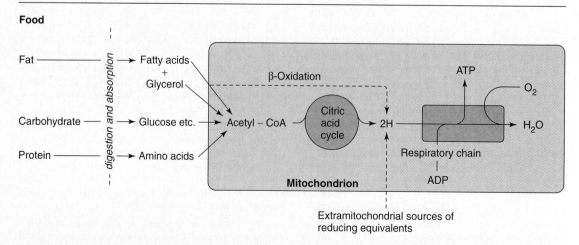

Figure 5–3. The mitochondrial respiratory chain. Oxidation of food molecules generates reducing equivalents (2H) that are transported into the mitochondrion and collected by the respiratory chain. Further oxidation is coupled to synthesis of ATP. (Modified and reproduced from Murray RK: *Harper's Biochemistry,* 24th ed. Appleton & Lange, 1996.)

Glycolysis

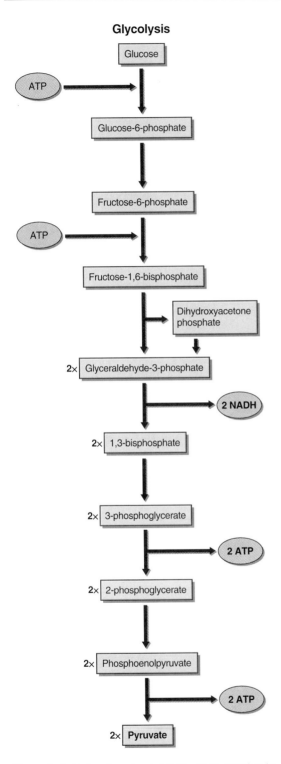

Figure 5–4. Major steps in glycolysis. Each reaction in the glycolytic pathway is catalyzed by a separate enzyme. Following cleavage of fructose 1,6-bisphosphate (a six-carbon sugar), two three-carbon sugars are produced at each of the subsequent steps in the pathway. (Modified and reproduced, with permission, from Alberts B et al: *Molecular Biology of the Cell,* 3rd ed. Garland, 1994.)

phate to 1,3 bisphosphoglycerate, a molecule of oxidized NAD (NAD^+) is changed to NADH (Figure 5–4). NAD plays a pivotal role in metabolism; the reduced molecule (ie, NADH) is formed when a hydride ion (a hydrogen nucleus plus two electrons) are taken up by NAD. This reaction yields a "high-energy intermediate," in that NADH readily donates the electrons to the electron-transport chain (see below) that produces ATP.

Although the glycolytic cycle is not a major source of cellular ATP, it is important under anaerobic conditions (ie, when oxygen is absent, limiting, or too low for ATP synthesis by mitochondrial oxidative phosphorylation), because it then becomes the main source of ATP for the cell. For example, during intense exercise, when breathing or heart rate cannot supply sufficient oxygen to muscles for oxidation of pyruvate in mitochondria, the pyruvate can be reduced (accept electrons) by NADH to produce lactic acid, which is eventually excreted from the cell. The now oxidized NAD^+ can then recycle to act as an electron acceptor (ie, be reduced to NADH) in the glycolytic cycle from glyceraldehyde-3-phosphate. Because the production of lactate simultaneously regenerates NAD^+, glycolysis continues and produces ATP even in the absence of oxygen. When levels of oxygen are restored, the reaction

pyruvate + NADH → lactate + NAD^+

is reversed, and the pyruvate is fed into the citric acid cycle.

PRODUCTION OF ACETYL CoA

As outlined above, during lipid metabolism, fatty acids are acetylated to fatty acyl CoA in the mitochondrial matrix, where β-oxidation and the citric acid cycle generate high-energy electrons for transport down the electron-transport chain. The energy generated during fatty-acid and carbohydrate oxidation is made available in the form of reducing equivalents (ie, there is gain in electrons) in mitochondria. Pyruvate and fatty acids are selectively transported from the cytosol into the mitochondrial matrix, where a series of enzymes known as the **respiratory chain** transport the liberated reducing equivalents, thereby allowing them to react with oxygen to form water. The enzymes that produce the reducing equivalents (ie, those of the citric acid cycle and of β oxidation) are present in the matrix space, and the free energy generated during transport is coupled to the generation of ATP (Figure 5–3).

Pyruvate, produced by glycolysis in the cytoplasm, and fatty acids are transported from the cytosol into the mitochondrial matrix. Pyruvate is then converted in the matrix to **acetyl CoA;** this process occurs via the enzyme complex pyruvate dehydrogenase. Acetyl units "carried" via acetyl CoA are oxidized to CO_2 in the **citric acid cycle,** or Krebs cycle (named after Sir Hans Krebs, who elucidated many of these reactions and received the Nobel Prize in 1953). In this series of reactions, the overall products are CO_2, ATP, NADH, and the reduced form of flavin adenine dimicleotide ($FADH_2$). Because NAD^+, FAD, and their reduced forms are regenerated at each turn of the citric acid cycle, the net result is the formation of one ATP molecule. More importantly, in terms of energy production much of the energy released by the oxidation reactions in the citric cycle is "stored" in electrons carried by NADH and $FADH_2$. NADH is soluble in the matrix, whereas $FADH_2$ is bound to the enzyme acyl-CoA dehydrogenase and can deliver high-energy electrons directly to **ubiquinone** (also known as coenzyme Q) in the electron-transport system (see below). The electrons "held" transiently by both these compounds are rapidly transferred to the respiratory chain in the mitochondrial inner membrane (Figure 5–5).

Chemiosmotic Coupling

In the early 1960s, Mitchell realized that the orientation of an enzyme in a membrane can confer directional properties on the reactions involved. He proposed that the results of a reaction on the inside of a membrane would be different from those on the outside if the enzymes involved are membrane proteins that release their products only on one side of the lipid bilayer. He suggested that production of ATP by mitochondria might occur through (1) reversal of an ATPase reaction because of its orientation in the membrane or (2) the effect of proton charge separation, which occurs at the oxidation-reduction steps during electron transport. This hypothesis eliminated many then-prevailing ideas, which had suggested a direct link between phosphorylation of ADP to generate ATP with each oxidation-reduction step. Mitchell postulated several major ideas to explain the obligatory coupling of oxidative-phosphorylation to ATP synthesis:

1. Energy released from metabolite oxidation is made available in mitochondria as reducing equivalents (—H or e^-), which are channeled into the respiratory chain. Here, electrons pass down a redox gradient of electron carriers to their final reaction with molecular oxygen to form water.
2. The redox carrier complexes are grouped together in the inner mitochondrial membrane. The energy released in the passage of electrons at various stages of the redox gradient is used to pump protons out of the matrix, thereby generating an electrochemical potential across the inner mitochondrial membrane.
3. The mitochondrial "ATP synthase" (a large multisubunit membrane protein) translocates protons

across the membrane. In the presence of an electrochemical proton gradient, protons will flow from the intermembrane space back into the matrix, which causes the enzyme to function as an ATPase in reverse to generate ATP from ADP and P_i.
4. The inner membrane is impermeable to protons and other ions. Consequently, exchange carrier proteins are present in the membrane, thereby allowing the selective passage of ions and metabolites without collapsing the electrochemical gradient across the inner membrane.

This chemiosmotic process couples the energy of metabolite oxidation to the production of ATP on the inner mitochondrial membrane. The energy that results from oxidation of pyruvate in citric acid, which leads to the production of NADH and $FADH_2$ from NAD^+ and FAD, is therefore stored as electrons or reducing equivalents. These electrons ultimately combine with oxygen to produce ATP in the process of oxidative phosphorylation. As the electrons stored in NADH and $FADH_2$ are released, they are transported down the respiratory chain housed in the inner mitochondrial membrane. Energy released in passing from one carrier complex to the next pumps H^+ from the matrix space across the inner membrane to the intermembrane space (Figure 5–6). This process creates the electrochemical proton gradient across the inner mitochondrial membrane. Because the concentration of protons is now higher in the intermembrane space, protons flow down the proton gradient (driven in part by the negative charge on the matrix side of the inner membrane) back into the matrix. This "powers" the membrane-bound ATP synthase, which converts ADP + P_i to ATP.

Electron Transport

The electron-transport system comprises three large protein complexes (I, III, IV) and ubiquinone, which are responsible for the sequential delivery of high-energy electrons carried by NADH and $FADH_2$ to molecular oxygen (Figure 5–6). Each complex possesses the following: (1) a major multisubunit enzyme complex that catalyzes electron transfer; (2) nonprotein organic (prosthetic) groups, which are bound to the enzyme and accept and release electrons; and (3) proteins that facilitate proton movement. Two small, mobile electron carriers (cytochrome *c* and ubiquinone) that oscillate among the three major complexes are also present (Figure 5–6). Table 5–1 summarizes the major properties of each complex.

Electron transport begins when two electrons released from NADH are passed to the first of some 15 electron carriers in the respiratory chain. The electrons that are initially released have the highest energy. This energy gradually dissipates as the elec-

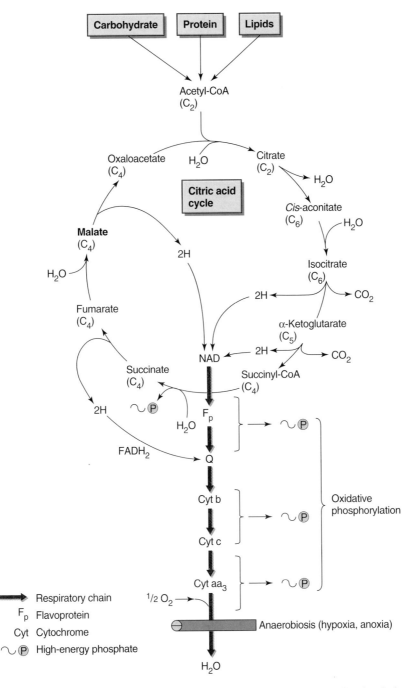

Figure 5–5. The citric acid cycle. Under aerobic conditions, pyruvate molecules produced by glycolysis enter the mitochondria and are converted into acetyl CoA. Acetyl CoA and one molecule of water enter the citric acid cycle and are oxidized to two CO_2 and reducing equivalents (2H). Oxidation of the reducing equivalents in the respiratory chain is coupled to formation of ATP. Note that the enzymes of the citric acid cycle are in the mitochondrial matrix, and the enzymes of the respiratory chain are located in the mitochondrial inner membrane. (Modified and reproduced from Murray RK: *Harper's Biochemistry,* 24th ed. Appleton & Lange, 1996.)

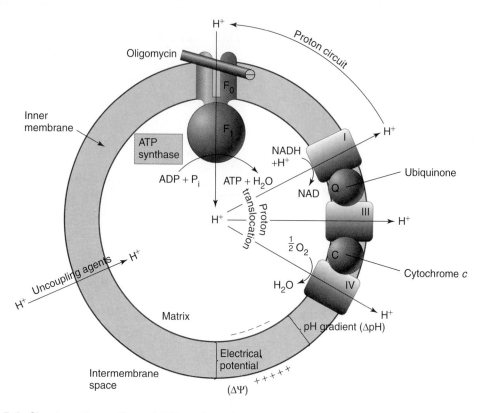

Figure 5–6. Chemiosmotic coupling and ATP synthesis. Formation of ATP by ATP synthase is associated with proton entry through the inner membrane (top). Oxidation in the respiratory chain involves proton translocation out of the matrix, preserving the proton gradient (right). F_1 and F_0 are the protein subunits that promote phosphorylation. The respiratory chain complexes I, III, and IV act as proton pumps. Researchers use compounds that disturb this chemiosmotic coupling to study the normal processes. Dinitrophenol, an uncoupling agent, makes the inner membrane permeable to protons (left). Oligomycin acts on ATP synthase to block proton entry into the matrix (top). (Modified and reproduced from Murray RK: *Harper's Biochemistry,* 24th ed. Appleton & Lange, 1996.)

trons are transferred along the chain; the acceptors at the end of the chain therefore have a higher affinity for electrons than do those at the beginning. The electrons actually pass from metal atoms in the prosthetic groups attached to proteins in each complex of the respiratory chain, and each complex has a greater affinity for electrons than the preceding complex.

The electrons pass down the chain until they are transferred to molecular oxygen, which has the highest affinity for electrons. The electron carriers in the respiratory chain absorb visible light and have a characteristic spectrum when oxidized or reduced. This property has allowed the behavior of the various complexes to be analyzed spectroscopically in re-

Table 5–1. Major properties of each complex.

Complex	Function	Total Molecular Weight	Polypeptide Subunits	H+ Transport
I (NADH dehydrogenase complex)	Electron transport from NADH to ubiquinone	~850,000	16–26	Yes
II (FAD-mediated)	Carries electrons from oxidation of succinate in citric acid cycle to ubiquinone	97,000	4–5	No
III (Cytochrome *b-c* complex)	Electron transfer from ubiquinone to cytochrome *c*	~300,000	8	Yes
IV (cytochrome oxidase *a/a₃* complex)	Transfer of electrons from cytochrome *c* to oxygen	~200,000	10–13	Yes

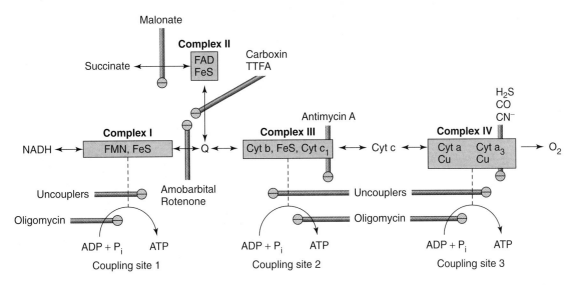

Figure 5–7. Inhibition of the respiratory chain by various compounds. This diagram shows the four respiratory-chain complexes and possible sites of action for various chemical inhibitors. Note that TTFA is an iron-chelating agent. ($\ominus$ = proposed site of inhibition; Complex I = NADH:ubiquinone oxidoreductase; Complex II = succinate:ubiquinone oxidoreductase; Complex III = ubiquinol:ferricytochrome c oxidoreductase; Complex IV = ferricytochrome c:oxygen oxidoreductase.) (Modified and reproduced from Murray RK: *Harper's Biochemistry,* 24th ed. Appleton & Lange, 1996.)

sponse to inhibitors or stimulators of oxidative phosphorylation. In particular, the use of specific antibiotics, chemicals, and drugs that interfere with different steps along the electron-transport chain have helped define the sequence of electron transport (Figure 5–7). Further, some of these membrane-bound complexes can be solubilized by mild detergent, and their spectroscopic properties analyzed. A brief description of the major electron carriers is given below; however, a biochemistry text would provide a more detailed account, which is beyond the scope of this chapter.

With the exception of ubiquinone, all the prosthetic groups that transport electrons are linked to proteins. The prosthetic groups cycle between an oxidized and reduced state as electrons are donated or gained along the pathway. One type of prosthetic

group (in complex II) consists of FAD, which accepts electrons from succinate oxidized in the citric acid cycle. Unlike NAD, FAD is tightly membrane bound to the inner mitochondrial membrane and feeds its electrons directly to the ubiquinone complex (Figures 5–5 and 5–7). FAD has the structure:

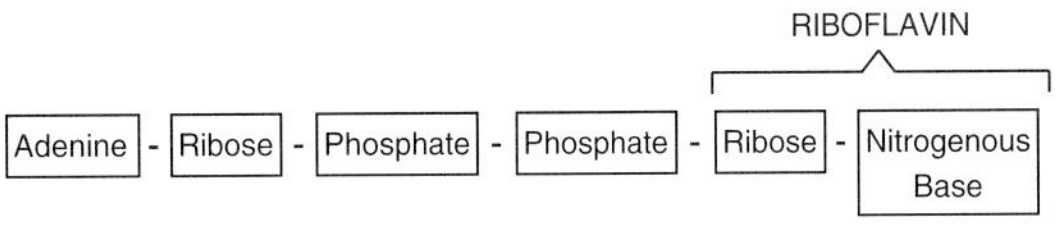

RIBOFLAVIN

| Adenine | - | Ribose | - | Phosphate | - | Phosphate | - | Ribose | - | Nitrogenous Base |

The oxidized or reduced part of the molecule in both FAD and flavin mononucleotide (FMN), which is present in complex I phosphate-ribose-nitrogenous base, is derived from riboflavin (Figure 5–8). These

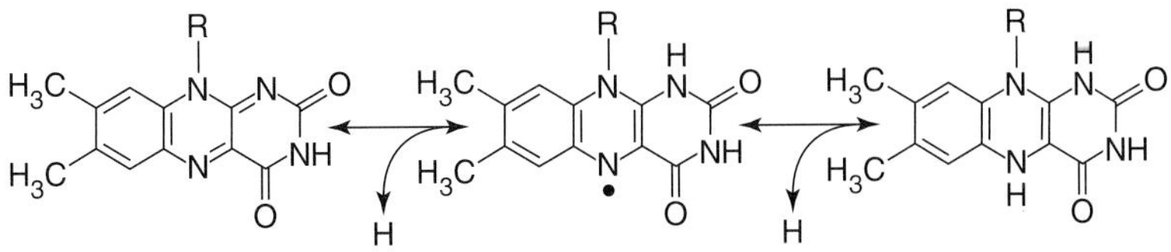

Figure 5–8. Oxidation-reduction in flavin nucleotides. Oxidation-reduction reactions in FAD and FMN involve changes in the isoalloxazine ring (center ring of the three-ring structure). (FAD = flavin adenine dinucleotide; FMN = flavin mononucleotide.) (Modified and reproduced from Murray RK: *Harper's Biochemistry,* 24th ed. Appleton & Lange, 1996.)

carriers transport pairs of electrons and bind two hydrogen atoms to form $FMNH_2$ during reduction; the linkages between FAD and FMN and their proteins form complexes known as flavoproteins. A second group of carriers are the cytochromes, which comprise a family of related colored proteins that all possess a bound "heme group" whose central iron atom alternates between the ferrous (Fe^{3+}) oxidized and ferric (Fe^{2+}) state. The heme group consists of a "porphyrin" ring with a tightly bound central iron atom held by four nitrogen atoms at each corner of a square. (Figure 5–9).

The third group of electron carriers are the "iron-sulfur proteins," in which two or four iron atoms are covalently bound to an equal number of sulfur atoms, thereby forming an iron-sulfur center. Some sulfur atoms are part of cysteine residues in the polypeptide chain of an iron-sulfur protein. As do the cytochromes, the iron atoms alternate between Fe^{2+} and Fe^{3+} states as the complex gains and loses electrons (Figure 5–10). The fourth type of prosthetic group that acts as an electron carrier is the copper (Cu) center. At present, however, little is known about the structure of these proteins, except that copper atoms oscillate between the Cu^+ and Cu^{2+} states as the complex is reduced and oxidized. Copper may participate in a bimetallic center, with a heme-linked iron atom at the final stage of the electron-transport pathway.

Ubiquinone, which is a small hydrophobic molecule that is not protein associated and is dissolved in the lipid bilayer, is the simplest of the electron carriers. Ubiquinone can accept one H^+ for each electron it accepts and can carry either one or two electrons.

When the electrons are transferred to the next carrier in the chain, the protons are released. Both ubiquinone and cytochrome c can diffuse very rapidly in the plane of the inner mitochondrial membrane and collide randomly with each of the carrier complexes approximately once every 10 ms. The three major complexes apparently exist as separate entities in the lipid bilayer, and electron transfer is dictated by the specificity of the interactions within each component (ie, their relative affinities for electrons). This view of how the electron-transport complexes are arranged is somewhat different from earlier models. In those models, it was assumed that there was a structurally ordered chain of electron-transport proteins, which were tethered together in a raft-like structure within the membrane. Electron transfer was therefore thought to be determined by the affinity of the next component along the chain for the donated electron (ie, its redox potential) rather than by formation of a specific structural complex.

Proton Pumping by the Electron-transport System

As outlined above, the electron-transport system pumps H^+ from the mitochondrial matrix into the intermembrane space as electrons flow from NADH to oxygen. The carrier complexes I, III, and IV have been solubilized from mitochondrial membranes and shown to pump H^+ in vitro. Both in vitro and in vivo measurements have demonstrated that a minimum of three protons are translocated as a pair of electrons move through the complex. Although the evidence supports Mitchell's hypothesis, the actual mechanism

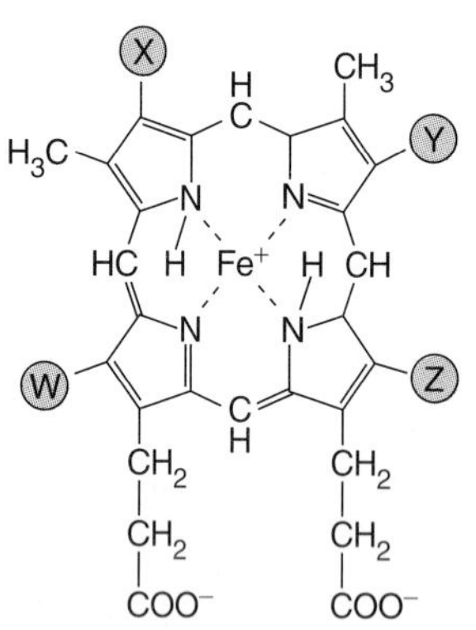

Figure 5–9. The cytochrome prosthetic group. The complete molecule, including the central iron atom (Fe) and the tetrapyrrole ring, is called a heme group. The iron atom alternates between the Fe^{2+} and Fe^{3+} states during a cytochrome's oxidation-reduction cycle. Various cytochromes possess different side groups attached to each of the positions designated as W, X, Y, and Z in the core ring structure.

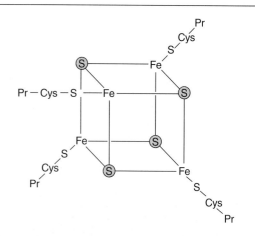

Figure 5–10. An iron-sulfur protein. The structure and geometry of the iron-sulfur protein Fe_4S_4 is shown. Other sulfur-iron proteins exist that have a geometry based on a center of Fe_2S_2. (Ⓢ = acid-labile sulfur; Pr = apoprotein; Cys = cysteine residue.)

as to how the electron-transport complexes translocate protons across the inner membrane is still unclear. The most widely accepted idea is that the major carrier complexes transport H⁺ as an active transport process, which is powered by alternating oxidation-reduction cycles. According to this idea, reduction of a carrier complex induces a conformational change that activates a high-affinity proton-binding site on the matrix side of the inner membrane. Oxidation of the carrier alters the conformation of the carrier such that the H⁺ binding site faces the opposite side of the membrane. The affinity of the site for proton binding is simultaneously reduced, and, consequently, the proton is released to the intermembrane compartment. There are examples in which active transport of ions across membranes can be explained by this kind of model. Indeed, bacteriorhodopsin, which is the most well-understood example of proton pumping, is considered the model that most accurately explains the experimental data.

ATP SYNTHESIS & THE RESPIRATORY CHAIN

As discussed above, transport of protons down their concentration gradient from the intermembrane space back into the matrix via the enzyme ATP synthase generates ATP from ADP + P_i (Figure 5–6). Many details of how this process occurs come from

experiments performed in the late 1960s by Racker and colleagues, who isolated submitochondrial particles by sonicating mitochondria stripped of their outer membrane and reconstituted ATP synthesis in vitro (Figure 5–2). When such particles are prepared, inside-out vesicles are formed in which the matrix-facing molecules are now on the outside. If NADH, ADP, and P_i are added to such preparations, electron transport occurs and the particles synthesize ATP. The ATPase involved in this process is designated the F_0F_1 ATPase, because the enzyme complex can be readily separated into F_0 and F_1 subunits. The F_1 subunits comprise many polypeptides that can be solubilized from the inner membrane by mild detergents and consist of at least six separate subunits, several of which are present in multiple copies. The F_0 ATPase comprises three separate polypeptides, which are also present in multiple copies, that can be removed from the inner membrane only by harsh detergent treatment. With the use of negative-stain electron microscopy, Racker noted that the ATPase had a lollipop shape, with a spherical head region. If these spherical particles were removed from the inside-out mitochondrial vesicles, the residual particles could oxidize NADH but could not synthesize ATP. In the absence of membranes, however, the isolated spheres could hydrolyze ATP to ADP + P_i (ie, they had ATPase activity). Most importantly, when the spherical particles were added back to the stripped inner mitochondrial membrane vesicles, the reconstituted

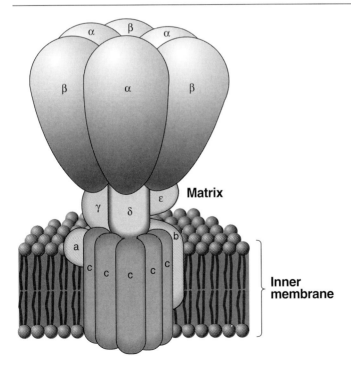

Figure 5–11. The mitochondrial F_0F_1 ATPase. This model shows the chief F_1 and F_0 components. The F_1 component comprises the α, β, γ, δ, and ε subunits. The F_0 component consists of the a, b, and c subunits, which are embedded in the lipid bilayer of the inner mitochondrial membrane. This model is based on the *E coli* F_0F_1 ATPase, whereas the mitochondrial enzyme has three additional subunits in the membrane. The ring of c subunits probably makes up the H⁺-conducting channel. (Adapted and reproduced, with permission, from Wolfe SL: *Molecular and Cellular Biology*. Wadsworth, 1993.)

particles acted as an ATPase in reverse and generated ATP from ADP and P_i. Since this classical experiment, it has been shown that the F_1 ATPase corresponds to the "spherical blob," is part of a much larger complex that has a molecular weight of approximately 500,000, and is composed of at least nine subunits. This enzyme is now referred to as ATP synthase. The F_0 component of ATP synthase consists of at least six separate subunits, most of which are thought to span the membrane bilayer. The F_0 complex cannot synthesize ATP in the absence of the F_1 spherical head complex. It is therefore thought that the F_0 complex provides the H^+-conducting channel of ATP synthase (Figure 5–11).

MITOCHONDRIA & DISEASE

Even though mitochondria have their own DNA, it is of limited coding capacity, and most of the mito-

chondrial proteins are encoded by nuclear genes. Many mutations in the enzymes of oxidative phosphorylation have been described in human beings. For example, several rare genetic diseases have been attributed to pyruvate metabolism at the step where pyruvate is converted to acetyl CoA to enter the citric acid cycle. This step is mediated by the enzyme complex pyruvate dehydrogenase, which actually consists of three separate enzymes designated E_1, E_2, and E_3. E_1 and E_3 have been linked to several genetic disorders in which metabolic imbalances can lead to severe developmental defects. A severe form of neonatal lactic acidosis, which causes neurologic abnormalities, has been linked to a defect in one of the three subunits that constitute the E_1 enzyme. Patients who are very severely affected do not usually survive beyond early infancy, whereas those who are less severely affected can be treated with bicarbonate, dialysis, or both to control the level of acidosis. Nevertheless, mild forms of the disease can lead to progressive degeneration of the nervous system.

As discussed above, oxidative phosphorylation is the major source of energy production in the cells. Consequently, defects in any of the steps in this path-

Table 5–2. Disorders of oxidative phosphorylation that result from defects in nuclear DNA (nDNA).[1]

Disorder	Complex Subunits	Clinical Phenotypes
Deficiency of complex I (NADH:ubiquinone oxidoreductase)	At least 35 polypeptides; seven encoded by mtDNA	1. Myopathy 2. Fatal infantile multisystem disorder 3. Encephalomyopathy
Deficiency of complex II (succinate:ubiquinone oxidoreductase)	Four components, encoded only by nDNA	1. Encephalomyopathy 2. Myopathy
Deficiency of complex III (ubiquinol: ferrocytochrome *c* oxidoreductase)	11 subunits; one encoded by mtDNA	1. Myopathy 2. Histiocytoid cardiomyopathy of infancy 3. Multisystem encephalomyopathy a. Fatal infantile form b. Milder disorder
Deficiency of complex IV (cytochrome *c* oxidase)	13 subunits; three encoded by mtDNA	1. Myopathic form a. Fatal infantile myopathic form b. Benign infantile myopathic form 2. Encephalomyopathic form a. Leigh syndrome b. MNGIE syndrome c. Alpers syndrome
Deficiency of complex V (ATP synthase)	12–14 subunits; two encoded by mtDNA	1. Myopathy 2. Multisystem disorder
Deficiency of coenzyme Q_{10} (CoQ$_{10}$)		1. Myopathy and seizures
Defects in intergenomic signaling Depletion of mtDNA		1. Congenital infantile mitochondrial myopathy 2. Fatal infantile hepatopathy 3. Infantile or childhood myopathy
Multiple mtDNA deletions		1. AD form of CPEO

[1]From Seashore MR, Wappner RS: Lactic acidosis & mitochondrial oxidative phosphorylation. Chapter 16 in: *Genetics in Primary Care & Clinical Medicine.* Appleton & Lange, 1996, p. 212, with permission.
AD = autosomal dominant; CPEO = chronic progressive external ophthalmoplegia; Leigh syndrome = subacute necrotizing encephalomyopathy; MNGIE = mitochondrial neuropathy, gastrointestinal disorder, encephalopathy syndrome; mtDNA = mitochondrial DNA.

Table 5–3. Disorders of oxidative phosphorylation associated with mutations in mitochondrial DNA (mtDNA).[1]

Disorder	Clinical Phenotypes	Inheritance Pattern
Large-scale rearrangements (deletions or duplications) of mtDNA	Kearns-Sayre syndrome Variants of Kearns-Sayre syndrome (CPEO and CPEO Plus) Pearson syndrome Diabetes mellitus and deafness	Sporadic, not inherited Sporadic, not inherited Sporadic, not inherited Maternal

Point mutations of mtDNA
  Structural mtDNA genes
 	
  Synthetic mtDNA mutations [point mutations in mtDNA that affect transfer RNA (tRNA)]
	LHON; Leber hereditary optic neuropathy
	NARP; neuropathy, ataxia, and retinitis pigmentosa
	MELAS; mitochondrial encephalomyopathy with lactic acidosis and stroke-like episodes
	MERRF; myoclonic epilepsy and ragged-red fibers
	MiMyCa; maternally inherited disorder with adult onset myopathy and cardiomyopathy
	Maternally inherited diabetes mellitus and deafness
		Maternal
		Maternal
		Maternal
		
		Maternal
		Maternal
		
		Maternal

[1]From Seashore MR, Wappner RS: Lactic acidosis & mitochondrial oxidative phosphorylation. Chapter 16 in: *Genetics in Primary Care & Clinical Medicine.* Appleton & Lange, 1996, p. 215, with permission.
CPEO = chronic progressive external ophthalmoplegia.

way could have profound effects on muscle or brain function. The cases of children who have had defects in complexes I, II, and IV have therefore been described. These patients have multiple phenotypes, including weakness, inability to tolerate exercise, my-opathy, encephalopathies, and cardiomyopathies. Some of these genetically characterized defects are summarized in Tables 5–2 and 5–3. For a complete description of these complex diseases, however, the reader is referred to a genetics text.

SUGGESTED READING

Alberts B et al: Energy conversion: mitochondria and chloroplasts. Chapter 14 in: *Molecular Biology of the Cell,* 3rd ed. Garland, 1994.

Hatefi Y: The mitochondrial electron-transport system and oxidative phosphorylation. Annu Rev Biochem 1985; 54:1015.

Leningher AL: Glycolysis. Chapter 16 in: *Principles of Biochemistry,* 2nd ed. Worth, 1978.

Leningher AL: The tricarboxylic acid cycle and phosphogluconate pathway. Chapter 17 in: *Principles of Biochemistry,* 2nd ed. Worth, 1978.

Leningher AL: Oxidative phosphorylation, mitochondrial structure, and the compartmentation of respiratory metabolism. Chapter 19 in: *Principles of Biochemistry,* 2nd ed. Worth, 1978.

Mitchell P: Chemiosmotic coupling in oxidative and photosynthetic phosphorylation. Biol Rev 1966;41:445.

Mitchell P: Coupling of phosphorylation to electron and hydrogen transfer by a chemiosmotic type of mechanism. Nature 1961;191:144.

Mayes PA: The respiratory chain & oxidative phosphorylation. Chapter 14 in: Murray RK et al (editors): *Harper's Biochemistry,* 24th ed. Appleton & Lange, 1996.

Mayes PA: The citric acid cycle: the catabolism of acetyl-CoA. Chapter 18 in: Murray RK et al (editors): *Harper's Biochemistry,* 24th ed. Appleton & Lange, 1996.

Seashore MR, Wappner RS: Lactic acidosis & mitochondrial oxidative phosphorylation. Chapter 16 in: *Genetics in Primary Care & Clinical Medicine.* Appleton & Lange, 1996.

Wolfe SL: Energy for cell activities: cellular oxidations and the mitochondrion. Chapter 9 in: *Molecular and Cellular Biology.* Wadsworth, 1993.

6

The Cell Cycle & Cell Division

KEY TERMS

Mitotic phase
Interphase
G_1 phase
G_0 phase
S phase
G_2 phase
Maturation promotion factor
Cyclins
Tumor suppressor
p53 protein
Retinoblastoma
Apoptosis
Chromatin

It is a sine qua non of biology that cells reproduce by cell division. With progressive advances in microscopy in the 19th and 20th centuries, biologists have acquired ever-more-powerful tools to study cell reproduction in greater detail. One result is the increasingly precise description of the events of cell division.

There are two major phases of the life of a cell: the M phase or **mitotic phase** and the **interphase.** During the M phase, the following biological events can be observed:

- chromosome condensation
- spindle formation and alignment of chromosomes onto an equatorial plane
- separation of chromatids toward the poles of the cell
- formation of a cleavage furrow
- final separation of one cell into two daughter cells.

Biological events of the **interphase** are equally fascinating. The principal tools to examine these events include such techniques as labeling specific components of the cell with radioactive tracers, growing cells in defined culture conditions, and developing molecular probes to identify specific molecules that prepare the cell for the M phase. Research

with these and other advanced procedures has revealed many dramatic events of the cell cycle during interphase.

Our discussion begins by describing the signals and the processes that take place within the cell, preparing it to undergo division. Study of the biochemical events of the cell cycle has revealed many specific molecules that must be regulated precisely in order to keep the cells from overdividing, leading to the formation of tumors. Many of these regulatory molecules have a brief half-life and are made or activated only after they have received a biochemical signal.

GENERAL PRINCIPLES OF THE CELL CYCLE

PHASES OF THE NORMAL CELL CYCLE

Figure 6–1 illustrates the four phases of the cell cycle:

A. M Phase. This is the mitotic cycle, which typically requires 30–60 minutes to complete. The separation of two daughter cells concludes the M phase.

B. G_1 (Gap 1) Phase. This is the interval between the end of the M phase and the beginning of deoxyribonucleic acid (DNA) replication. The duration of this phase varies according to cell type. For most cycling mammalian cells, G_1 phase is about 12 hours.

C. S Phase or Synthesis Phase. DNA is synthesized and replicated during this period in the cell cycle in preparation for mitosis.

D. G_2 (Gap 2) Phase. This is a period of preparation before the cell enters mitosis. During G_2, replicated DNA is monitored to ensure that is has doubled. This is also a period of cell growth and

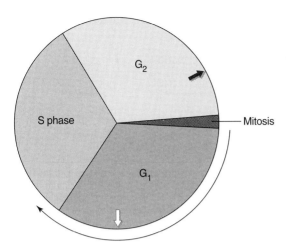

Figure 6–1. The cell cycle. The four phases of the cell cycle are G_1, S, G_2, and mitosis. Note that in a typical mammalian cell, mitosis is by far the shortest phase. The S phase (for DNA *s*ynthesis and replication) is divided from mitosis by G_1 and G_2 (for *g*ap periods). The open arrow indicates the point at which the cell becomes committed to entering the S phase; the closed arrow, committed to entering mitosis. (Modified and reproduced, with permission, from Murray RK et al: *Harper's Biochemistry*. Appleton & Lange, 1996, p. 412.)

finalization of cellular contents before proceeding into the M phase.

DURATION OF THE CELL CYCLE

The duration of the cell cycle varies depending on the type of cell and the stage of development of the organism. For example, the cell cycle time of a fertilized egg is usually very brief. A fertilized frog egg undergoes very rapid division—about 30 minutes to complete a cell cycle. Most of this time is spent in the S phase and M phase—and very little time is spent in G_1 and G_2. Because a large supply of proteins and other components needed for division already exist in the frog egg, almost no new protein synthesis is required. Therefore, the Gap phases are very brief.

The goal in the early stages of development is to form as many cells as possible in a relatively short time. For example, a fertilized frog egg undergoes 12 doublings within 6 hours to form an embryo of 8192 cells. Although the cells divide rapidly, they do not increase significantly in size. Nevertheless, by sheer number and some asymmetric cleavages, the cells form an embryo within a few hours. Once the embryo is formed and the three basic tissues are established, the time required for a cell cycle increases because of lengthened Gap phases. As new essential proteins are made, the cell increases in size and volume.

Progressive Nature

The cell cycle is progressive. When cells enter G_1, a series of molecular events "instruct" the cell to approach and enter the S phase. If these biochemical events do not occur, the cell does not progress to replication and remains in the G_1 compartment.

When cell cycle progression in the G_1 phase slows down, the cell can express proteins that do not include molecules required for cell division. In this instance, the G_1 phase becomes greatly extended. This extended G_1 phase is called the **G_0 phase,** and it is a special condition of the cell cycle.

All cells in the body are in some phase of the cell cycle. Fully differentiated neurons or cardiac myocytes, eg, are in a G_0 compartment, which means they have left the dividing cycle and do not return to it. Cells of the bone marrow or the lining of the gut, on the other hand, are almost constantly in a cycling process and rarely enter the G_0 compartment. Cells in most tissues of the body can re-enter the dividing cycle, but this usually occurs in only a few cells at a time in any given tissue—unless there is tissue damage or an irregular molecular event forces mature differentiated cells back into the dividing compartment.

The biochemical events that cause a cell to progress through the cycle cell cycle are the same for all eukaryotic cells. In fact, much has been learned about the molecules that underlie and drive cell division by studying lower organisms. Thus, although this chapter focuses on events in the vertebrate cell cycle, it is important to emphasize that studies of budding and fission forms of yeasts, for example, have greatly clarified cellular and molecular events in each stage of the cell cycle. Research with lower vertebrates such as the African clawed frog (*Xenopus laevis*) or invertebrates such as sea urchins or nematodes (*Caenorhabditis elegans*) have also provided many essential insights.

LESSONS FROM THE FROG EGG

MATURATION EVENTS

Major breakthroughs in deciphering the molecular processes of the cell cycle have come from studies involving eggs of *X laevis*. These cells are quite large—approximately 1 mm in diameter—and contain thousands of times the amount of cytoplasmic proteins of cells in developing tadpoles. The secreted frog egg progresses through a specialized type of mitosis, called meiosis, in which the chromosome number and hence DNA are reduced by one half (Figure 6–2). The reduction in chromosome number occurs by two unique cell divisions in which the DNA is not

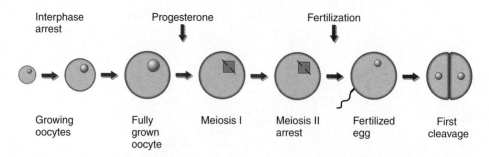

Figure 6–2. Oocyte development and fertilization. After DNA is synthesized, a frog oocyte arrests in G$_2$ phase and grows to full size. Under the influence of progesterone, the mature oocyte completes the first meiotic division and enters the second. The oocyte then arrests in metaphase of the second division. Fertilization is the trigger for completion of the second meiotic division and for the beginning of embryonic development (shown as the first cleavage of the fertilized egg). (Modified and reproduced, with permission, from Murray A, Hunt T: *The Cell Cycle*. Freeman, 1993.)

replicated. In the first stage, the eggs, which are still in the ovary, arrest in the G$_2$ phase (the first meiotic division) and remain in this arrested state. When the female reaches the point for the eggs to be fertilized, a steroid hormone, progesterone, is secreted into the blood of the animal and causes the eggs arrested in G$_2$ to move through mitosis. The resulting daughter cells are of two types. One, an oocyte, contains one half the chromosome number, whereas the other daughter cell is called a **polar body.** The polar body is no longer functional and is lost. The oocyte reenters M-phase but arrests in this phase. It is secreted from the oviducts of the female. These haploid cells are now ready for fertilization by sperm which have also undergone meiotic reduction in chromosome number in the male. When the sperm fertilizes the egg, the chromosome number (DNA content) doubles and sets in motion all the subsequent cell divisions and developmental processes.

Maturation-Promotion Factor

When the oocytes are fertilized, other ovarian cells secrete progesterone, which induces the G$_2$-arrested oocytes to (Figure 6–2)

1. enter meiosis I and proceed through a second round of division
2. arrest in the second meiotic cycle in the M phase, with the haploid chromosomes aligned in a metaphase configuration.

Under natural conditions during amplexus, the haploid sperm fertilizes the egg, and mitosis proceeds rapidly through 12 cycles, forming the body of the tadpole. Of interest is that the oocytes that are arrested either in G$_2$ or at meiosis II can be isolated in large numbers and used for in vitro experiments. In a study in which cytoplasm isolated from meiotic II (M phase) cells was injected into oocytes that were ar-

rested in G$_2$, the injected cells progressed from G$_2$ into mitosis and through one round of cell division. Such findings led to the identification of a substance that was present in the cytoplasm of cells arrested in metaphase but not in cells arrested in G$_2$. This substance is called the **maturation-promotion factor** or **mitosis-promoting factor** (MPF). This factor stimulates G$_2$-arrested cells to progress through mitosis. Progesterone can also drive G$_2$ cells into mitosis, because this steroid stimulates the production of MPF.

When mammalian cells grown in culture are treated with a reagent that blocks the formation of spindle microtubules—eg, colchicine—cells arrest in **prophase.** When cytoplasmic extracts are taken from cells treated with colchicine and are injected into frog oocytes that are in G$_2$, cells overcome the block and progress into mitosis. This finding suggests that MPF is also present in mammalian cells. Indeed, mammalian MPF has been found to be effective in stimulating mitosis in amphibian cells.

MPF: REGULATOR OF MITOTIC EVENTS

Role of Cyclin B

In nearly all eucaryotic cells that have been studied—including those of yeast, worms, and flies—MPF appears to control the entry of cells into mitosis. An appreciation of how this molecule is expressed in the cell is essential to understanding the molecular events of mitosis. Toward this end, two types of in vitro experiments have been instrumental and are described below.

A. A frog oocyte that is arrested in G$_2$ has a full complement of proteins and ribonucleic acid (RNA) molecules (including messenger RNAs or mRNAs) necessary to carry out multiple rounds of cell division. However, if an inhibitor of protein synthesis (ie, cycloheximide or puromyocin) is added to frog oocyte G_2 cells, progression of the cell cycle is blocked. This indicates new proteins must be synthesized for the cell to complete the cycle.

B. If radiolabeled amino acids are added to oocytes—eg, to media containing sea urchin eggs—the labeled amino acids are rapidly transported into the cytoplasm of the oocytes and are incorporated into new proteins. If during this process the cycling oocytes are lysed at various times and the cytoplasmic proteins are separated by electrophoresis, many proteins will be found to contain the radioactive amino acid. One protein in particular, however, will appear in the G_1 phase and will continue to increase in amount during the S and G_2 phases. It will suddenly disappear, however, when the cell enters mitosis. These results will recur if the experiment is carried through several rounds of the cell cycle.

Findings like these, confirmed that a protein is made and degraded, which follows closely the events of the cell cycle. This particular protein was called **cyclin** and has now been isolated. It is now understood that cyclin is synthesized continuously throughout the cell cycle but is abruptly destroyed at the beginning of anaphase.

It is now known that several types of cyclins exist in the cell. Because the rise and fall of the protein—called **cyclin B**—coincided precisely with events of the cell cycle, cyclin B is now considered the key component of MPF.

Structure of Cyclin B

Cyclin B has two subunits:

1. One subunit carries a **kinase domain** capable of phosphorylating particular substrates within the cell.
2. The other subunit of cyclin B is called the regulatory subunit and its synthesis rises and falls during the cell cycle.

Cyclin B synthesis begins in G_1 and reaches its highest level in early prophase before ending abruptly at the beginning of anaphase. When the concentration of the **regulatory subunit** is sufficient, the kinase domain is activated. When this occurs, specific proteins are phosphorylated by the cyclin B kinase, thereby changing their function and leading to **chromosome condensation, nuclear envelope breakdown,** and **spindle assembly.**

CELL CYCLE ENGINE

Studies with frog oocytes suggest that the early embryonic cell cycle behaves like a **biochemical oscillator** that periodically drives the cell into and out of the cell cycle (Figure 6–3). The oscillator is actually a series of biochemical events in which MPF plays an important role. Biomolecular events during the rise and fall of MPF levels parallel several mor-

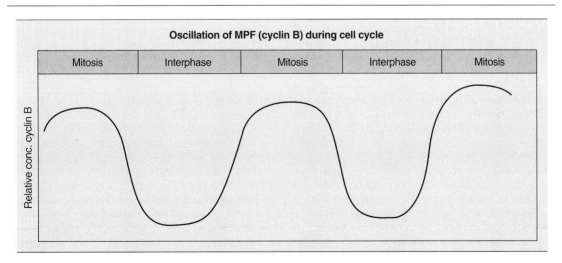

Figure 6–3. Concentration of cyclin B and movement through the cell cycle. The relative concentration of cyclin B in fertilized sea urchin eggs was determined electrophoretically. For the three cell cycles studied, the concentration of cyclin B rose rapidly in late metaphase, was relatively stable during mitosis, and fell abruptly at the beginning of interphase. Studies such as this led to the conclusion that cyclin B is the principal component of mitosis-promoting factor (MPF). (Modified and reproduced, with permission, from Evans T et al: Cyclin: a protein specified by maternal mRNA in sea urchin eggs that is destroyed at each cleavage division. Cell 1983;33:389.)

Table 6–1. Biomolecular events of MPF synthesis parallel mitotic events.

High Levels of MPF Lead To
Chromosome condensation
Nuclear envelope breakdown
Spindle assembly
Low Levels of MPF Lead To
Chromosome segregation
Chromosome decondensation
Nuclear envelope reassembly
DNA replication
Centrosome duplication

Cyclin degradation by ubiquitination

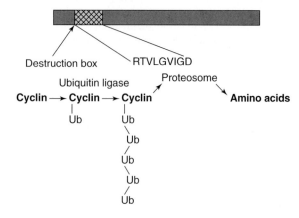

Figure 6–4. Degradation of cyclin B. The rapid destruction of cyclin B associated with the beginning of interphase is accomplished through ubiquitination. A specific sequence near the amino terminal of cyclin B (the destruction box) is recognized by an enzyme called ubiquitin ligase. The enzyme links ubiquitin protein molecules (Ub) to lysine residues in the cyclin B sequence. The modified protein is recognized by a proteosome, taken into the proteolytic complex, and destroyed.

phological events in mitosis. These events are summarized in Table 6–1. The **cell cycle engine** involves biochemical events that lead to the expression of proteins affected in the steps listed in this table.

In embryonic cells and during development, control of MPF expression is critical. Control of the events of the cell cycle engine varies. Fertilization of the egg starts the engine in oocytes; but different events can start the engine in somatic cells.

CYCLIN B DEGRADATION

Destruction Box & Ubiquitin

Proteins are synthesized and degraded continually within the cytoplasm. Most often degradation occurs within a specified compartment such as the lysosome, where most degradative enzymes and the environment for their activity can be controlled (see Chapter 4). However, a second method of protein degradation has been identified for proteins that are part of cellular *regulatory* processes. This type of regulatory proteins includes the cyclins. What singles out these proteins for this special degradation process is a stretch of 8–10 amino acids located near the amino terminus and called the **destruction box.** When proteins containing this motif are to be degraded, a second protein (a **recognition protein**) binds to the amino acids in the destruction box. This provides a site where a third protein, called a **ubiquitin ligase,** can attach several copies of a small, 76–amino acid protein, called **ubiquitin,** to lysine residues located just downstream of the destruction box motif. Interestingly, ubiquitin itself has several other ubiquitin residues attached to it. Once a protein has been polyubiquitinated, it passes into a larger protein-RNA complex called a **proteosome,** in which proteases reside. It is in this complex that destruction of the original regulatory protein occurs (Figure 6–4).

The signals that trigger degradation of cyclin B during anaphase are still being elucidated. It is thought that the destruction box recognition protein is activated by phosphorylation. During most of the buildup of MPF (cyclin B) a phosphatase appears to render the recognition protein inactive. When the

level of cyclin B reaches its highest state in mitosis, MPF phosphorylates the recognition protein much faster than the phosphatase can remove the phosphate, and the recognition protein binds to the destruction box motif on cyclin B—thus leading to its destruction. This model describes, in part, the rise and fall of MPF levels during the cell cycle.

MPF IN MITOTIC EVENTS

The increase in MPF (cyclin B) during late G_2 drives the cell from G_2 into M, and its rapid destruction induces the exit from mitosis. Entry into mitosis is a consequence of phosphorylation of specific proteins by the MPF kinase (or cyclin B). It is these phosphorylated proteins that induce the dramatic morphological changes that occur when the cell enters mitosis (Figure 6–3).

The basic molecular structure of the nuclear envelope has been described previously (Chapter 3). The protein structure that stabilizes the lipid bilayer of the inner membrane of the envelope is the **nuclear lamina,** a meshwork of lamin filaments located on the inner surface of the nuclear membrane. The proteins that comprise this layer are the nuclear lamins A, B, and C.

Lamins A and C are products of the same gene, and they arise by alternate splicing of the lamin mRNA. Lamin A has an extension of 113 amino acids at its C terminus. Lamin B is derived from a different gene and is associated with the internal lipid leaflet by a hydrophobic isoprenyl anchor.

The three nuclear lamins form dimers that contain rod-like α-helical coils with globular domains at each end. The dimers, as basic units, polymerize and form the mesh-like structure on the inner surface of the nuclear envelope. In early prophase, MPF phosphorylates specific serine and threonine residues on the lamins and causes them to depolymerize, leading to the disintegration of the nucleus.

MPF also phosphorylates **histone H1** and other proteins of the chromosome scaffold, leading to their condensation. Together with other kinases, MPF is likely involved in phosphorylations that block **vesicle trafficking** and cause the endoplasmic reticulum and Golgi complex to break down.

Cytokinesis is blocked in early mitosis because MPF phosphorylates a site in myosin's light chain that inhibits its adenosine triphosphatase (ATPase) activity and association with actin filaments. When MPF (cyclin B) is degraded at the onset of anaphase, the action of continuously acting phosphatases that remove phosphates is unopposed, and the proteins are dephosphorylated. This allows the reversal of many effects of MPF.

In summary, the MPF complex contains a catalytic kinase subunit and a cyclin regulatory subunit. These subunits are the major initiating molecules of the events of mitosis. Their removal brings the cell back to interphase configuration.

REGULATED PASSAGE OF MAMMALIAN CELLS THROUGH THE CELL CYCLE

ROLE OF MULTIPLE CDKs & CYCLINS

It is now recognized that MPF is the major regulator of entry into M phase in frog and mammalian cells. Recall that MPF is composed of two polypeptides, a kinase subunit and a regulatory (cyclin) subunit. It turns out that mammalian cells have a small family of cyclin-dependent (or binding) kinases called Cdk—for **cyclin-dependent kinases.** Cdks 1 through 5 are numbered on the basis of their order of discovery. Likewise, several different cyclins are involved in different phases of the cell cycle (Figure 6–5).

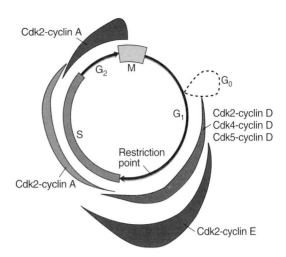

Figure 6–5. Cdk-cyclin complexes and the mammalian cell cycle. The diagram reflects the activity of different Cdk-cyclin complexes during the four phases of the cell cycle. The varying width of each band representing a specific Cdk-cyclin complex is roughly proportional to the activity of the complex at different points of the cell cycle. For example, Cdk2-cyclin E appears during G_1, reaches maximal activity late in G_1, and rapidly disappears during early S phase. (Adapted and reproduced from Sherr CJ: Mammalian G_1 cyclins. Cell 1993;73:1059. Copyright © 1993 by Cell Press.)

Role of Cdk-Cyclin Complexes

When cells are stimulated by growth factors to leave the G_0 compartment, the first Cdk that appears is Cdk2-cyclin D. This cyclin apparently recognizes substrates that regulate enzymes involved in synthesis of proteins that are required to generate pools of precursors for DNA replication. As long as the cells continue to be stimulated by the growth factor, Cdk2-cyclin D will be active. However, both the mRNA and the proteins of cyclin D are unstable, and if the level of growth factor falls, Cdk2-cyclin D disappear.

Shortly after the appearance of Cdk2-cyclin D, two other members are also detected: Cdk4-cyclin D and Cdk5-cyclin D. Cdk2-cyclin E makes its appearance in G_1 and reaches its greatest concentration at the G_1/S boundary, after which it falls off dramatically. Cdk2-cyclin A also appears at the G_1/S boundary and is in high concentration for the duration of the DNA replication phase (S phase).

Near the end of the G_2 phase, manufacture of Cdk2-cyclin B begins. The complex increases in concentration through the G_2/M boundary, then decreases precipitously by degradation. These different kinases and cyclins are necessary for the orderly recruitment and expression of genes whose products are essential for the cell to replicate. Most genes that are regulated by the Cdk-cyclins fall into two categories:

1. early response genes
2. delayed response genes.

Usually the early response genes encode proteins that function as transcription factors, which are involved in regulating other genes. The products of delayed response genes are typically involved in executing a metabolic event, including the expression of cyclin subunits (Table 6–2).

CHECKPOINTS IN CELL CYCLE REGULATION

p53 Protein: Selected Clinical Correlates

Accurate replication and partitioning of the genetic material of a cell is fundamental to its survival. There are four positions in the cell cycle where accuracy of replication, sequence fidelity, and equal separation of the DNA is monitored by cellular quality control mechanisms.

A. The G_1 Checkpoint: When damaged DNA is detected during G_1, the **p53 protein** functions as a transcription factor and causes G_1 arrest. An unstable protein, p53 is normally short-lived. However, when abnormal DNA is present in the cell, p53 binds and stabilizes itself to the DNA. This causes an accumulation of p53 in the nucleus and leads to the induction of the expression an inhibitor protein of Cdk-2.

The cell remains arrested in the G_1 compartment while the DNA **repair enzymes** reconstruct damaged nucleotides. The arrest in G_1 prevents copying of damaged bases that would lock a mutation into the DNA. When p53 dissociates from the DNA, its concentration diminishes; the inhibitor of Cdk is released, and Cdk is once again expressed.

In many human metastatic cancers, both alleles of p53 are inactive. The normal surveillance exerted by p53 is lost, and damaged DNA can replicate. In some cases, this leads to transformed metastatic tumors.

B. The S Phase Checkpoint: It is during the S phase that DNA is replicated. If mistakes occur in DNA synthesized during the replicative process and then are incorporated into the genome, a number of serious consequences will likely occur, including possible cell death. If replication errors happen (and they do) and if they are not fixed by the repair enzymes, the cell does not proceed out of the S phase. Ensuring the fidelity of the replicated DNA is an important checkpoint for the cell.

C. The G_2 Checkpoint: Unreplicated DNA blocks the cell from moving out of G_2 into M. Catastrophic damage occurs if the cell progresses through a phase of the cycle without completing the required molecular events in preparation for cell division. For example, if MPF is injected into cells in S phase, the incompletely replicated chromosomes will condense, then fragment. Occasionally MPF expression reaches the critical level in S phase, rather than in late G_2 or M. When this happens, serious biological consequences occur.

Apparently there are substances that regulate the expression of MPF activity—either of the kinase or cyclin subunit. The substance(s) prevents MPF action before completion of DNA replication. However, if MPF is degraded before chromosomal kinetochore microtubules are aligned properly, the chromosomes will fail to move from the metaphase plate, leading to **chromosomal nondisjunction.** Although some genetic mistakes are not detected by the cell's surveillance systems, the cell has developed a number of mechanisms that help to ensure the correct synthesis and replication of its genetic heritage (see Figure 6–6 and Table 6–3).

INHIBITORY PROTEINS OF CDK-CYCLIN COMPLEXES

A number of specific proteins inhibit the activity of the Cdk-cyclin complexes, thereby providing an additional level of regulation and further complexity to cell cycle control. At least seven inhibitory molecules have been identified. These are grouped into two major families of inhibitors:

1. p21 family
2. p15 and p16 family

p21 Family

The p21 family of inhibitors has three distinct gene products: **p21, p27,** and **p57.** The gene products have homologous amino-terminal regions that interact with the Cdk-cyclin complexes.

p21 is (1) a Cdk-binding protein that is up-regulated in senescent (aging) cells and (2) a gene product that can be induced by tumor suppressor p53.

p21 inhibits a number of different Cdk-cyclin complexes by blocking their interaction with the downstream substrate of the complex. The observation that p21 expression is up-regulated by p53 sug-

Table 6–2. Cyclins and cyclin-dependent kinase involved in cell cycle progression.[1]

Cyclin	Kinase	Function
D	Cdk4, Cdk6	Progression past restriction point at G1/S boundary
E, A	Cdk2	Initiation of DNA synthesis in early S phase
B	Cdk1	Transition from G2 to M

[1]Reproduced, with permission, from Murray RK et al: *Harper's Biochemistry,* 24th ed., Appleton & Lange, 1996, p. 412.

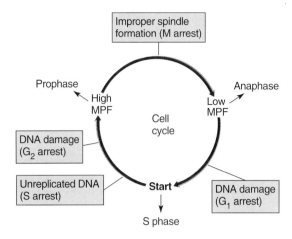

Figure 6–6. Checkpoints in cell cycle regulation. Four points exist where recognition of errors involving DNA triggers arrest of the cell cycle. Arrest prevents progeny cells with DNA composition different from that of the parent cell from being formed. The cell's surveillance systems recognize DNA damage during G_1 or G_2, unreplicated DNA during S phase, and improper spindle formation during mitosis. (Modified and reproduced, with permission, from Murray A, Hunt T: *The Cell Cycle.* Freeman, 1993.)

gests a possible mechanism for the induction of cell cycle arrest by the related actions of these two proteins. p21 can block other proteins, such as DNA polymerase subunits, and likely has other important substrates.

Another member of the p21 family—p27—also interacts with several Cdk-cyclin complexes. p27 has been implicated in the mediation of **contact inhibition of cell growth,** which causes cells to leave the

Table 6–3. Types of damage to DNA.[1]

I. Single-base alteration
  A. Depurination
  B. Deamination of cytosine to uracil
  C. Deamination of adenine to hypoxanthine
  D. Alkylation of base
  E. Insertion or deletion of nucleotide
  F. Base-analog incorporation
II. Two-base alteration
  A. UV light–induced thymine-thymine dimer
  B. Bifunctional alkylating agent cross-linkage
III. Chain breaks
  A. Ionizing radiation
  B. Radioactive disintegration of backbone element
IV. Cross-linkage
  A. Between bases in same or opposite strands
  B. Between DNA and protein molecules (eg, histones)

[1]Reproduced, with permission, from Murray RK et al: *Harper's Biochemistry,* 24th ed., Appleton & Lange, 1996, p. 413.

dividing cycle. When they achieve a critical population density, contact inhibition of growth occurs in vitro when normal cells reach confluence, the point at which all cells have contacted each other and the cells have stopped dividing. The **cell-cell contact** sends a signal that stimulates the expression of p27.

p15 & p16 Family of Inhibitors

p15 and p16 target exclusively to Cdk4 and Cdk6. These inhibitors can disrupt binding to the D cyclins, or they can bind to the cyclin's monomeric kinase subunit and prevent association.

Both p15 and p16 map to human chromosome 9p21, a region frequently deleted in **hereditary melanoma** and other tumors. This finding suggests the potential clinical significance of characterizing and regulating molecules and signaling pathways that drive the cell through the cell cycle. It has been suggested, eg, that p15 and p21 may be important as mediators of proliferation arrest induced by negative growth factors such as transforming growth factor-β (TGF-β). (See Chapter 10.)

TUMOR SUPPRESSOR PROTEINS: CLINICAL CORRELATES

p53 & Rb

Two proteins, p53 and retinoblastoma (Rb), function as tumor suppressors. A mutation in the gene encoding either protein can lead to unregulated cell proliferation and malignancy. If either protein is inactivated by a mutation affecting its structure or by a viral protein that binds to it and prevents its function, then uncontrolled cell replication will occur. It is now known that several viruses have evolved proteins that can inactivate each tumor suppressor.

The basic function of p53 and Rb is to block proteins involved in inducing the cell cycle. p53 is sequence-specific, which means it binds to a specific sequence of nucleotides in the control regions of a gene that is involved in regulating events of the cell cycle. Various genes are involved in the control of cell growth and are known to have a **p53 binding domain** in their promoter regions. Thus, when p53 is bound to the regulatory region of the gene, it is not able to be expressed—and the required cell cycle protein is not made.

Rb works in a different way. It inhibits the activity of a family of transcription factors known as E2F. E2F binding sites are present in several genes that are involved in initiating DNA synthesis. When in the hypophosphorylated state, Rb blocks these transcription factors.

Hyperphosphorylation of Rb by cyclin-dependent kinases inactivates it at the G_1/S transition and allows the cells to enter the S phase. It has been shown that p53 controls the expression of p21. Recall that p21 is a potent inhibitor of Cdk-cyclin complexes, and this inhibitor prevents the phosphorylation of Rb, thereby allowing it to sequester the transcription factors (E2F).

APOPTOSIS

From the foregoing discussion, it is evident that contol of cell replication is essential for survival of the organism. For this reason the cell has a number of proteins that act as a cell cycle brake. Loss of activity of these important proteins often leads to the formation of tumors.

One can think of the rate of cell growth or proliferation as the result of **cell proliferation minus cell death.** The cell proliferation component of cell growth has two factors: (1) the rate of stimulation and (2) the rate of inhibition of proliferation. The two components in the rate of cell death include (1) the rate of stimulated cell death and (2) the rate of inhibition of cell death.

A normal process in an organism is the orderly removal of cells by cell death. This process is termed **apoptosis** (the term is derived from Greek and means dropping of leaves or petals from flowers). This word was coined in 1972 to describe a type of cell death that exhibits very characteristic morphological properties. The cascade of events includes:

- condensation of chromatin
- breaking up of the nucleus
- blebbing of the plasma membrane
- fragmentation of the cell into discrete **apoptotic bodies.**

This process has also been called **programmed cell death,** which describes one type of apoptosis but not all types. One might think of apoptotic cell death as arising from external signals such as noxious stimuli, and programmed cell death as arising from signals within the cell. Signals that induce the cascade of events leading to cell death—including activation of a family of death genes—can occur through several mechanisms. Some are programmed, whereas others arise from nonprogrammed sources.

The triggering event of apoptosis is not the same in all cells. The orderly elimination of cells during apoptosis occurs in

- development
- normal cell turnover
- cytokine-induced atrophy, eg, through tumor necrosis factor
- viral induced processes, eg, in acquired immunodeficiency syndrome
- some neurodegenerative diseases, such as Huntington's disease and Alzheimer's disease.

Several molecular events play a role in initiating apoptosis, in particular:

1. action of divalent cations (Ca^{2+} and Zn^{2+})
2. changes in the membranes of apoptotic cells
3. signal transduction pathways for apoptosis.

Importance of Divalent Cations

Calcium ions appear to play a key role in the early signaling events leading to apoptosis. Findings from various studies suggest that sustained increases in intracellular free calcium precedes apoptosis. In many instances of apoptosis, if the amount of free calcium can be reduced, the onset of apoptosis can be delayed. The potential sites of calcium activation are numerous; however, two enzymes are activated during apoptosis:

1. endonucleases, which cleave DNA at internucleosomal sites
2. tissue transglutaminase, which covalently links proteins to the membrane through the formation of isopeptide bonds.

Zinc has been described as an inhibitor of apoptosis. One mechanism of this inhibition may be that zinc suppresses endonuclease activity.

Changes in the Membranes of Apoptotic Cells

It is important to emphasize that cells undergoing apoptosis—eg, cells in necrosis—do not pose a threat to surrounding cells. Apoptotic cells are readily phagocytosed, and it appears that changes in the membrane make the cell more "palatable" to the macrophage.

One feature that occurs on the membrane is a loss of sialic acids as the terminal sugar on glycoproteins and glycolipids. This seems to make the cell more available for engulfment by the resident phagocyte. It also appears that the presence of **vitronectin receptors** on the cell's surface attracts the macrophage. Other membrane changes—eg, lipid rearrangement of its phosphatidyl serine to be more externally exposed—are also characteristic of some apoptotic cells.

Signal Transduction Pathways in Apoptosis

Proliferation, differentiation, and apoptosis are closely related cellular responses that appear to share many molecular mechanisms. It has already been mentioned that free cytosolic calcium is an important component in the induction of apoptosis of many cell types. Activation of various isozymes of phospholipase C is a consequence of ligand binding to several specific cell surface receptors (Chapter 9). When this occurs, the generation of second messengers follows, eg, diacylglycerol and inositol 1,4,5-trisphosphate (IP_3).

Diacylglycerol promotes the activation of a family of serine and threonine kinases, collectively known as protein kinase C (PKC). IP_3 promotes the release of Ca^2 from internal stores. Thus, agents that ordinarily generate the signaling cascade involving PKC also stimulate the release of calcium into the cytosol from internal stores. Moreover, certain chemical toxins may stimulate apoptosis by disrupting normal calcium homeostasis. Other steps involving protein tyrosine kinases in signal transduction cascades may be involved in initiating apoptosis.

Apoptosis is an essential cellular process for the organism; this is especially true during development. For example, when the central nervous system is developing, many more neurons are formed than will be used. Only those neurons that form competent connections with other neurons will survive—all others will undergo apoptotic death. Apoptosis is also an essential event in the immune response. One host-defense mechanism is to greatly expand the number of lymphocytes producing antibodies to an invading organism. Once the invading organism has been eliminated, most of these specific lymphocytes are eliminated through apoptosis. One can readily recognize that a mechanism to eliminate unwanted cells is a necessity for survival of the organism.

CELL SENESCENCE & AGING

Senescence of Cells in Tissue Culture: Lessons Learned From Research

Normal cells—ie, nontransformed cells—have a finite capacity to proliferate. After going through a number of population doublings, they enter into a state of replicative **senescence.** The cells do not die; rather, they can be maintained for long periods in culture if their media are renewed frequently. If cells—eg, skin fibroblasts—are removed from a young individual and from an older person and placed in culture under identical conditions, the younger person's cells replicate longer than do the cells from the older individual. It has been suggested that a limited number of population doublings—approximately 50—is possible for any given cell type. This phenomenon has been observed for some time. It was originally described by Professor L. Hayflick, and is often referred to as the **Hayflick phenomenon.** The biological principle is that cells seem programmed to undergo a certain number of rounds of division and then cease to divide.

Cells can withdraw from the dividing cycle for a number of reasons that do not necessarily reflect replicative senescence. Other factors—such as damage to DNA or a terminal differentiation—can cause a cell to leave the replicative cycle. Melanocytes, for example, can be grown in culture for extended periods without producing any melanin. If they are treated with agents that stimulate the production of cyclic adenosine monophosphate (cAMP), which in turn induces enzymes for producing melanin, melanocytes divide only one or two more times. They then begin to make large quantities of the pigment—and never re-enter the dividing cycle. The number of cell replications such experimental melanocytes undergo is only a small fraction of the replications experienced by their uninduced counterparts.

There are many examples of the in vitro biochemical dissection of processes that lead to replicative senescence. Findings from the biochemical comparison of terminally differentiated cells and replicative senescent cells suggest they have a common alteration in gene expression. Both types of cells are unable to phosphorylate Erb2; phosphorylation of this kinase leads to activation of the mitotic signaling cascade. Moreover, both types of cells have an elevated expression of p21, the Cdk inhibitor. In addition, only terminally senescent cells produce large quantities of p27.

Information gained from such studies clearly suggests there are programmed events that drive a cell from replicating to nonreplicating conditions. Interestingly, cells taken from organisms that have lived a long time—such as the Galapagos tortoise with a life span of more than 100 years—will undergo 130 cell doublings before becoming senescent, whereas cells taken from a mouse—life span of 3 years—undergo 10 doublings before becoming senescent.

Findings & Implications

Within the context of the cell cycle, it is appropriate to note two emerging concepts regarding the molecular basis of senescence and aging:

1. Aging is not simply a stochastic event. Rather, there are specific predictable genetic components involved, and these components can be studied.
2. There is strong evidence that oxidative stress and caloric restriction are key factors in the aging process.

A large number of studies on the biochemical and cellular processes of aging have been performed in various species, including yeast, fruit flies, mice, and the nematode *Caenorhabditis elegans. C elegans* has been especially useful in studies of development, since all the cells of this worm can be identified early and their differentiation fate can be followed easily. The average life span of *C elegans* is 20 days. Findings from the genetic analysis of these animals suggest that a mutation in a cell (hx546) may confer a survival benefit. Nematodes that carry this mutation—appropriately labeled Age-1—appear to live an average of 65% longer than those without the mutation. Also, no morphological, embryological, or postembryo phenotypes are distinguishable from organisms that lack the mutation.

Moreover, worms with the mutation appear to have a greater tolerance to environmental oxidative stress. When worms carrying the mutation are exposed to hydrogen peroxide (H_2O_2) or paraquat, both of which promote highly reactive hydroxyl radicals, the worms live longer and show fewer deletions in their mitochondrial genome. Age-1 mutants show a corresponding increase in levels of the antioxidants' copper and zinc dismutase enzyme. These nematodes also have greater levels of catalase, the enzyme that detoxifies hydrogen peroxide and paraquat. Moreover, the Age-1 mutants show greater thermotolerance.

These findings suggest that the greater life span of Age-1 mutant nematodes may be due to their enhanced capacity to tolerate environmental stress. This implication has been reinforced by results that suggest the *daf* family of genes in Age-1 nematodes regulate the expression of other genes needed to defend the organism against environmental stress, eg, heat shock genes. Taken together, these experimental results strongly imply that the molecular events underlying the action of stress-response genes help to determine the life span of *C elegans*.

Salient Hypotheses on Aging: Oxidative Stress

One hypothesis on the cause of aging postulates that as cells age, they lose their capacity to counteract oxidative damage to key molecules. This hypothesis is based on the observations that (1) excessive **oxygen** is potentially toxic and (2) required use of oxygen by aerobic organisms may be detrimental to long-term survival.

Recall that oxygen is a biradical. When a single electron is added, a partially reduced molecule is generated. By further reaction, a number of additional **reactive oxygen metabolites** (ROMs) are produced. Recent findings suggest that ROMs can cause extensive oxidative damage to cell molecules—DNA, proteins, and unsaturated fatty acids in lipids of the bilayer.

This oxidant challenge is not trivial, since it has been estimated that 2–3% of the oxygen consumed by organisms is diverted to generate these deleterious compounds. Moreover, research findings strongly suggest that oxidative damage can increase with age. Thus, the study of mechanisms that regulate the expression of genes and proteins that protect against oxidative stress can help to elucidate the molecular basis of aging.

CONTROL OF THE CELL CYCLE IN TISSUES

Role of Platelet-Derived Growth Factor

The availability of cellular nutrients is an essential external cue for lower organisms to enter into the S phase of the cell cycle. If nutrients are insufficient, the cell will not divide. In higher organisms, the availability of essential nutrients is not usually a limiting factor. However the "signal" that tells quiescent cells to undergo division is often brought to the cell rather than being generated within the cell. Evidence for this came from early in vitro studies of mammalian cells in culture.

When mammalian cell culture techniques were first being developed it was noted that cells grew better if they were suspended inside blood clots. Because of the inconvenience of examining the growing cells inside a clot, investigators would allow the blood to clot and then remove the clot by removing blood cells. The resultant fluid is known as serum. If all the cells are removed from whole blood prior to clotting and this solution is used to grow cells, it is unable to support growth. These findings indicated that some factor is released by blood cells during clotting and that this factor is necessary for cells to divide.

This material has been shown to be derived from platelets and is called **platelet-derived growth factor** (PDGF). Normal cells in mammalian tissue appear to have sufficient nutrients to undergo cell division. Thus, the positive signal for proliferation must originate elsewhere. In the case of PDGF, this protein is secreted by the platelet at the time of blood clotting, after some wounding event. To replenish cells damaged by tissue injury, PDGF—one of the body's principal growth factors—signals cells around the wound to leave the nondividing phase of the cell cycle and enter the division cycle.

Growth Factors

A large number of **growth factors** have been isolated and characterized and will be discussed in detail in Chapter 10. Growth factors fall into two general categories:

1. those with broad cell and tissue specificity
2. those that are quite specific to certain types of cells.

Among the growth factors that exhibit broad cell and tissue specificity are

- PDGF
- epidermal growth factor (EGF)
- fibroblast growth factors (FGF) (These have nine isotypes and show some cell type specificity but are still regarded as a member of the broad spectrum group.)

- nerve growth factor (NGF) (This growth factor is restricted to cells of the nervous system.)
- erythropoietin (EPO) (This growth factor stimulates cells in the bone marrow to produce erythrocytes.)
- interleukin-2 and interleukin-3.

All of these growth factors act primarily on specific target cells. Each growth factor is also known as a **ligand** that binds to a specific cell surface receptor, with concomitant activation of a signal pathway (see Chapter 10).

NONDIVIDING COMPARTMENT OF THE CELL CYCLE

Role of G_0 Phase & Genetic Switching

Most cells that comprise mammalian tissues and organs are in the special part of the cell cycle called the G_0 or cell differentiation compartment, which, as discussed, is an extended G_1 phase of the cell cycle. This means that genes that encode the proteins that trigger cells to divide and proliferate are in the "off" position. In this state, the cell's metabolic energy is used to produce specialized proteins needed for differentiated cellular tasks. Also, by implication, genes for these proteins are in the "on" position.

In most types of cells, genes for cell proliferation can be reset to the "on" position. However, in some cells, once proliferation genes are switched off, they can never be restarted. When cardiac muscle cells have completed their proliferation and the cyclins and Cdks are switched off, they do not turn on again. The same appears true for neurons of all types.

Under suitable conditions, however, many cells retain the capacity to move back into the dividing cycle. In fact, there is cell "turn-over" in most tissues of the body. However, the rate of this turnover is usually slow—except in certain cells, such as blood cells and cells that line the intestine. In these tissues, the rate of cell renewal is substantial.

As indicated above, one of the main types of signal that can activate the Cdks-cyclins are generated by growth factors. But even when such a signal is triggered, the body must regulate the response so as to maintain the precise number of cells and their spatial organization. Were this not to occur, huge changes would ensue and ultimately lead to the organism's demise.

Findings from studies of normal cells growing in tissue culture suggest that cells have various factors that determine the number of cells that must be made to maintain tissue architecture and the integrity of cell attachments to their basal lamina. Salient findings from research involving fibroblasts are briefly described below.

Cell-Cell Contact: When Normal Cells Stop Dividing

If fibroblasts are grown in vitro until they completely fill a culture plate, the cells stop dividing and appear to move from the cycling phase to a quasi-G_0 stage of the cell cycle. Under sterile conditions, the scraping of cells with a spatula in a diagonal line across the plate kills the cells along the diagonal line—and a **cell-free diagonal** remains. The cells immediately next to the "wounded" area begin to divide and proliferate, and thus fill the vacant space. As soon as the space is filled, the cells again stop dividing.

This observation has contributed to the understanding that normal cells stop dividing after they reach a certain density. It is believed that after a cell makes contact with other cells on a substratum, a signal is relayed to the cell interior that confirms all contact points have been satisfied—and genes that signal proliferation are apparently turned off.

In another type of in vitro experiment, if the cell is not prevented from attaching to the surface of the dish, it remains in a rounded-up shape and fails to undergo mitosis. If on the other hand the cell is allowed to attach and spread, it forms contacts with the surface—called **focal contacts and focal adhesion plaques** (Chapter 7). Important cytoskeletal components—including actin filaments, microtubules, and other structural proteins—are part of the focal adhesion plaque. After a suitable period, these cells undergo mitosis.

Findings from these two types of experiments—as well as from similar research studies—suggest that molecules of the external environment—eg, those involved in cell-cell contacts and cell-matrix contacts—are a necessary part of the signal that drives cells to proliferate. (See Chapter 10.)

UNREGULATED CELL GROWTH: CLINICAL CORRELATES

Proto-oncogenes

So far in our discussion of the cell cycle, we have defined the molecules that drive the cell through the phases of the cell cycle, including G_1, the G_1/S boundary, the S phase, and the S/G_2 boundary. These are complicated interacting molecules that are poised to phosphorylate and be dephosphorylated as the principal biochemical signal that starts the processes. Of course, the availability of subunits of the complexes (Cdk-cyclin) and the presence of various inhibitor proteins are critical for the cell to traverse the cycle.

Under normal circumstances, we observe rapid cell proliferation during embryogenesis and development. We know all too well that cells can lose their capacity to control the cell cycle, and when this occurs unregulated cell growth—ie, cancer—can occur.

Table 6–4. Oncogenes related to cancer.[1]

Oncogene	Related Cancer
c-raf	Lung cancer, parotid gland
c-kit	Lung cancer
myc	Small cell lung cancer, colon cancer, lymphoma
N-myc	Neuroblastoma
k-ras	Colon cancer
erbA	Lymphoma, small cell lung cancer
bcr-abl	Chronic myelogenous leukemia
ras	Colon, pancreas, bladder, lung

[1]Reproduced, with permission, from Seashore MR, Wappner RS: Genetics in *Primary Care & Clinical Medicine,* Appleton & Lange, 1996, p. 60.

There are many places where control of the cell cycle can be lost. Genes whose products are involved in controlling cell proliferation are called **proto-oncogenes,** meaning that if the gene is mutated, it gives rise to uncontrolled cell proliferation and has potential to become an oncogene. The intense study of cancer cells in the past three decades has led to many insights into specific molecules involved in directing cell proliferation.

As more is learned about molecular events that help to regulate growth factors, protein synthesis, and protein degradation, additional insight into the pathogenesis of various cancers will undoubtedly be gained with the liklihood of being able to control cell division in certain types of tumors (Tables 6–4 and 6–5 and Figure 6–7).

KEY MECHANISMS OF CELL DIVISION

Mitosis

In mammalian cells, mitosis lasts only about 30 minutes. During this brief time, the following series of events lead to the segregation of genetic material:

1. Chromatin condenses.
2. The nuclear envelope dissociates.
3. A spindle apparatus forms.
4. Chromosomes move to an equatorial plane of the cell.
5. Sister chromatids separate and move to the poles.

These mitotic events usually occur in the order listed and most often without a sharp demarcation between events.

Chromatin Condensation

Chromosomes are huge macromolecular complexes of DNA plus many types of nuclear proteins. The average human chromosome contains 130×10^6 base pairs and is about 45 mm long. The DNA must be packaged into a much smaller bundle—the chromatin—to fit on the metaphase plate. In fact, the chromosome is condensed an estimated 10,000-fold, which reduces the risk that DNA will become entangled or DNA strands will break during the mitotic process. Condensation of the chromosome is one of the first visual signs that mitosis is under way. Chromatin condensation is first visible by light microscopy as occurring around the middle of the G_2 phase (Figure 6–8).

The most abundant proteins that associate with chromosomal DNA strands are a family of small, highly basic proteins, the **histones.** Four types of his-

Table 6–5. Tumor suppressor genes.[1]

Gene	Protein	Protein Function	Disease	Map Location
p53	p53	DNA binding protein	Sporadic acquired cancer, all kinds; germline mutations, Li-Fraumeni, osteosarcoma	17p13.1
WT1	WT1	Zinc finger DNA binding protein	WAGR, Denys-Drash, Wilms tumor	11p13
WT2	Unknown	Wilms tumor	Wilms tumor	11p13
APC	β-catenin	Cell adhesion molecule	Familial adenomatous polyposis	5q21
NF1	Neurofibromin	G-protein, GTPase activity	Neurofibromatosis 1	17q11
p16	p16	Binds proteins that regulate cell cycle	Familial melanoma	9p21
RB1	RB1	DNA binding	Retinoblastoma, osteosarcoma, other sarcomas	13q14

[1]Reproduced, with permission, from Seashore MR, Wappner RS: *Genetics in Primary Care & Clinical Medicine,* Appleton & Lange, 1996, p. 60.

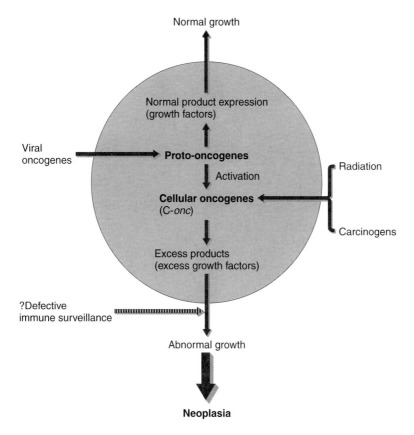

Figure 6–7. Loss of cell cycle regulation and the development of cancer. This diagram shows two relationships between genetic composition and cell cycle: maintenance of proto-oncogenes and normal cell growth (top) and activation of onco-genes and abnormal cell growth (bottom). (Modified and reproduced from Chandrasoma P and Taylor CR: *Concise Pathology,* 2nd ed. Appleton & Lange, 1995.)

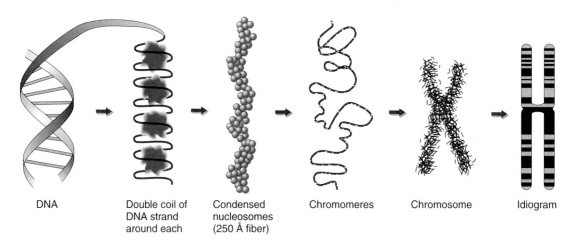

Figure 6–8. Formation of visible chromosomes. Chromosomes are formed as the chromosomal components (DNA, nu-clear proteins) condense approximately 10,000-fold in size. The smallest human chromosome consists of roughly 50 mil-lion base pairs; the largest, roughly 250 million base pairs. (Modified and reproduced, with permission, from Chandra-soma P, Taylor CR: *Concise Pathology,* 2nd ed. Appleton & Lange, 1995, p. 273.)

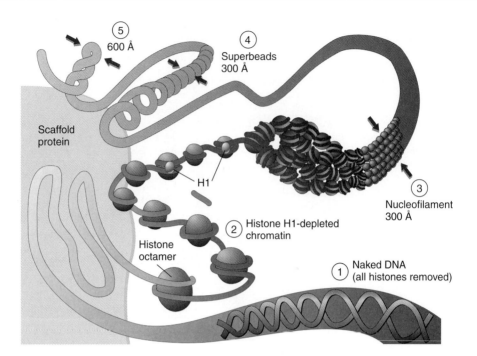

Figure 6–9. Organization of chromosomal material. The increasingly complex levels of DNA-histone protein organization are shown. Naked DNA (①) associates with histone octamers to form nucleofilaments (③), which then wrap into solenoid-like superbeads (④). The superbeads subsequently form large loops off the central scaffold protein (⑤). (Modified and reproduced, with permission, from Devlin T: *Textbook of Biochemistry with Clinical Correlations,* 3rd ed. Wiley-Liss, Inc. 1992.)

tones associate with each other to form an octad complex. DNA strands wrap around the octad twice, and in the process take up 160 bp of DNA. This arrangement is called a **nucleosome.** At the electron microscopic level, the nucleosome looks a little like a string of pearls. The nucleosome wraps in a solenoid-like structure, and the solenoids form large loops off the central chromosomal scaffold (Figure 6–9). The physical and chemical mechanisms and the critical proteins that drive this process are being intensely investigated. An enzyme in the nucleus, topoisomerase II, untangles DNA, breaking one DNA duplex and passing another duplex through the break, then reforming the original strand of DNA. Topoisomerases are essential enzymes that help to keep the DNA from becoming irreversibly entangled during condensation. Of course, many additional and subtle events are involved in the segregation of genetic material during mitosis. The student interested in more on this topic is referred to articles and texts listed at the end of this chapter.

Breakdown of the Nuclear Envelope

The fibrillar network lining the inner surface of the

nuclear envelope is made up of two major proteins: lamin A and lamin B, as described earlier. Nuclear pores embedded in the nuclear envelope provide a gated channel for movement of material into and out of the nucleus from the cytosol. At the onset of mitosis, a wave of phosphorylation occurs within the nucleus. Both lamins become phosphorylated, causing them to dissociate from each other. Lamin A forms its monomer, and lamin B remains associated with the lipid vesicles of the nuclear envelope by a tether to a lipophilic isoprenyl group. The entire nuclear envelope dissociates; the nuclear pores remain as larger complexes, but they still are soluble in the cytosolic milieu—although there is some change in the subunits that make up the complex. During disassembly, membranes of the nuclear envelope change from a sheet of lipid bilayer into smaller vesicles, as does the endoplasmic reticulum, Golgi apparatus, and other membrane components of the cell.

At the end of mitosis, after separation of the chromatids to their respective pole, vesicle fusion begins around the decondensing chromosomes. Lamins undergo a series of dephosphorylations that initiate the reformation of the proteinaceous coating of the inner surface of the forming nuclear envelope.

Role of Microtubules, Microtubule Motors, & Kinetochores

Microtubules (Figure 7–3) play an essential part in mitosis. They form the spindle apparatus and provide both the track and electromotive force that separates the chromatids. That microtubules are a part of the mitotic apparatus has been recognized for several decades, but the mechanisms underlying the role of microtubules in mitosis are still being discovered.

Fundamental to understanding how the mitotic spindle is formed and how chromosomes are separated is to recognize that the mitotic spindle (composed primarily of microtubule proteins) is not a stable polymer. The seeming chaotic movement of the dynamic microtubules in the spindle—the pushing and pulling of the chromosomes and the eventual final separation of chromatids—is necessary for the chromatids to separate accurately, which is essential for cell viability. When the microtubule is elongating faster than it is shrinking, the microtubule increases in length and the concentration of free tubulin in the cytoplasm decreases. During mitosis, microtubules undergo abrupt and unpredictable transitions from the growing state to the shrinking state—known as catastrophe—or from the shrinking state to the growing state—known as rescue (discussed in more detail in Chapter 7).

MICROTUBULES, SPINDLE FORMATION, & METAPHASE

Centrioles

The centrosome is an amorphous body that lies near the nuclear envelope and contains **centrioles,** a pair of cylindrical structures that reside at right angles to each other. During interphase, the centrosome is where cytoplasmic microtubules are formed and thus is known as the **microtubule organizing center (MTOC).** The centrosome, including its paired centrioles, duplicates in the late G_1 phase, but the centrioles do not separate. During interphase, the cytoplasmic microtubules are continually forming and disintegrating. However, as the cell moves into early prophase, the longer cytoplasmic microtubules begin to break down. As new shorter microtubules form around the centrosome, these microtubules are very unstable, forming and breaking down at a faster rate than in the interphase.

The shorter microtubules that form around the centrioles are called **astral microtubules.** Also during this period, the two centrosomes become more apparent, and a few astral microtubules from each centrosome begin to overlap; in so doing, they stabilize. As assembly continues, these increase in length and push the centrioles to the opposite poles of the cell. The microtubules that connect opposite poles form a second subtype of microtubule, the **polar microtubule.** This subtype is also active in the gain and loss of

tubulin at the positive and negative ends, respectively, but is more stable than other subtypes.

Kinetochore

The duplicated chromosome is joined lengthwise and possesses a special region called the centromere, where the chromatin is more condensed. Within the centromere, a specialized protein complex is organized, forming a plate-like structure called the **kinetochore.** This serves as a microtubule organizing center for the chromosome and is likely involved in creating the conditions required for pulling the chromosomes to the pole during anaphase. Each duplicated chromatid has a kinetochore that is located precisely opposite and faces the opposite poles of the spindle.

During early prometaphase, kinetochores are capable of binding to the side of a growing microtubule and sliding along it toward the spindle pole. The initial binding to the side of the microtubule is converted into end-on binding. In time, the opposite kinetochore finds a spindle microtubule and forms a pole to the kinetochore microtubule. Sufficient attachment of all of the chromosome to microtubules and orientation for eventual movement take time. During this period, much pulling and pushing of the duplicated chromosomes occurs. The dynamics of microtubules (rescue and catastrophe) provide the dynamics of this process.

Alignment of all the chromosomes on the metaphase plate marks the beginning of metaphase. By the time all the chromosomes have positioned themselves on the metaphase plate, all the forces required to move the chromatids to the opposite pole are already active. No additional special force is required. Yet why must the chromosomes line up on the equatorial plane before separation occurs? Two hypothesis have been suggested.

One hypothesis proposes that a greater tension is exerted by longer kinetochore microtubules, thus a stronger pull would be exerted on a chromosome by the more distant pole and would have more force to pull the chromosome to that pole. A second hypothesis suggests that the astral exclusion force exerts a strong influence on aligning the chromosomes at the metaphase plate. Experiments using laser beams to cut selected microtubules indicate that both types of forces are involved and are important in the equatorial alignment of the chromosomes. Alignment at the metaphase plate is *essential* for the correct distribution of genetic material to the daughter cells.

Up to now, we have emphasized the dynamic state of the tubulin subunits in the various subtypes of microtubules (kinetochore, spindle, astral), indicating they are in a constant state of flux—forming and disintegrating. Once the final structure has been assembled and the mitotic spindle is in place—with the chromosomes lined up on the metaphase plate—does the apparatus stabilize or are there continual changes of tubulin monomers in the various microtubule fibers?

Many approaches have been taken to answer this question, including treating the cell with drugs to block addition of new subunits to the microtubule and using immunofluorescent tubulin monomers. Results suggest that the fully assembled spindle is still quite dynamic and that a constant disassembly and assembly process occurs. The overall structure of the spindle, however, remains essentially unchanged.

Microtubule Motors

Microtubule motors are enzyme complexes that use the energy of adenosine triphosphate hydrolysis to move along the surface of the microtubule (Chapter 7). There are two types of motors; one is a large enzyme complex composed of multiple subunits called **dynein.** This motor can move along the tubule toward the minus end. The second type of motor is called **kinesin.** This is a smaller complex—only two subunits—and its direction of movement on the microtubule is toward the plus, or growing, end.

Both motors have the capacity to attach firmly to the chromosome and are capable of pulling the chromosome. These complexes can move along the microtubule at rates that suggest they are capable of rapidly moving the chromosome toward the poles during anaphase.

Anaphase

Anaphase signals the end of mitosis, occurs suddenly, and is triggered by the degradation of Cdk-cyclin B (MPF). Cyclin B is proteolytically destroyed by means of the ubiquitin-proteosome digestive complex discussed earlier. Other proteolytic events, in addition to the degradation of MPF, are also likely involved in sister chromatid separation.

When a proteolytic-resistant MPF is injected into a cell and the cell is treated with Ca^{2+}, the endogenous cyclin is degraded, but levels of undegradable cyclin remain high. The sister chromatids, however, move away from each, toward poles, suggesting that complete degradation of MPF and cyclin is insufficient to achieve chromatid separation. If peptides derived from the amino-terminal region of cyclin are injected into the cytoplasm and the cell is treated with Ca^{2+}, sister chromatid movement is delayed. These findings suggest the presence of a protease in the cytoplasm that can be inhibited by peptides derived from cyclin.

Telophase

Telophase is the final stage of mitosis. In telophase, a nuclear envelope reassembles and a series of reversal steps occur, leading to an interphase cellular morphology.

Cytokinesis

Cytokinesis, the process of a cell dividing into two daughter cells, occurs by contraction of a ring of actin and myosin that resides just under the inner surface of the membrane, in the plane of the mitotic spindle. Usually the location of this contractile ring divides the cell into two daughter cells of equal size. There are many instances during embryonic development in which cells divide asymmetrically. In these cases, two cells are created that are of different size and are destined to develop along divergent paths.

The actin-myosin contractile ring assembles during early anaphase. The contraction process is similar to skeletal muscle contraction, but it has important differences. The actin-myosin contractile ring contains a bundle of about 20 actin filaments. During contraction, the ring does not get thicker as the cleavage furrow increases, indicating that it reduces its volume by losing filaments. The contractile ring is lost as the cleavage furrow narrows and the membranes fuse, leaving a remnant of the spindle apparatus in a structure known as the midbody.

SUMMARY

This chapter focuses on the molecular events that occur during cell division, in particular, during the two phases of a cell's life—the period of mitosis (M phase) and the period that prepares the cell for division and carries out all other differentiated tasks (interphase). The two major types of proteins that drive the cell during these two phases have been described. Levels of these proteins—the cyclins and their kinase subunits—rise and fall at precise times during the cycle. Cyclin B, with its attendant kinase, is synonymous with the MPF. Cyclin B reaches its greatest concentration in the cell in early prophase, triggering many of the morphological and biochemical events that allow the chromosomes to condense and separate. A sudden proteolytic event occurs within the cell, which degrades cyclin B and causes the onset of anaphase and the rebuilding of the internal cytostructure of the cell.

Cells have developed an elaborate system to carefully control the expression of the cyclins. The forward side of the cycle is controlled by growth factors that induce signal pathways, which in turn lead to the expression of the cyclins and their kinases. The reverse side is controlled by inhibitory proteins that either prevent the expression of the cyclins or block at other sites molecules required to carry out the forward signal. Both tumor suppressors and other inhibitory proteins maintain a precise balance for regulated cell growth.

A regulatory pathway helps to balance the number of normal cells by activating a pathway that leads to their self-destruction. This process, apoptosis, is especially active during development, when the organism is producing cells rapidly to form its organs. Often, too many cells are made, thus apoptosis has developed, allowing for the controlled demise of these cells. Apoptosis is also important in the clonal expansion of antibody-producing cells. If these cells cannot be systematically eliminated, the organism is soon overpopulated with normal antibody-producing cells that are no longer needed.

Evidence that cell senescence and aging are regulated was presented. Research findings suggest the importance of genes that encode for stress-relieving proteins—eg, superoxide dismutases, catalase, and other proteins that can reduce oxygen radicals effectively.

REFERENCES

Alberts B et al: *Molecular Biology of the Cell.* Garland, 1994.

Coleman TR, Dunphy WG: Cdc2 regulatory factors. Curr Opin Cell Biol 1994;6:877.

Deshaies RJ: The self-destructive personality of a cell cycle transition. Curr Opin Cell Biol 1995;7:781.

Draetta G: Mammalian G_1 cyclins. Curr Opin Cell Biol 1994;6:842.

Elledge SJ, Harper JW: Cdk inhibitors: on the threshold of checkpoints and development. Curr Opin Cell Biol 1994;6:847.

Evan GI et al: Apoptosis and the cell cycle. Curr Opin Cell Biol 1995;7:825.

Glotzer M et al: Cyclin is degraded by the ubiquitin pathway. Nature 1991;349:132.

Kerr JFR: Neglected opportunities in apoptosis research. Trends Cell Biol 1995;5:55.

La Thangue NB: DRTF1/E2F: An expanding family of heterodimeric transcription factors implicated in cell-cycle control. Trends Biochem Sci 1994;19:108.

Lees E: Cyclin dependent kinase regulation. Curr Opin Cell Biol 1995;7:773.

Lock LF, Wickramasinghe D: Cycling with CDKs. Trends Cell Bio 1994;4:404.

Martin SJ, Green DR, Cotter TG: Dicing with death: Dissecting the components of the apoptosis machinery. Trends Biochem Sci 1994;19:26.

McConkey DJ, Orrenius S: Signal transduction pathways to apoptosis. Trends Cell Biol 1994;4:370.

Muller R: Transcriptional regulation during the mammalian cell cycle. Trends Genet 1995;11:173

Murray A: Cell cycle checkpoints. Curr Opin Cell Biol 1994;6:872.

Nigg EA: Cyclin-dependent protein kinases: Key regulators for the eucaryotic cell cycle. BioEssays 1995;17:471.

O'Connell MJ, Nurse P: How cells know they are in G-1 or G-2. Curr Opin Cell Biol 1994;6:867.

Peitsch MC, Mannherz HG, Tschopp J: The apoptosis endonucleases: Cleaning up after cell death? Trends Cell Biol 1994;4:37.

Picksley SM, Lane DP: p53 and Rb: Their cellular roles. Curr Opin Cell Biol 1994;6:853.

Sherr CJ: Mammalian G-1 cyclins. Cell 1993;73:1059.

SUGGESTED READING

Bassett DE, Boguski MS, Hieter P: Yeast genes and human disease. Nature 1996;379:589.

Border WA, Noble NA: Mechanisms of Disease: Transforming growth factor B in tissue fibrosis. N Engl J Med 1994;331:1286.

Krontiris TG: Molecular medicine: Oncogenes. N Engl J Med 1995;333:303.

Oliver SG: From DNA sequence to biological function. Nature 1996;379:597.

Papavassiliou AG: Molecular medicine: Transcription factors. N Engl J Med 1995;332:45.

7

The Cytoskeleton

KEY TERMS

Cytoskeleton
Microtubules
Actin filaments
Intermediate filaments
Centrosome
Centrioles
Microtubule organizing center
Saltatory movement
Myosin
Kinesins
Dyneins
Axoneme
Actin
Actin-binding proteins
Contractile bundles
Sarcomere

Eukaryotic cells have the ability to change their shape transiently, move organelles within the cytoplasm, migrate or crawl, and segregate chromosomes during mitosis. This property is conferred by the **cytoskeleton,** a set of proteins that constitute the major cytoarchitecture of the cell. The cytoskeleton was originally defined during early cell fractionation experiments as a detergent-insoluble complex of proteins that, when viewed under the microscope, maintain a certain degree of structural organization. We now know that the cytoskeleton consists of three major units—microtubules, actin filaments, and intermediate filaments–and that each unit contains hundreds of accessory proteins (Table 7–1).

All three major cytoskeletal elements can self-assemble into polymers because they have the ability to polymerize, ie, many thousands of identical actin subunits assemble into linear arrays that can be sufficiently long to traverse the length of a cell ~ 10–15 μm long. These large elongated filamentous structures then function as the internal cell scaffolding on which organelles are supported; they also provide the "railroad" tracks along which organelles move. In addition to the major components of the cytoskeleton, accessory proteins play a critical role in cytoskeletal

assembly, organization, and functional integration. These accessory proteins are responsible for

- attaching organelles to the cytoskeleton, eg, secretory vesicles to microtubules
- providing directionality to organelle movement
- linking and coordinating cytoskeletal function (Figure 7–1).

MICROTUBULES & THE CENTROSOME

The main cytoskeletal proteins can polymerize into long filaments; this process occurs in one direction (ie, protein subunits are not added uniformly to each end of a particular growing filament). Filaments, however, have **polarity** with respect to subunit addition; this means that one end of a filament must differ structurally from the other. In the case of microtubules, one end—designated the **plus end**—can grow rapidly, whereas the other—designated the **minus end**—loses tubulin subunits unless it is stabilized. Microtubule stabilization is achieved when the minus end of the microtubule is attached to or imbedded in the **centrosome,** also known as the **microtubule organizing center (MTOC),** which is located at the center of the cell near the nucleus. In contrast, free tubulin subunits can be added at the plus ends. Microtubules are dynamic structures; consequently, at any one time some microtubules are growing in length while others are shortening. The MTOC is therefore constantly producing growing microtubules that emanate from it and can extend as far as the cell periphery, whereas other microtubules are shortening and shrinking back into the MTOC.

Compared with actin filaments, microtubules are rather rigid structures that function not only as "support beams" in the cytoplasm but also as tracks along which organelles move. The organized directional movement of organelles is referred to as **saltatory movement,** which is mediated by **molecular motors.** These are proteins that bind to microtubules or actin filaments, and their movement is powered by the en-

Table 7–1. Major units of the cytoskelton and their main proteins.

Unit	Major Protein	Properties
Microtubules	Tubulin	Long cylinders of tubuin ~ 25 nm in diameter. One end is attached to the microtubule organizing center (MTOC), which is located near the Golgi apparatus
Actin filaments	Actin	Actin forms two stranded flexible helical polymers ~ 5–9 nm in diameter. Mostly concentrated in the cell cortex beneath plasma membrane
Intermediate filaments	Vimentin Keratins Lamins	Rope-like fibers ~ 10 nm in diameter; located in the cytoplasm and nucleus (nuclear lamina). These filaments impart mechanical strength on the cell and, by spanning from cell to cell, confer resistance to shearing forces

ergy liberated from adenosine triphosphate (ATP) hydrolysis.

Molecular Motors

Many different species of motor protein have been identified in recent years; these can be broadly categorized based on (1) the filament along which they move and (2) the components that are moved. The principal molecular motors are

1. **Myosin:** Originally discovered as one of the major proteins of skeletal muscle, myosin moves along actin filaments and is a key component in muscle contraction. We now know that several nonmuscle myosin molecules also exist; however, all myosins appear to share similar **motor domains** (ie, myosin head groups that mediate ATP hydrolysis).
2. **Kinesins:** These proteins move along microtubules in the direction of the plus end (ie, away from the centrosomal MTOC and toward the cell periphery).
3. **Dyneins:** These proteins move toward the minus ends of microtubules (ie, toward the centrosome [MTOC]).

Keep in mind that each of these motor molecules is responsible for moving different "cargo" components, as discussed later in the chapter.

The Actin Cortex

In contrast to microtubules, which are organized into individual polymers whose function is coordinately regulated, actin filaments are organized into cross-linked networks or **bundles** by different **actin-binding proteins (ABPs).** Actin filaments located just beneath the plasma membrane constitute part of the **cell cortex,** and the location of the cortical actin cytoskeleton is controlled by **nucleation sites** in the plasma membrane. Similar to microtubules, actin filaments are highly dynamic structures, and extracellular signals received at the plasma membrane by receptors can lead to the local reorganization of the actin cytoskeleton. The actin cortical cytoskeleton

can affect the morphology of the plasma membrane; eg, in association with myosin, actin filaments can form a **contractile bundle** that causes invaginations of the cell surface during cell division.

INTERMEDIATE FILAMENTS

Intermediate filaments confer tensile strength on the cell because (1) they are strong, rope-like fibrous polypeptides that resist stretching and (2) they extend throughout the cytoplasm and form a meshwork that provides mechanical strength. The designation **intermediate filaments** is derived from the fact that their diameter is intermediate between actin filaments and microtubules. Intermediate filaments are very prominent (eg, in epithelial cells subject to mechanical stress and shearing forces). In addition, intermediate filaments are present in the cell nucleus and constitute the **nuclear lamina** of the nuclear envelope (see Chapter 3).

Structure of Intermediate Filaments

Many different types of monomer proteins constitute the subunits of intermediate filaments; some consist of only a single protein species, whereas others (eg, neurofilaments) consist of three distinct proteins.

Regardless of cell type, the basic organization of intermediate filament proteins consists of elongated fibrous polypeptides with an N-terminal **head domain,** a C-terminal **tail domain,** and a central **rod domain.** The latter domain consists of an alpha-helical (α-helical) region that contains tandem repeats of a 7–amino acid motif; this motif is responsible for the formation of **coiled-coil dimers** between two parallel α-helices (ie, one α-helical coil twists around another to form a stable structure like a twisted wire).

In the formation of intermediate filaments, two coiled-coil dimers bind in an antiparallel manner to form a tetramer; ie, the N-terminus of one dimer and the C-terminus of the other are oriented in the same direction. Because the N- and C-termini of the intermediate filament proteins differ and the dimers and

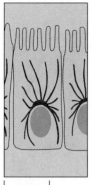

Microtubules are long and straight and typically have one end attached to a single microtubule organizing center (MTOC) called a *centrosome*, located near the Golgi apparatus.

25 μm

A

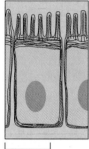

Actin filaments are dispersed throughout the cell, they are most highly concentrated in the *cortex*, just beneath the plasma membrane.

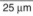25 μm

B

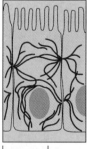

Intermediate filaments are ropelike fibers with a diameter of around 10 nm. They impart mechanical strength in an epithelial tissue by spanning the cytoplasm from one cell-cell junction to another.

Figure 7–1. Elements of the cytoskeleton. Microtubules (A) are elongated structures within the cell that have one end attached to a microtubule organizing center (MTOC). In this panel, the MTOC, or centrosome, is located just above the nucleus, near the Golgi apparatus. Actin filaments (B) are scattered throughout the cytoplasm, but they are most dense in the region beneath the cell membrane, which is often referred to as the cell cortex. Intermediate filaments (C) cross the cytoplasm from one intercellular junction to another, mechanically strengthening the tissue. In terms of relative size, microtubules are 25 nm in diameter, actin filaments 5–9 nm in diameter, and intermediate filaments 10 nm in diameter. (Modified and reproduced, with permission, from Alberts BA et al: *Molecular Biology of the Cell,* 3rd ed. Garland, 1994, p. 789.)

tetramers are arranged in antiparallel fashion, the filament is not polarized; rather, it is identical at each end. Recall that this contrasts with the polarized structure of microtubules and actin filaments; this is one reason that intermediate filaments have quite different properties.

The tensile strength of these filaments is achieved in part because the dimers of each tetramer are staggered with respect to one another; this arrangement allows the tetramers to associate with each other. The mature intermediate filament is assembled when tetramers align along the filament axis and bind to the free ends; this results in the formation of a helical array in which the filaments are packed together. This packing is stabilized by lateral binding interactions between adjacent tetramers, which are conferred by the structurally similar motifs in the central rod domain of each intermediate filament. Seven or eight elongated tetrameric complexes (each is called a protofilament) are intertwined to form the mature intermediate filament (Figure 7–2).

Intermediate Filament Proteins

At least four classes of intermediate filament proteins have been described (Table 7–2):

- **keratin filaments**
- **vimentin-related filaments**
- **neurofilament (NF) proteins**
- **lamins.**

Keratins. The keratins, also known as cytokeratins, are the most diverse family of intermediate filament proteins; at least 20 different keratins have been identified in human epithelial cells. In addition, at least eight isoforms of so-called **hard keratins,** which are specific to hair and nails, have been described. The keratins can be subdivided into two types:

- type I (acidic): 16 isoforms
- type II (neutral/basic): 13 isoforms.

Intermediate filaments that comprise types I and II keratins can form in vitro, but homodimers cannot, which is consistent with the observation that keratin filaments are heteropolymers. Indeed, epithelial cells express several different keratin polypeptides that can co-polymerize into a single keratin filament system; however, the simplest epithelia (eg, in developing embryos) express only type I and type II keratins, whereas cells of other tissues may express multiple forms of different keratins.

Vimentin & related proteins. Examples of vimentin-related proteins include desmin, peripherin, and vimentin. Vimentin is the most widely distributed of cytoplasmic intermediate filament proteins and is present in many cell types, including fibroblasts and endothelial cells; moreover, copolymers of

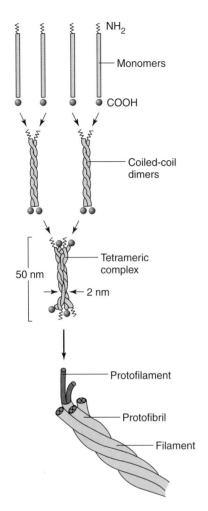

Figure 7–2. Structure of neurofilaments. Two pairs of monomers associate with each other to create two coiled-coil dimers. The two dimers twist around each other to generate a single tetrameric complex in which the N- and C-termini of each dimer are oriented in the same direction, giving rise to a symmetric structure. In the third assembly step, each tetramer acts as an individual protofilament. After two protofilaments twist around each other, generating a protofibril, a third protofilament interacts with them to form the final helical filament. (Modified and reproduced, with permission, from Kandel ER et al: *Essentials of Neural Science and Behavior.* Appleton & Lange, 1995, p. 66.)

vimentin and vimentin-related proteins are found in numerous cell types. Unlike keratins, vimentin can also form polymers of a single protein species. Although intermediate filament proteins can copolymerize, when the complementary deoxyribonucleic acids (cDNAs) that encode keratins and vimentin are coexpressed in cells, separate filaments are formed. In muscle cells, the major intermediate filament pro-

tein is the 53-kDa molecule **desmin** (Table 7–2), which acts to link myofibrils together. In the central nervous system, several types of intermediate filament–related proteins have been described; eg, glial filaments formed by **glial fibrillary acidic protein** are the intermediate filaments of astrocytes.

NF Proteins. Three NF proteins that form the major cytoskeletal element of nerve cells have been described (Table 7–2):

- NF-L: low molecular weight
- NF-M: medium molecular weight
- NF-H: high molecular weight.

Neurofilaments extend along the length of the neuron. It is believed that cross-linking mediated by the C-terminal tails of the NF-M and -H NF proteins generates **cross-bridges** that impart tensile strength to the long neuronal cell processes. Among other specialized functions in various cell types, intermediate filaments play an essential role in attaching epithelial cells to (1) cell junctions called **desmosomes,** which anchor adjacent cells together, and (2) **hemidesmosomes** (see Figure 8–4), which tether cells to the **basal lamina** on which they reside.

Nuclear lamins. The nuclear lamina, or fibrous lamina, comprises a net of intermediate filaments on the inner surface of the nuclear membrane and is associated with the nuclear pores. In mammalian cells, the nuclear lamina consists of at least three related intermediate filament polypeptides called **lamins,** which have a molecular weight of 65,000–75,000 (Table 7–2). In addition to the conserved motifs present in other intermediate filament proteins, the lamins also possess **karyotypic signals,** ie, motifs that facilitate and confer transport into the nucleus (see Chapter 4). Unlike other intermediate filaments, the lamins disassemble during mitosis—when the nucleus and nuclear envelope fragment—and reassemble when mitosis ends. **Phosphorylation** on specific serine residues in the lamin polypeptides allows these normally insoluble molecules to **solubilize** during mitosis. At the end of mitosis, dephosphorylation—mediated by specific phosphatases—presumably reestablishes the insolubility of the lamins, which in turn facilitates re-formation of the nuclear lamina.

As discussed in Chapter 8, intermediate filaments engender cells with considerable tensile strength and therefore allow cells to resist mechanical stress. In several diseases, mutations in selected keratin genes alter the organization of the keratin filaments that are normally expressed in the basal layer of the epidermis. Such genetic abnormalities increase the sensitivity of the cell to mechanical damage. In certain diseases—eg, pemphigus vulgaris and bulloid pemphigus—the skin of affected patients is particularly sensitive to blistering (see Chapter 8).

Table 7–2. Classes of intermediate filaments of eukaryotic cells and their distribution.[1]

Proteins	Mass (kDa)	Distribution

Keratins
    Type I (acidic)
    Type II (basic)
	
	40–60
	50–70
		
		Epithelial cells, hair, nails

Vimentin-like
    Vimentin
    Desmin
    Glial fibrillary acid protein
    Peripherin
	
	54
	53
	50
	66
		
		Various mesenchymal cells
		Muscle
		Glial cells
		Neurons

Neurofilaments Low (L), medium (M), and high (H)[2]	 60–130	 Neurons
Lamins A, B, and C	 65–75	 Nuclear lamina

[1]Modified from Murray RK et al: *Harper's Biochemistry,* 24th ed. Appleton & Lange, 1996, p. 705, with permission.
[2]Refers to their molecular masses.

MICROTUBULES

Present in all eukaryotic cells, microtubules are elongated filamentous structures that extend throughout the cytoplasm and form a framework that facilitates the structural organization and location of some organelles. This has been particularly well documented for the endoplasmic reticulum. Microtubules also have important functions in

- cell division
- intracellular transport, especially in movement of synaptic vesicles
- recycling of components from the Golgi apparatus to the endoplasmic reticulum
- cell motility.

Basic Structure

Two globular polypeptides, α- and beta (β)-tubulin (MW ~ 54,000), form the tubulin dimer and comprise the basic subunits of microtubules, which are cylindrical structures in which 13 tubulin α/β heterodimers are arranged around the circumference of a hollow cylinder approximately 25 nm in diameter (Figure 7–3).

In many cells, **tubulin polypeptides** are extremely abundant proteins; in the brain, which has a vast number of microtubules involved in synaptic vesicle transport, up to 20% of the total soluble protein is tubulin. To date at least six different forms of α- and β-tubulin have been described; although each is encoded by a separate gene, individual tubulin molecules are quite similar. Microtubules are quite labile structures that are in a continuous state of dynamic flux: the α/β tubulin subunits are rapidly added to the growing end—the **plus end**—of the tubule and removed from the slow-growing one, the **minus end.**

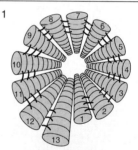
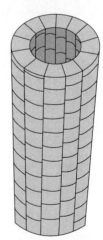

Figure 7–3. Microtubule structure. Tubulin is the building block of microtubules. Each tubulin molecule is a dimer consisting of one α-tubulin and one β-tubulin polypeptide. Tubulin molecules associate in linear arrays called protofilaments. Each microtubule (1) is composed of 13 protofilaments interacting to form a helical cylinder. A side view (2) shows the characteristic alternating pattern of α-tubulin and β-tubulin. (Modified and reproduced, with permission, from Kandel ER et al: *Essentials of Neural Science and Behavior.* Appleton & Lange, 1995, p. 66.)

The assembly of microtubules can be perturbed by drugs that bind tightly to free tubulin monomers but not to polymerized tubulin, eg, colchicine; this type of binding prevents incorporation of the monomer into the growing microtubule.

Microtubule Assembly in Vitro

An enormous amount of information on microtubule assembly has been learned by studying the formation, assembly, and behavior of microtubules in vitro. In the presence of only guanosine triphosphate (GTP) and Mg^{2+} ions, purified α- and β-tubulin polymerize into microtubules at 37 °C (physiologic temperature) but not at 4 °C. This reaction can be followed by various techniques, including electron microscopy of negatively stained microtubules, biophysical methods, and use of recombinant DNA procedures, that generate mutant tubulin subunits (Figure 7–4). The kinetics of this process are complex but can be divided into three distinct phases that correspond to different steps in microtubule polymerization:

A. Lag phase (nucleation): In this step, tubulin subunits associate to form small oligomeric structures, a process termed **nucleation.** This initial assembly is less efficient than adding subunits to existing microtubules and is therefore slow kinetically—hence the term "lag phase."

B. Polymerization phase (elongation): Here the high concentration of free tubulin results in a faster rate of polymerization vs depolymerization, and subunits are added to free plus ends of existing microtubules. As the concentration of free tubulin decreases because of incorporation into microtubules, the rate of polymerization decreases, as polymerization is proportional to the concentration of free tubulin.

C. Steady state phase: Tubulin subunits also dissociate from microtubules, and at steady state free tubulin is present as a consequence of this **depolymerization.** At steady state, polymerization and depolymerization are in equilibrium, and this concentration of tubulin is called the **critical concentration.**

This rapid elongation rate of tubulin polymerization manifests itself when purified tubulin is added to pre-existing microtubules. On electron microscopic examination, one end of the microtubule appears to have elongated more rapidly than the other; as mentioned earlier, this end is defined as the plus end, whereas the other is the minus end. The plus end of microtubules can also be defined at the electron microscopic level by the binding of high molecular weight molecules, like dynein, that bind to the plus end.

Microtubules & Dynamic Instability

In eukaryotic cells, the organelle known as the **centrosome** acts as the MTOC. From the MTOC, located near the nucleus, microtubules grow toward the

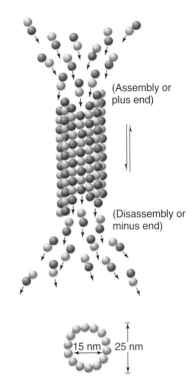

Figure 7–4. Assembly and disassembly of microtubules. The dynamic state of microtubules results from ongoing polymerization and depolymerization at opposite ends of the structure. The dimers, consisting of α- and β-tubulin are incorporated into the microtubule at the plus end and are released at the minus end. The dimensions of the microtubule cylinder (15 nm inner diameter, 25 nm outer diameter) are shown at the bottom. (Modified and reproduced from Sloboda RD: The role of microtubules in cell structure and cell division. Am Sci 1980;68:290. Reprinted with permission of *American Scientist,* journal of Sigma Xi, the Scientific Research Society.)

cell periphery. A pair of cylindrical structures called **centrioles** are found within the centrosomal region and are composed of small fibers. The centrosome matrix surrounds the centriolar pair of microtubules, and it is this region that nucleates microtubule polymerization.

By using sophisticated fluorescence or video enhanced microscopy to follow the fate of fluorescently tagged tubulin subunits, researchers have shown that microtubules in tissue culture cells are continuously polymerizing and depolymerizing. Individual microtubules grow toward the cell periphery then suddenly shrink—either partially or completely—in the direction of the centrosome, only to repolymerize later. This process, known as **dynamic instability,** can be reproduced in vitro by using purified tubulin and microtubules.

Energy in the form of GTP hydrolysis is required for dynamic instability to occur; the main features of this process are as follows:

1. Tubulin molecules bind both GTP and guanosine diphosphate (GDP); however, those subunits that contain GTP have a much higher affinity for the growing plus end of the microtubule than do those that contain GDP.
2. The growth of the plus end is dependent on the binding of new tubulin-GTP before the previously added subunits have hydrolyzed their GTP. After incorporation into the growing microtubule, the GTP at some point is hydrolyzed to GDP. If at this point the tubulin subunit containing GDP is present at the plus end—ie, no additional tubulin dimers have become attached to the growing chain—that tubulin subunit will dissociate.
3. If, however, another tubulin that contains GTP is incorporated at the plus end before the previous subunit has hydrolyzed its GTP, that first subunit cannot hydrolyze its GTP and will dissociate from the complex. Again, this occurs because it is no longer at the plus end but rather has become incorporated into the microtubule.
4. The hydrolysis of GTP is thought to cause dynamic instability. The rapid tubulin assembly precedes GTP hydrolysis at the plus growing end; this leads to a GTP cap at the plus end. GTP-tubulin polypeptides bind each other with higher affinity than GDP-tubulin; consequently a GTP "cap" forms, and this promotes tubulin polymerization. On GTP hydrolysis, the rate of polymerization slows and the microtubule begins to depolymerize. This is thought to occur as a consequence of change in the conformation of the tubulin β protofilaments. It is believed that GDP-protofilaments are more curved, thereby leading to inefficient assembly and progressive disassembly of those protofilaments, and that this in turn generates free tubulin dimers (Figure 7–4).

Dynamic instability has important physiologic significance. During cell division, for example, the rate of microtubule formation and depolymerization is enhanced enormously; this enables chromosomes to bind microtubules and form a mitotic spindle. Conversely, during differentiation microtubule depolymerization can be suppressed by microtubule binding proteins that stabilize the microtubules, as discussed below. After polymerization, tubulin subunits are covalently modified. In particular α-tubulin molecules are modified by:

• acetylation of lysine residues
• cleavage of tyrosine residues, or detyrosination.

These modifications occur only on α-tubulin subunits that are polymerized into microtubules and not on free tubulin molecules. Because these reactions occur relatively slowly and are reversed rapidly on depolymerization, they can be used as an index to determine how long a particular microtubule has been polymerized. Generally, the longer the time since polymerization, the higher the number of acetylated and detyrosinated subunits. Depending on the cell type, this can range from about 20 minutes—eg, in fibroblasts—to several hours, eg, in nerve axons.

Microtubule-associated Proteins

In addition to GTP capping and covalent modification of tubulins that stabilize microtubules, the properties of microtubules are also modified by interactions with specific **microtubule-associated proteins (MAPs).** These molecules are involved in

1. Regulating microtubule disassembly
2. Linking microtubules to specific organelles.

Moreover, specialized MAPs are microtubule motors that move along microtubules. Furthermore, some MAPs are cell type specific; in the brain, for example, two classes of MAPs have been isolated:

• **High molecular weight MAPs** that weigh 200,000–300,000, eg, MAP-1 and MAP-2
• **Tau** proteins that weigh 55,000–65,000.

Both classes of MAPs possess a **microtubule binding domain** and have regions that link microtubules to other intracellular components. Perhaps the best characterization of MAP function has occurred in nerve cells. The distribution of particular MAPs can be followed with fluorescence microscopy, by using antibodies specific for a particular MAP. Neurons, which can be up to 1 meter long, move synaptic vesicles many centimeters from their site of biogenesis in the neuronal cell body to the periphery; this movement is achieved along microtubules. In axons, microtubules are very elongated, and their plus ends extend from the cell body toward the terminal branches of the axon. It appears that some tau proteins are present only in axons; whereas MAP-2 is present in the cell body and dendrites but not in axons. Consequently, it is thought that in neurons MAPs may play a role in mediating intracellular compartmentalization by sequestering particular components—eg, secretory and synaptic vesicles—to different regions of the cell.

This type of local compartmentalization is not restricted to neurons, although it is less pronounced in other cell types. The minus ends of microtubules are anchored to the MTOC and radiate from it in various directions toward the cell periphery. Polymerization and depolymerization of tubulin molecules is regulated, however, so that microtubules oriented in a particular direction can predominate; this can impart a certain degree of polarity with respect to the distribution of organelles in a cell. Although precisely how this is achieved remains uncertain, it is thought that particular microtubules can be stabilized by MAPs, which prevents depolymerization, whereas uncapped microtubules are in a continuous state of flux between assembly and disassembly. Consequently, if a set of capped microtubules is oriented in a particular direction, this will establish a polarity with respect to the MTOC.

MICROTUBULES: SELECTED CLINICAL CORRELATES

An important treatment regimen for patients who have cancer is the disruption of the mitotic spindle by drugs that interfere with tubulin polymerization (eg, colchicine, vinblastine, and vincristine). The rationale for using such drugs is that the mitotic spindle that facilitates chromosome segregation during mitosis consists of microtubules. Antimitotic drugs that target these microtubules and inhibit formation of the mitotic spindle prevent segregation of chromosomes and therefore should preferentially kill rapidly dividing cancer cells. Another antimicrotubule drug that has been used to treat breast cancer is taxol. Although the mechanism of action of taxol is the opposite of that of colchicine—taxol stabilizes microtubules by preventing their depolymerization—the pharmacologic result is similar to that of colchicine: the arrest of rapid cell division.

MOLECULAR MOTORS: MOVEMENT ALONG MICROTUBULES

If isolated microtubules are placed on a glass microscope slide, they can be seen to slide along the surface in the presence of ATP and a cytosolic cell extract. Indeed, by using sophisticated light microscope techniques (eg, video-enhanced light microscopy), single microtubules can be seen to slide on glass surfaces, or small particles can be observed to move along the microtubules if the microtubules are first tethered to the surface. By reconstituting these motility reactions in vitro and purifying cytosolic components that enhance movement, investigators have been able to identify two types of microtubule motor proteins:

- **cytoplasmic dyneins**
- **kinesins.**

Cytoplasmic dyneins are involved in organelle transport and mitosis and are related to ciliary dynein, the motor protein present in cilia and flagella. Kinesins are a large diverse family of related proteins

involved in organelle transport, mitosis, and meiosis. These molecules are members of a large family of **molecular motors** that interact with multiple components of the cytoskeleton (Table 7–3).

Both these motor proteins are high molecular weight molecules that consist of two heavy chains and several light chains. Because the heavy chains are particularly large molecules (MW ~ 300,000), they can be observed in the electron microscope by using rotary shadowing techniques. The heavy chains can be divided into two major regions: (1) a head domain that has a globular shape and possesses the ATP-binding domain and (2) a rod-like tail domain that interacts with specific components such as secretory vesicles. The two head domains bind to microtubules and are the ATPase motors, whereas the tail regions bind to specific organelles and cell components that will be transported by the motor (Figure 7–5). These motor molecules are restricted in the direction of their movement along microtubules because they move in only one direction.

- Dynein moves organelles toward the minus end of microtubules, ie, from the cell periphery toward the centrosome.
- Kinesins move toward the plus end of microtubules, ie, from the centrosomal region toward the cell periphery.

Some of the most compelling results on movement along microtubules have come from studies on transport along nerve axons. *Both in vitro and in vivo, it has been observed that organelle movement away from the cell body is driven by kinesin, whereas traf-*

Table 7–3. Molecular motors from eukaryotic cells.[1]

Motor	Effect
Actin-based	
Myosin-I	Moves vesicles on actin filaments; moves one actin filament on another
Myosin-II	Causes muscle contraction, cortical tension, capping surface molecules, cell polarity, cytokinesis
Microtubule-based	
Axonemal dynein	Causes sliding of one flagellar microtubule on another, moves particles toward "minus" end of microtubule
Cytoplasmic dynein	Moves particles and vesicles toward "minus" end of microtubule
Kinesin	Moves particles and vesicles toward "plus" end of microtubule
Dynamin	Drives active sliding of one microtubule on another; involved in endocytosis

[1]Modified and reproduced, with permission, from Scholey JM: Multiple microtubule motors. Reprinted by permission from *Nature* 343:118, 1990. Copyright © 1990. Macmillan Magazines Ltd.

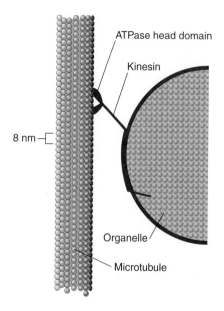

Figure 7–5. Model of kinesin cross-bridging between organelles and microtubules. The kinesin molecule is shown as the connector for the organelle and the microtubule. The ATPase head domain of the kinesin molecule acts as the motor, enabling the organelle to move along the microtubule. (Reproduced, with permission, from Howard J: One giant step for kinesin. Nature 1993;365: 696. Copyright © 1993 Macmillan Magazines Limited.)

their sperm. The movement of cilia and flagella, which are essentially elongated cilia, have been examined in considerable detail by studying unicellular organisms, such as the protozoan *Chlamydomonas*, in which it is possible to generate flagella mutants. Researchers have gained an extensive understanding of how these organelles work through the use of (1) electron microscopic analysis of native and mutant flagella coupled with biophysical and biochemical techniques and (2) mathematical analysis of ciliary beat frequency and motion. The carefully orchestrated movement of cilia, ie, their beating, occurs in unidirectional waves: Each cilium moves in a whip-like fashion according to the following pattern:

- The forward stroke extends the cilium and causes it to beat against the surrounding medium.
- In the recovery phase, the cilium returns to its original position by an unrolling movement that minimizes viscous drag from the medium.
- Adjacent cilia are not quite synchronous in their movement, and this creates a wave-like pattern that can be seen under the microscope as the cilia beat.

Cilia and flagella project from the cell surface; consequently, their outer surface corresponds to the plasma membrane. If this membrane is solubilized by treatment with non-ionic detergents, the inner ciliary structure and organization are preserved, thereby re-

ficking from the nerve terminal region toward the cell body is dynein driven.

CILIA & CENTRIOLES

Cilia are beating microscopic hair-like structures about 250 nm in diameter that extend from the cell surface of many different cells, including protozoa (Figure 7–6). The main functions of cilia are to

- move fluid and particles over the cell surface
- propel unicellular organisms through fluids
- move ova along the oviduct
- propel sperm.

Cilia possess a bundle of microtubules at their center that is approximately 10 times the size of the large ribosomal subunit.

Epithelia lining the respiratory tract have vast numbers of cilia that move layers of mucus, trapped particles, and dead cells toward the mouth, where they are eliminated by swallowing. Patients who have defects in ciliary structure have a tendency toward respiratory infection, and male patients can be infertile because of the diminished swimming ability of

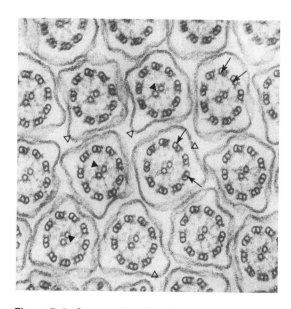

Figure 7–6. Cross section through clam-gill cilia. In this electron micrograph, note the following structures: outer doublet microtubules (→), central doublet microtubules (▲), and plasma membrane (△). (Courtesy of Dr P Satir.)

vealing the **axoneme.** This structure consists exclusively of microtubules and their associated proteins. The microtubules are arranged in a distinct, highly ordered, regular repeating structure along the length of the cilium. Nine doublet microtubules are arranged in a circle around a central pair of single microtubules (Figure 7–7).

This so called "9 + 2" arrangement of microtubules is present in virtually all eukaryotic cells. Each of the nine outer doublets consists of a complete

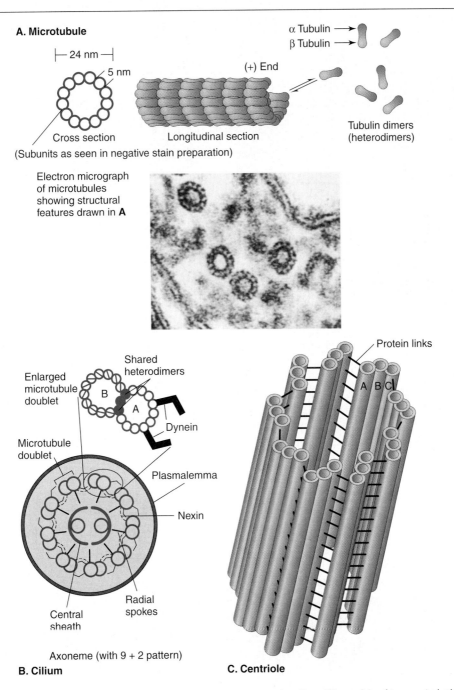

Figure 7–7. Microtubules and ciliary structure. The core, or axoneme, of a cilium (B) consists of two central microtubules surrounded by nine outer doublets (9 + 2 pattern). Microtubule structure is shown in diagram form (A) and as seen in an electron micrograph. The microtubular structure of centrioles is also depicted (C). (From Junqueira LC et al: *Basic Histology,* 8th ed. Appleton & Lange. 1995, p. 43, with permission.)

and a partial microtubule that are fused together. In cross section, the complete tubule (termed the "A" tubule) consists of 13 tubulin subunits; whereas the incomplete "B" tubule possesses 11 subunits. Each microtubule of the central pair is complete, and the two tubules of the central pair are tethered by accessory proteins.

If the polypeptides of the axoneme are analyzed by two-dimensional electrophoresis, approximately 200 spots are apparent. By generating antibodies to individual polypeptides and studying the morphologic structure of mutants that are defective in particular components, it has been possible to map many of the protein interactions within the axonemal microtubules. Some of these proteins are **cross-linkers** that hold the microtubules together, whereas others act to generate and regulate the bending and movement of the microtubules (Figure 7–8).

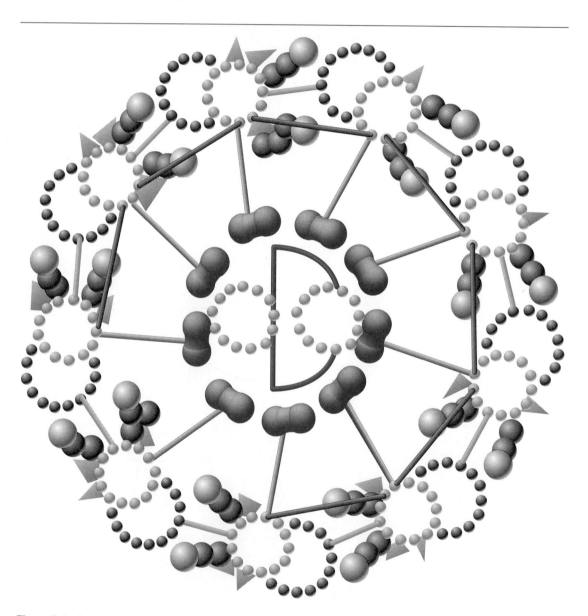

Figure 7–8. Axoneme structure in *Tetrahymena*. This computer model depicts a ciliary axoneme in cross section. The tubulin subunits of microtubules are shown as small shaded balls. Associated proteins, including cross-linkers and molecular motors, are shown as bars and globular forms. (Modified and reproduced from J Cell Sci 1991;98:cover, with permission from the Company of Biologists, Ltd.)

Dynein Is the Molecular Motor of Cilia & Flagella

Cilia and flagella grow from **basal bodies,** which are structures similar to **centrioles.** Basal bodies are cylindrical structures from which the doublet microtubules grow during cilia formation. The centrosome has a centriolar pair of microtubules. During doubling, these microtubules separate, and a daughter centriole is formed perpendicular to each original centriole. The nascent centriole contains a ninefold symmetric array of single microtubules, each of which acts as a template for assembling the triplet microtubule of mature centrioles.

Ciliary dynein is the biochemical motor that generates the sliding and bending forces between adjacent microtubules. Ciliary dynein has a domain structure that comprises

- a motor domain that hydrolyses ATP
- a tail region that interacts with adjacent microtubules.

A more complex protein than cytoplasmic enzyme, ciliary dynein possesses two or three heavy chains, each of which is approximately 450 kDa; the molecule has an overall molecular weight in excess of 2,000,000. The head domain of ciliary dynein interacts with adjacent microtubules, and its hydrolysis of ATP generates a mechanochemical force that results in its movement toward the minus end of the microtubule. This also generates a sliding force between microtubules; because the microtubule doublets are held together by multiple cross-links, however, this force is converted into a bending motion (Figures 7–7 and 7–8).

Selected Clinical Correlates: Ciliary Dysfunction in Human Beings

A number of rare defects that cause patients to be susceptible to respiratory diseases and be infertile have been attributed to the so-called **immotile-cilia syndrome.** Sterile male patients have been found to have immotile sperm; ultrastructural analysis has revealed that their sperm possessed axonemes that lacked dynein arms. These same patients also have a history of chronic respiratory infections since childhood. A combination of these and related diseases is known as **Kartagener's syndrome.**

This syndrome has a familial basis, as siblings are sometimes affected. However, because the axoneme is a complex structure and multiple gene products are required for its assembly, the affected genes have not been isolated and characterized. In fact, several defects can cause a similar phenotype. In some affected patients, cilia are missing their central pair of microtubules; others have a transposition of a peripheral doublet microtubule to the center; and in a third group of patients, cilia lack radial spokes. Clearly, this is a complex set of diseases in which the genes encoding many ciliary components are likely to be affected.

ACTIN FILAMENTS

Actin is probably the most abundant protein in eukaryotic cells and comprises about 5% of the total protein; in skeletal muscle, actin constitutes approximately 20% of the cell mass. Actin filaments assemble spontaneously—both in vivo and in vitro—and consist of actin subunits, each of which is a single polypeptide (375 amino acids) that contains a tightly bound molecule of ATP. In some texts, the actin molecules are referred to as **G-actin** or **globular actin** to distinguish it from the polymerized or filamentous actin, which is sometimes designated **F-actin.** Numerous studies have demonstrated that, like tubulin subunits, actin molecules add to and dissociate from the ends of the helical filament.

Some of the basic properties of actin filaments are outlined below; note that actin filaments are

- linear helical arrays, the subunits of which are oriented in the same direction
- about 8 nm in diameter
- more flexible, thinner, and shorter than microtubules
- essential components of the contractile apparatus in muscle cells
- the core of microvilli.

Each actin filament consists of a helix of actin polypeptides; like microtubules, actin filaments are polarized structures. The faster growing end is the **plus end** and the slow-growing end is the **minus end.** Actin filaments can be "decorated" with myosin (see below), and because of the size, shape, and orientation of the myosin head groups that resemble arrow heads, each end of the filament has a characteristic morphology. The plus end is referred to as the **barbed end,** whereas the minus or slow-growing end is designated the **pointed end.** The two ends can have different rates for their interaction with incoming and leaving actin subunits. Mammals have multiple actin genes that encode six different actin isoforms that are expressed in different tissues. Overall, however, the sequence of these different forms is highly conserved, and all assemble into similar helical filaments. Table 7–4 lists actin isoforms and their associated tissues.

ACTIN POLYMERIZATION

Like microtubule assembly, actin polymerization can be studied in vitro by (1) measuring changes in fluorescence spectrum response to fluorescently labeled actin incorporation into filaments or (2) monitoring the changes in viscosity of an actin solution on polymerization. Actin polymerization requires:

- ATP, which is hydrolyzed to adenosine 5′-diphosphate (ADP) after each subunit is incorporated into the filament
- K^+ and Mg^{2+} ions.

As with the kinetics of tubulin polymerization, several distinct stages of actin filament formation can be discerned:

1. An initial lag phase in which new filaments are nucleated.
2. Rapid polymerization in which short filaments elongate.
3. Actin polymerization at each end of the filament is quite different; the plus (barbed) end of the filament polymerizes up to 10 times faster than the minus (pointed) end.

It appears that the spontaneous polymerization of actin involves actin subunits linked as a trimer; this conclusion follows the observation that the polymerization rate of actin in the initial phase is related to the cube of actin concentration. By contrast, elongation of actin filaments appears to occur by the progressive accretion of single actin molecules and thus appears to be governed by the local concentration of free actin monomers.

After polymerization, ATP bound to each actin subunit is hydrolyzed to ADP plus phosphate; this results in formation of an actin ADP polymer. On the basis of data from its x-ray crystallographic structure, we know that actin is clam shaped and that it binds ATP in a slot between the two halves of the clam shell; like a clam, actin can open and close. On polymerization, the shell closes, which results in ATP hydrolysis; the generated ADP is then trapped between the two halves of the actin molecule, which has become incorporated into the filament.

ATP Hydrolysis in Actin Polymerization

The function of ATP hydrolysis is similar to that of GTP in tubulin polymerization. In both cases, nucleotide triphosphate hydrolysis weakens the bonds in the polymer, thereby enhancing depolymerization, which then allows a new cycle of assembly to begin. The rate of ADP-ATP exchange on free G-actin, however, is relatively slow (minutes); consequently, there is a relatively long lag before a liberated actin monomer rebinds ATP and can be reused in filament assembly. This property theoretically enables the cell to maintain a high concentration of unpolymerized ADP actin monomers in the cytoplasm. Although this property no doubt plays a role in regulating the level of subunit incorporation into filaments, it seems that **ABPs** play a crucial role in this process.

As outlined above, the concentration of G-actin in the cell is very high (~ 200 µM), yet its **critical concentration**—ie, the level of free actin monomer that helps determine the amount of actin in polymer—is quite low: approximately 0.2 µM. This is obviously far lower than the concentration of unpolymerized actin in the cell. Consequently, the cell has evolved a mechanism that regulates filament assembly and prevents most of the G-actin from being assembled into filaments; in part this is mediated by ABPs that prevent polymerization.

Control of Actin Polymerization & Actin-binding Proteins

Actin is involved in forming various structures in the cell, eg, (1) extensions of the cell surface, the leading edge of mobile cells, and (2) the actin cortex, which is a region below the plasma membrane. These are discussed below. Because the actin filaments are identical and the different actin monomers are quite similar, variation in the actin cytoskeletal structure results from

- filament stability
- filament length
- geometry of filament attachment.

ACTIN-BINDING PROTEINS

The modulation of actin properties and the amount of G-actin that is polymerized into filaments is mediated by a large number of ABPs several of which are discussed below.

Profilins

Profilins are a family of actin monomer-binding

Table 7–4. Actin isoforms and associated tissues.

Actin Isoform	Tissue
α-actin	Different muscle cells
β-actin	Nonmuscle cells
γ-actin	Nonmuscle cells

proteins. In many cells, profilin is associated with the plasma membrane and binds actin with a 1:1 stoichiometry. It was originally thought that because of this binding, profilin regulates the level of filamentous and soluble actin by simple mass action effects. It is now known, however, that insufficient profilin exists in the cell to bind all the G-actin. At least in platelets and neutrophils **thymosin-β4** is the most likely protein that binds actin monomers. Profilin does, however, modulate actin assembly by catalyzing the exchange of ADP-actin for ATP-actin and by shuttling actin monomers from thymosin to the growing end of actin filaments.

Thymosin-β4

Thymosin-β4 is a small, 43-amino acid polypeptide that is widely distributed in vertebrate cells. It is a potent inhibitor of actin polymerization and is present in some cells (human platelets) at sufficiently high concentration (~ 200 μM) to bind most of the monomeric actin. The mode of actin binding is unclear, but one can envision two possible mechanisms: thymosin-β4 either sterically blocks the site where actin monomers bind to each other or prevents ADP-ATP exchange between subunits.

Spectrin

Although thymosin and profilin prevent actin monomer binding to the barbed end of the actin filament, one of the first ABPs to be studied in detail is **spectrin,** also called **fodrin.** Spectrin is associated with the erythrocyte membrane and is a pointed-end binding protein. In these cells, which are essentially a bag of hemoglobin, the plasma membrane is the only major membrane. It is supported by a network of spectrin tetramers that are connected by short actin filaments of uniform length. In the red blood cell, spectrin is also linked to the cytoplasmic tail of one of the major membrane proteins, **band III,** by **ankyrin bridges.** Isoforms of spectrum-like proteins are found in a wide range of cells, and it is thought that they function as actin filament **cross-linking proteins.** In many cases, the actin filaments of the **cell cortex** are much longer than in erythrocytes and project into the cytoplasm to form a three-dimensional network of filaments. The cortical actin network determines the shape and mechanical properties of the plasma membrane (Figure 7–9).

Actin Cross-linking Proteins

In addition to the ABPs that regulate either the polymerization or binding of actin to other components, **actin cross-linking proteins** organize cortical actin filaments into distinct patterns that have specific functions (Table 7–5).

Actin cross-linking proteins can be divided into two major types:

1. **Bundling proteins,** which cross-link actin filaments into parallel arrays
2. **Gel-forming proteins,** which cross-link actin cross-wise to generate a loose gel-like organization.

Among the best characterized bundling proteins are **fimbrin** and **α-actinin.** Fimbrin is enriched in the

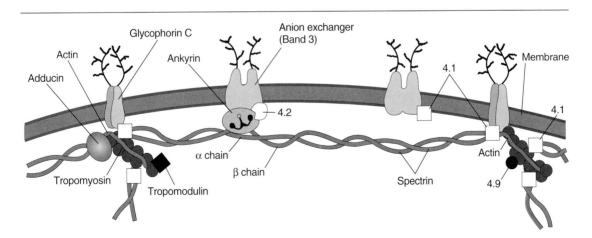

Figure 7–9. Role of actin in stabilization of erythrocyte structure. Actin is one of the most important proteins involved in the cell membrane-cytoskeleton interaction in red blood cells. Actin microfilaments are anchored to the cell membrane by a variety of associated proteins. Note that some of these proteins have names, whereas others are identified by numbers (eg, 4.1, 4.2, 4.9). (Reproduced, with permission, from Luna EJ, Hitt AL: Cytoskeleton-plasma membrane interactions. Science 1992;258:955. Copyright 1992 American Association for the Advancement of Science.)

Table 7–5. Actin cross-linking proteins organize actins in distinct patterns.

Cortical Actin Filaments	Functional Patterns
Parallel bundles	Present in microspikes, filopodia. Actin filaments have same polarity; closely spaced ~10–20 nm apart
Contractile bundles	eg, stress fibers; contractile ring that divides cells during mitosis. Filaments in opposite polarities; loosely spaced ~60 nm apart. Contain myosin-II
Gel-like networks	Filaments in loose, open arrays, many orthogonal connections

leading edge of motile cells where there are abundant parallel filament bundles. Found in contractile bundles called **stress fibers,** which are transient bundles of actin and myosin-II, α-actinin cross-links actin filaments loosely to these contractile bundles and also helps anchor the ends of stress fibers to the plasma membrane at **focal contacts** where the cell attaches to the extracellular matrix (Chapter 8). **Filamin** is an abundant actin cortex protein found in many cells; it is a gel-forming protein that promotes the formation of a dense, viscous network by cross-linking actin filaments that crisscross each other into a three-dimensional, gel-like network.

Function of Actin Filaments: Clinical Correlates

Much has been learned about the role of actin filaments in mediating movement and cell shape by using drugs that either stabilize or disrupt these filaments. **Cytochalasins** are drugs that prevent actin polymerization by binding to the plus end; **phalloidins** are mushroom toxins that bind actin filaments and prevent depolymerization. Prolonged exposure of cells to either drug is toxic: The actin filaments are in dynamic equilibrium between the F-actin and monomeric actin, and disruption of this equilibrium is lethal to cells. By disrupting the movement of mobile cells with cytochalasin, investigators have observed that the "leading edge" of cells contains actin filaments that are constantly forming and depolymerizing—and consequently are sensitive to cytochalasin.

Many vertebrate cells—in particular cancer cells—can migrate toward and then invade foreign tissues. In tissue culture, for example, fibroblasts extend processes from their cell surface termed **lamellipodia,** which is a dense network of actin filaments. Cells can also extend thin, stiff extensions or **microspikes;** these can be up to 10 μm long and have loose actin bundles with plus ends extending outward. An extreme example of a microspike is the growth cone of a developing nerve cell axon, where microspikes called **filopodia** can protrude for up to 50 μm.

A lamellipodium is an organized structure in which highly ordered actin filaments have their plus ends inserted into the leading edge of the plasma membrane. **Ruffling** of the plasma membrane occurs when the lamellipodium cannot attach to the substra-

tum; in this case, the microspikes and lamellipodia move backward over the top of the cell. Lamellipodia and microspikes are generated by rapid local actin polymerization at the plasma membrane, and this causes the plasma membrane to push forward or be extruded at the leading edge of the cell.

Actin is continuously being moved back toward the cell body; ie, actin is in a continuous state of polymerization near the tip of the leading edge and is continuously depolymerizing at internal sites. Cell mobility is directed by this dynamic behavior at the leading edge, where actin filaments are attached to the plasma membrane.

Regulation of Cell Cortex Actin Assembly: Selected Clinical Correlates

Actin polymerization is a highly regulated process that is controlled by cell surface receptors. Cortical actin filaments can rapidly rearrange their organization in response to extracellular signals. Moreover, some of the same cellular components that participate in signal transduction pathways (see Chapter 9) also regulate the actin cortex in a highly localized manner, ie, by affecting discrete areas of the plasma membrane. For example, neutrophils, which are chemotactic, can move in response to chemotactic peptides in bacteria. Neutrophils polymerize their actin locally; this enables these cells to migrate rapidly in the direction of the attractant peptide and destroy the invading bacteria.

Signaling molecules, such as **heterotrimeric G proteins,** (see Chapter 9) appear to be involved in regulating this response, as are two **Ras-related** small GTP-binding proteins **Rho** and **Rac,** which act downstream of the receptor to mediate rapid formation of lamellipodia. In addition to participating at the biomolecular level in the body's immune response to selected extracellular stimuli—eg, certain bacteria—it appears that the actin cytoskeleton plays a key role in helping prevent some cells from becoming cancerous.

ACTIN CYTOSKELETON & CANCER

Prolonged exposure of cells to drugs that disrupt the polymerization or depolymerization of actin filaments is lethal to those cells. Consequently, given the essential role that actin plays in the cell, it is very likely that gross abnormalities in actin can produce a lethal phenotype. Indeed, research has shown that in certain malignant cancer cells, changes in cell shape that accompany the transformed phenotype can result from diminished expression of actin assembly proteins. In particular, differences in the organization of the actin cytoskeleton have been linked to the potential for certain transformed cells to metastasize. In model studies using rat sarcoma cells, for example, cells with short, fine actin filaments have been found to be more motile than nontransformed cells—and thus have a greater probability of metastasizing. Also of note, the level of **thymosin-β4,** the actin monomer-binding protein, is diminished in transformed cells that are metastatic. In addition, levels of thymosin-β4 are lower in metastatic tumors compared with tissue tumors without metastases.

Related research suggests that fibroblast cells transformed with a tumor virus (SV-40) can have diminished levels of α-actinon; however, when these cells are transfected with cDNA encoding α-actinin, the tumorigenicity is repressed. Although these studies have used model experimental systems, the findings raise the possibility that assays based on the relative expression level of proteins that regulate the actin cytoskeleton may provide important diagnostic indicators for potential metastatic tumors in human beings. For example, if levels of thymosin-β4 are found to be diminished in other types of tumor, measuring the expression of thymosin-β4 could constitute a useful prognosticator of metastatic tumors that involve this kind of actin dysfunction.

CELL SIGNALING, CALCIUM, & GELSOLIN

Solation

When actin is incubated with purified filamin in the presence of ATP at 37 °C, the actin polymers can be cross-linked into a gelatinous, viscous solution. If a cell extract is used instead of filamin and the Ca^{2+} ion concentration is increased to greater than 0.1 μM—the approximate physiologic level of free calcium in the cytoplasm—the gel becomes more liquid rather than gelatinous. This process is known as **solation.** On microscopic examination, the material that has changed from a gel to a sol shows a streaming pattern characteristic of the **cytoplasmic streaming** seen when ameboid cells move.

Gelsolin

Several proteins that promote solation in the presence of Ca^{2+} have been isolated: One is **gelsolin.** In the presence of Ca^{2+}, gelsolin severs cross-linked actin filaments in the cell cortex and "caps" the exposed plus ends; this breaks the highly cross-linked actin filament network and prevents further polymerization. Several related proteins are activated when the local concentration of Ca^{2+} is increased transiently 10-fold to about 1 μM, which is a reaction that occurs in response to activation of many receptors on ligand binding during signal transduction (see Chapter 9). For example, this transition of the cortical actin cytoskeleton from a gel to a sol is thought to be an important step in synaptic transmission in neurons.

Synaptic vesicles that contain neurotransmitters dock beneath the plasma membrane in a **prefusion** state. Vesicle docking is brought about by the cross-linked cortical actin filaments, which form a gel-like meshwork and thus physically prevent the synaptic vesicle membrane from fusing with the plasma membrane. Indeed, it is thought that synaptic vesicles are actually tethered to the actin filaments. During a transient influx of Ca^{2+}, the actin-severing proteins become activated, thereby reducing the gel to a liquid sol and severing the interaction between the synaptic vesicle membrane and the actin filaments. The released vesicle can then move, and the lipid bilayers of the vesicle and plasma membrane fuse, thereby allowing release of the neurotransmitter into the extracellular milieu.

MYOSINS & RELATED MOLECULES

The cell cortex is not only able to be transformed from a gel to a sol, and vice-versa, but is also continually moving. This movement is generated by a specific motor protein—**myosin**—which hydrolyzes ATP to ADP and P_i on binding to actin filaments. Investigators have recently devised direct motility assays in which the ability of myosin to impart mechanochemical movement can be observed. For example, if myosins are attached to a microscope coverslip and fluorescently tagged actin filaments are added, on addition of ATP the actin filaments can be seen to move over the myosin-coated surface. If, however, a nonhydrolyzable analogue of ATP is added instead of ATP, no movement occurs, thereby demonstrating that ATP hydrolysis by myosin is necessary to promote sliding.

It was originally thought that only a single myosin polypeptide exists, namely the skeletal muscle myosin from which much of the basic biochemistry and cell physiology of myosin-actin interactions were discovered, as discussed below. It is now apparent, however, that myosins are a multigene family and that nonmuscle cells have many different forms of nonmuscle myosins. Muscle myosin, designated **myosin-II,** consists of two heavy chains, each of about 2000 amino acids and four light chains. The light chains are of two types, a 190- and a 170-residue polypeptide and one molecule of each type is present on each myosin heavy chain N-terminus head domain.

The N-terminus of myosin-II—to which the light chains are bound—forms the motor domain, which has ATPase and motor activities. In electron micrographs, this domain can be seen as a globular structure. The C-terminal region of the myosin-II heavy chain forms an extended, elongated α-helix about 150 nm. A myosin dimer assembles by the association of the two heavy chains, thereby forming a coiled-coil extended α-helix; this is designated the **rod domain** (Figure 7–10).

Like actin, myosin-II is an abundant protein in the cell cortex and generates local movement by enabling oppositely oriented actin filaments to slide over each other. Indeed, this is the function of myosin-II in muscle contraction (see Figure 7–13).

In addition to myosin-II, nonmuscle cells possess nonmuscle myosins, the best characterized of which is myosin-I. This myosin isoform has a globular head motor domain present in myosin-II, but the remainder of the molecule, particularly the extended rod-like domain, varies considerably depending on the myosin isotype (Figure 7–10). A common feature of myosin molecules is that they hydrolyze ATP and move along actin filaments from the minus to the plus end. Depending on the arrangement of its C-terminal domain, myosins can play a diverse role in cell physiology; eg, myosin-like molecules are associated with Golgi membranes and have been shown to move vesicles along actin filaments. The earliest and perhaps best characterized role for myosin is its ability to cause two actin filaments to slide past each other, which is the basis for muscle contraction.

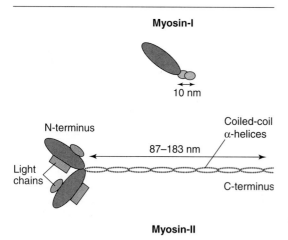

Figure 7–10. Myosin-II. Myosin-II, the protein found in muscle, consists of two heavy chains, each of which has two associated light chains. Note the long coiled-coil α-helical tail. The simpler, smaller structure of myosin-I is shown for comparison. (Modified from Pollard TD et al: Myosin-I. Annu Rev Physiol 1991;53:653. Reproduced with permission from the *Annual Review of Physiology,* Volume 53, © 1991, by Annual Reviews, Inc.)

MUSCLE-LIKE FUNCTION IN NONMUSCLE CELLS

Even in nonmuscle cells, actin filaments and myosin-II can form a transient muscle-like assembly to perform certain functions. This has been well documented in cell division, where the **contractile ring** composed of actin and myosin filaments forms during cell division and generates force on the plasma membrane, which in turn constricts the middle of the cell. This results in the eventual separation of the two daughter cells by a process called **cytokinesis.** The assembly and disassembly of the contractile ring is undergoing elucidation; it is known that both Ca^{2+} ions and calcium-dependent phosphorylation of myosin-II increase and that this interaction with actin promotes assembly of contractile ring components.

Stress fibers are readily discernible in fibroblasts grown in tissue culture, when the cells are stained with antibodies to actin or myosin-II. One end of these fibers is inserted into the plasma membrane at specialized sites—designated **focal contacts**—where the cell is attached to the **extracellular matrix** (see Chapter 8). The other end of the fiber can also be inserted into another focal contact site or into a meshwork of intermediate filaments that surround the nucleus. Stress fibers are formed when cells are subjected to tension generated across the cells—usually as a result of attachment to the substratum, as these fibers are not observed in cells that grow in suspension culture, ie, they are not attached to a matrix.

Adhesion belts found near the apical surface of epithelial cells are permanent assemblies of actin filaments and myosin in nonmuscle cells. Components of cell junctions, adhesion belts act to anchor cells together and are found in epithelial cells near the apical plasma membrane, where adjacent cells are attached to each other laterally (Chapter 8).

MICROVILLI

Microvilli are thin, finger-like projections on the surface of many cells and are particularly abundant in epithelia, where a large surface area is required for efficient function. For example, individual absorptive epithelial cells in the small intestine have thousands of apically disposed microvilli; these function to increase the absorptive surface area of the cell about 20-fold. Each microvillus has about 20–30 parallel actin filaments that extend from the tip into the cell cortex. In all the actin filaments, the plus ends point away from the cell body and are held together by actin-bundling proteins—the most important of which is **villin,** a protein that is specific to microvilli and cross-links actin filaments into tight bundles.

At the base of each microvillus, the actin filaments are anchored into a specialized region known as the **terminal web,** which contains a concentrated net-

Table 7–6. Types of muscle.

Type	Function
Skeletal	Contracts rapidly; voluntary movement
Cardiac	Heart pumping; involuntary movement
Smooth	Gut peristalsis; involuntary movement

work of spectrin molecules and a layer of intermediate filaments. It is thought that spectrin imparts rigidity to the cell cortex; because the actin filaments are anchored to the terminal web, this keeps the microvilli orientated perpendicularly to the apical surface of the cell. The actin filaments are attached to the plasma membrane by lateral bridges composed of myosin-I and several other molecules, including the Ca^{2+} binding protein **calmodulin.**

The actin cytoskeleton can simultaneously possess different properties in topologically separate areas of the cytoplasm. This most likely occurs because actin filaments can interact with several different binding proteins in different cellular locations. Just how these spatially segregated ABPs are regulated is still not well understood. By virtue of the differential interactions between various ABPs and actin filaments, it is possible to generate simultaneously an actin cytoskeleton with quite different properties. The combination of cooperative and competitive interactions between ABPs no doubt regulates these interactions, which themselves may be regulated by signaling proteins (monomeric GTPases) such as Rho and Rac.

MUSCLE

Muscle contraction is probably the best understood movement at the molecular level, and muscle cells represent the most evolutionary advanced and highly specialized tissue that facilitate mechanochemical mobility. Muscle is divided into three types, as shown in Table 7–6. Table 7–7 lists some differences between skeletal, cardiac, and smooth muscle.

SKELETAL MUSCLE

Muscle fibers constitute the basic unit of skeletal muscle; these are multinucleated, elongated cells approximately 50 μm long. Most of the cytoplasm consists of **myofibrils** that constitute the contractile machinery of the cell. These fibrils are cylindrical, elongated structures that transverse the length of the entire muscle fiber. Each myofibril (diameter, 1–2 μm) is composed of many repeating units called **sarcomeres,** which are the units of contraction for striated muscle. Sarcomeres are approximately 2 μm long, and their regular arrangement gives the myofibril its characteristic striated appearance in the microscope. Each sarcomere is a highly organized assembly of parallel and partially overlapping filaments (Figure 7–11).

A series of alternating light and dark bands called **A, I,** and **H bands** can be seen at high magnification;

Table 7–7. Some differences between skeletal, cardiac, and smooth muscle.[1]

Skeletal Muscle	Cardiac Muscle	Smooth Muscle
Striated.	Striated.	Nonstriated.
No syncytium.	Syncytial.	Syncytial.
Small T tubules.	Large T tubules.	Generally rudimentary T tubules.
SR well developed and Ca^{2+} pump acts rapidly.	SR present and Ca^{2+} pump acts relatively rapidly.	SR often rudimentary and Ca^{2+} pump acts slowly.
Plasmalemma lacks many hormone receptors.	Plasmalemma contains a variety of receptors (eg, α- and β-adrenergic).	Plasmalemma contains a variety of receptors (eg, α- and β-adrenergic).
Nerve impulse initiates contraction.	Has intrinsic rhythmicity.	Contraction initiated by nerve impulses, hormones, etc.
ECF Ca^{2+} not important for contraction.	ECF Ca^{2+} important for contraction.	ECF Ca^{2+} important for contraction.
Troponin system present.	Troponin system present.	Lacks troponin system; uses regulatory head of myosin.
Caldesmon not involved.	Caldesmon not involved.	Caldesmon is important regulatory protein.
Very rapid cycling of the cross-bridges.	Relatively rapid cycling of the cross-bridges.	Slow cycling of the cross-bridges permits slow prolonged contraction and less utilization of ATP.

[1]From Murray RK et al: *Harper's Biochemistry,* 24th ed. Appleton & Lange, 1996, p. 696, with permission.
SR, sarcoplasmic reticulum; ECF, extracellular fluid.

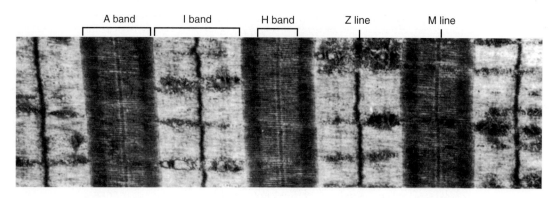

A band I band H band Z line M line

Figure 7–11. Skeletal muscle. This electron micrograph shows the characteristic banding pattern of striated muscle and the functional division into sarcomeres. The banding is due to the interaction of filaments made of myosin and filaments composed largely of actin. (× 13,500.) (Reproduced, with permission, from Ganong WF: *Review of Medical Physiology,* 17th ed. Appleton & Lange, 1995, p. 9. Courtesy of SM Walker and GR Schrodt.) See also the electron micrograph in Figure 1–4.

a densely staining band in the center of each lighter staining I-band separates each part of the sarcomere. This is designated the **Z-line** or **Z-disk.** Actin **thin filaments** are attached to the Z disk at each end of the sarcomere and extend inward toward the middle of the sarcomere. The plus ends of each actin filament are embedded in the Z-disk, whereas the minus end (pointed) is oriented in the direction of the myosin filaments. Within the Z disk, the actin filaments are tightly cross-linked to each other by the protein **α-actinin** (190 kDa). The A-band is at the center of the sarcomere and is composed of myosin-II. Here the myosin **thick filaments** overlap with actin filaments (Figure 7–12).

MUSCLE CONTRACTION

The **sliding filament** model of muscle contraction (first proposed in 1954 by Huxley) suggested that sarcomere shortening occurs by myosin filaments that slide past the actin filaments with no change in the length of either filament. On electron microscopic examination of the sarcomere, myosin thick filaments can be seen to possess side arms or cross-bridges that make contact with adjacent actin filaments—a distance of about 13 nm. The cross-bridges correspond to the head domains of myosin-II; during contraction, the myosin and actin filaments are pulled past each other by the cross-bridges. This is achieved by two complementary hexagonal lattices of actin and myosin sliding past each other (Figures 7–12 and 7–13).

Actin filaments in each half I-band therefore form a hexagonal lattice that is complementary to a similar lattice formed by myosin thick filaments in the A-band. Because of this arrangement, the thick and thin filaments do not collide when the I-band penetrates into the A-band. Moreover, when the I-band of each sarcomere penetrates into the A-band region, the distance between the Z disks is decreased; because this is repeated along the length of the myofibril, the muscle fiber shortens. This is known as the **sliding filament mechanism of muscle contraction.**

Basically, the globular head domain of myosin molecules within the A-band extend from the thick filament. These molecules bind to and form a cross-bridge with the thin filament actin of the A- and I-bands. On contact with the actin filament, the myosin head group changes its conformation, which pulls the actin filament further into the A-band (Figure 7–13).

The binding of the myosin-II head domain to adjacent actin filaments is the central feature of muscle contraction. ATP bound to the myosin head is hydrolyzed to ADP, and the dissociation of ADP and inorganic phosphate results in a series of conformational changes in the actin-bound myosin molecules. These structural changes—coupled to the energy of ATP hydrolysis—generate movement.

Contraction Cycle

The contraction cycle (Figure 7–14) that results in force generation by interaction of myosin head groups with actin filaments can be divided into five component steps:

1. Attachment: The myosin head groups are bound tightly to actin filaments. This is known as **rigor** and is very short lived because ATP rapidly binds to the myosin. Skeletal muscle has abundant mitochondria that provide the ATP neces-

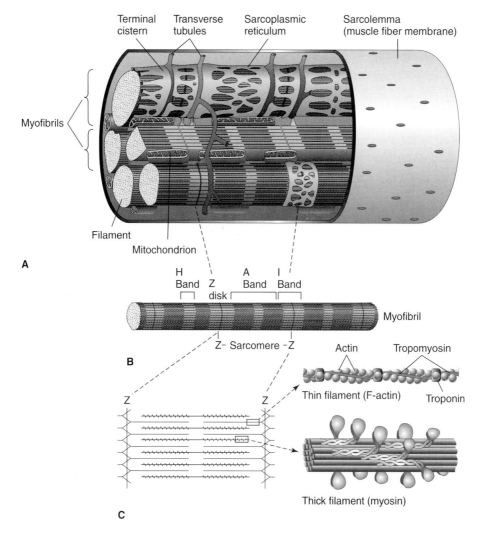

Figure 7–12. Levels of organization of skeletal muscle. A single muscle fiber (A) is composed of multiple myofibrils in close association with a tubular system. Examination of a myofibril (B) reveals the functional unit of muscle contraction, the sarcomere. Sarcomeres are defined visually as the distance between adjacent Z disks. At the macromolecular level (C), each sarcomere is composed of alternating thin and thick filaments. Thick filaments are made of myosin-II, and thin filaments are composed chiefly of actin. Note the globular heads that stick out from the surface of each thick filament; these are crucial in the filament interaction that produces contraction. (Modified and reproduced, with permission, from Kandel E et al: *Principles of Neural Science,* 3rd ed. Appleton & Lange, 1991, p. 549.)

sary for actomyosin interaction and the relative movement of these molecules.

2. Release: ATP binding induces a conformational change in the actin-binding site of myosin. This reduces the affinity of the myosin head group for the actin filaments.

3. Tilting: The ATP binding site in the myosin head domain closes, thereby resulting in a significant conformational change that causes displacement of the head group about 5 nm along the filament. During this step ATP hydrolysis occurs, but the ADP and P_i remain bound to myosin.

4. Force generation: The weak myosin that binds to a new site on the actin filaments releases the bound ADP as myosin binds tightly to the actin filament. With the release of ADP, force is generated, this results from the conformational change in myosin and allows myosin to return to its original conformation. During this **power stroke,** ADP is displaced from the myosin head group, and this causes myosin to initiate a new cycle of actin binding.

5. (Re)-Attachment: At the end of the cycle, the myosin head is tightly associated with the actin filament (**rigor conformation**) but has moved to

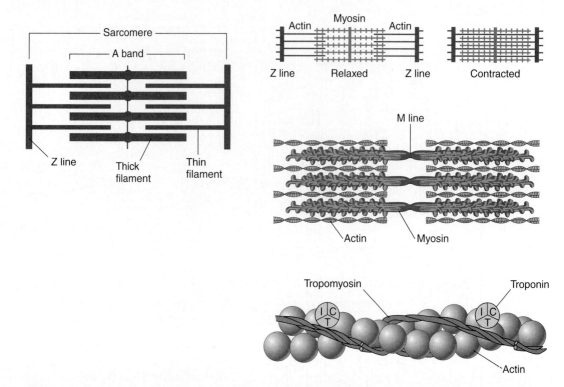

Figure 7–13. Actin-myosin interaction during muscle contraction. Thick filaments (myosin) and thin filaments (actin) are arranged in alternating fashion within a sarcomere (top left). During contraction, actin slides over myosin such that the Z lines are pulled toward the center of the sarcomere (top right). In closer view, the relationship between actin molecules and the globular myosin heads is clearly seen (middle right). The M line, which marks the sarcomere center, is the point toward which actin is pulled during contraction. A still closer view of a thin filament shows not only actin, but the proteins troponin and tropomyosin (lower right). (Top left and right, middle right, modified and reproduced, with permission, from Alberts BA et al: *Molecular Biology of the Cell,* 2nd ed. Garland, 1989. Bottom right modified and reproduced from Ganong WF: *Review of Medical Physiology,* 17th ed. Appleton & Lange, 1995.)

a new position along the actin filament—toward the plus end of the filaments.

In the above cycle, each myosin head domain is said to "walk" along the adjacent actin filament, thus causing it to slide against the myosin filament and toward the plus end. Although an individual myosin head may detach from the actin filament during this cycle, at any one time other myosin heads in the same myosin filament will attach to actin, thereby resulting in movement. Each thick filament has approximately 500 myosin heads, and each of these cycles about 5 times per second during rapid contraction.

Regulation of Muscle Contraction

The mechanochemical forces generated by actin-myosin interactions must be coordinated so that muscle contraction occurs in a regulated fashion. For example, one might think that the above cycle would continue until all the ATP is consumed; however, this does not happen because molecular switches regulate the cycle. In skeletal muscle, the interaction of actin and myosin and the changes in intracellular levels of Ca^{2+} are coordinated by switch proteins that control muscle contraction. Two of these are **tropomyosin** and **troponin.**

When the intracellular concentration of Ca^{2+} is at the resting level (~ 0.1 μM), tropomyosin and troponin form a complex whose conformation prevents the myosin head group from binding to actin; hence, the cross-bridges do not form. As the concentration of Ca^{2+} increases up to ~ 0.7 μM in response to a nerve impulse, the conformation of the tropomyosin-troponin complex changes; this allows the myosin head groups to bind actin, thereby turning on the cross-bridge cycle.

Tropomyosin is a rod-shaped, 70-kDa molecule that binds to the groove of the actin helix. **Troponin** is actually a complex of three polypeptide subunits that range in molecular weight from 18,000 to 35,000 Da. The key functions of troponin are summarized in Table 7–8.

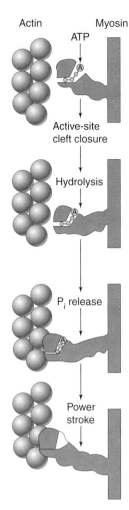

Actin   Myosin
ATP

Active-site
cleft closure

Hydrolysis

P_i release

Power
stroke

Figure 7–14. Mechanism of muscular contraction. This diagram shows a model for the action of the myosin head in moving a thin filament over a thick filament within the myofibril. After ATP is bound to the active site, it is hydrolyzed, releasing a phosphate group (P_i) and causing a change in the shape of the myosin head. The changed myosin head binds to actin and proceeds through the power stroke, moving the actin molecule over the myosin molecule. After the power stroke concludes, the myosin head is again in the shape that exposes the active site to ATP. (Modified from Rayment I et al: Structure of the actin-myosin complex and its implications for muscle contraction. Science 1993;261:58. Copyright 1993 American Association for the Advancement of Science.)

Stoichiometry of Troponin Subunits

The troponin subunits form an elongated complex; troponin I binds to actin and inhibits the interaction between actin and myosin, even in the presence of Ca^{2+}. Troponin C confers calcium sensitivity on the troponin complex and, in the process:

Table 7–8. Types of troponin and their key functions.

Troponin subunit	Function
Troponin T	Tropomyosin binding
Troponin I	Tropomyosin inhibitor
Troponin C	Tropomyosin calcium binding

1. Binds up to four Ca^{2+} ions
2. Abrogates the inhibition between actin and myosin that is mediated by troponin T and I.

It is believed that in any actin filament, every seven actin monomers are related to one troponin complex. It is thought that in actively contracting muscle, troponin I competes with the myosin-II heads for positions on the actin filaments, thereby inhibiting interaction between actin and myosin. As the intracellular concentration of Ca^{2+} increases, troponin C causes troponin I to dissociate from actin, thus allowing the troponin complex to alter its position on the actin filament. This in turn allows myosin head domains to bind actin (Table 7–9).

Role of Ca^{2+} in Muscle Contraction

As discussed above, calcium ions play a crucial role in regulating muscle contraction. With skeletal muscle, this is achieved when contraction occurs only in response to a neuronal signal that triggers an action potential in the muscle cell plasma membrane or **sarcolemma.** The electrical signal generated spreads rapidly throughout the length of the muscle cell by a series of membranous finger-like folds called **trans-**

Table 7–9. Sequence of events in contraction and relaxation of skeletal muscle.[1]

Steps in contraction
 (1) Discharge of motor neuron.
 (2) Release of transmitter (acetylcholine).
 (3) Binding of acetylcholine to nicotinic acetylcholine receptors.
 (4) Generation of action potential in muscle fibers.
 (5) Inward spread of depolarization along T tubules.
 (6) Release of Ca^{2+} from terminal cisterns of sarcoplasmic reticulum and diffusion to thick and thin filaments.
 (7) Binding of Ca^{2+} to troponin C, uncovering myosin binding sites on actin.
 (8) Formation of cross-linkages between actin and myosin and sliding of thin on thick filaments, producing shortening.
Steps in relaxation
 (1) Ca^{2+} pumped back into sarcoplasmic reticulum.
 (2) Release of Ca^{2+} from troponin.
 (3) Cessation of interaction between actin and myosin.

[1]Modified from Ganong WF: *Review of Medical Physiology,* 18th ed. Appleton & Lange, 1997, p. 65, with permission.

verse tubules, or T-tubules (Figure 7–12A). These are closely associated with the sarcoplasmic reticulum, the ramifying membrane-enclosed organelle that surrounds each myofibril and stores Ca^{2+}. Adjacent to each sarcomere, the T-tubules contact saccules called terminal cisternae of the sarcoplasmic reticulum to form a triad—ie, one T-tubule surrounded between two cisternae.

The electrical signal is relayed to the sarcoplasmic reticulum, where Ca^{2+} release channels contact the T-tubule membrane and become activated by the action potential. This causes some of the Ca^{2+} channels to open and release calcium from the sarcoplasmic reticulum into the cytoplasm, which initiates contraction of each myofibril. Because the electrical signal passes to every sarcomere within milliseconds, each myofibril is said to contract simultaneously (Table 7–9).

Other Proteins Required for Muscle Contraction: Dystrophin (Muscular Dystrophy)

To maintain the efficiency and speed of muscle contraction, the actin-myosin filaments in each myofibril must be precisely aligned and kept at an optimal distance from one another. Numerous proteins that govern this process have been described in recent years; one that has been characterized in detail—because its gene was isolated—is dystrophin. Dystrophin is a large, rod-shaped polypeptide (MW > 400,000). An ABP, dystrophin is thought to link muscle membrane proteins to actin filaments in the myofibril.

The characterization of the dystrophin gene has been very important clinically. Defects in the gene—or the absence of the ABP it encodes—are thought to result in loss of coordination during contraction, which is the cause of muscular dystrophy. Duchenne's muscular dystrophy affects about 1 in 3000 male infants and is frequently fatal by early adulthood.

Two other very high molecular weight proteins—titin ($\sim 3 \times 10^6$) and nebulin—form a fibrous network that associates with actin and myosin. Titin molecules are thought to be shaped like coiled springs; they extend from myosin thick filaments to the Z disk and may function to maintain myosin filaments in the sarcomere. Nebulin is associated with actin thin filaments and extends the complete length of the actin filament; this protein is thought to regulate the length of actin filaments during muscle development.

CONTRACTILE MACHINERY OF CARDIAC & SMOOTH MUSCLE

Like skeletal muscle, cardiac and smooth muscle cells contract and use the same actin–myosin-II sliding filament mechanism. These cells differ considerably, however, in their organization and function. Like skeletal muscle, heart muscle possesses cross-striations and is stimulated to contract by an action

Table 7–10. Actin-myosin interactions in striated and smooth muscle.[1]

	Striated Muscle	Smooth Muscle (and Nonmuscle Cells)
Proteins of muscle filaments	Actin Myosin Tropomyosin Troponin (Tpl, TPT, TpC)	Actin Myosin[2] Tropomyosin
Spontaneous interaction of F-actin and myosin alone (spontaneous activation of myosin ATPase by F-actin)	Yes	No
Inhibitor of F actin–myosin interaction (inhibitor of F actin–dependent activation of ATPase)	Troponin system (Tpl)	Unphosphorylated myosin p-light chain
Contraction activated by	Ca^{2+}	Ca^{2+}
Direct effect of Ca^{2+}	$4Ca^{2+}$ bind to TpC	$4Ca^{2+}$ bind to calmodulin
Effect of protein-bound Ca^{2+}	TpC · $4Ca^{2+}$ antagonizes Tpl inhibition of F actin–myosin interaction (allows F-actin activation of ATPase)	Calmodulin · $4Ca^{2+}$ activates myosin light chain kinase that phosphorylates myosin p-light chain. The phosphorylated p-light chain no longer inhibits F actin-myosin interaction (allows F-actin activation of ATPase).

[1]From Murray RK et al: *Harper's Biochemistry*, 24th ed. Appleton & Lange, 1996, p. 699, with permission.
[2]Light chains of myosin are different in striated and smooth muscles.

potential that triggers release of Ca^{2+}; contraction is regulated by the troponin-tropomyosin complex. In contrast to skeletal muscle cells, however, cardiac muscle cells do not form syncytia; moreover, they are joined by specialized units called intercalated disks, which serve three functions:

1. They attach adjacent cells to each other by desmosomes (see Chapter 8).
2. They connect myofibrillar actin filaments of adjacent cells.
3. They possess gap junctions, which allow the action potential to spread rapidly between cells. This process synchronizes muscle cell contraction.

In contrast to cardiac and skeletal muscle, smooth muscle

- has no cross-striations
- is responsible for contractile processes in blood vessels, the alimentary canal, the uterus, and respiratory tract
- is composed of elongated, spindle-shaped cells that contain actin and myosin II.

In smooth muscle cells, the filaments are loosely aligned along the long axis of the cell. Also, **dense bodies**—specialized junctions resembling disks—join smooth muscle cells to the plasma membrane.

The intermediate filaments and dense bodies of smooth muscle that contain α-actinin are thought to function similarly to Z disks in striated muscle. Bundles of actin and myosin-containing filaments are anchored to dense bodies on the plasma membrane at one end of the cell. At the other end, the filaments are attached to intermediate filaments. In contrast to striated muscle, although Ca^{2+} mediates contraction, release of the tropomyosin-troponin complex is not involved. Instead, the increase in concentration of Ca^{2+} mediated by the calcium-binding protein **calmodulin**—activates myosin light chain kinase, which in turn phosphorylates one of the two myosin light chains. On phosphorylation, the myosin head domain then binds to actin, and this initiates contraction. Table 7–10 summarizes the differences between striated and smooth muscle.

REFERENCES

GENERAL

Alberts BA et al: Molecular Biology of the Cell, 3rd ed. Garland Press, 1994.
Ganong WF: Review of Medical Physiology, 17th ed. Appleton & Lange, 1995.

ACTIN & ACTIN BINDING PROTEINS

Condeelis JC: Life at the leading edge. Ann Rev Cell Biol 1993;9:411.
Pollard TD et al: Structure of actin binding proteins. Ann Rev Cell Biol 1994;10:207.
Schafer DA, Cooper JA: Control of actin assembly at filament ends. Ann Rev Cell Dev Biol 1995;11:497.
Stossel T: On the crawling of animal cells. Science 1993;260:1086.

MICROTUBULES & ORGANELLE ASSEMBLY

Cole NB, Lippincott-Schwartz J: Organization of organelles and membrane traffic by microtubules. Curr Opin Cell Biol 1995;7:55.
Sugrue P et al: Computer modelling of tetrahymena axonemes at macromolecular resolution. J Cell Sci 1991;98:5.
Vallee RB, Sheetz MP: Targeting of motor proteins. Science 1996;271:1539.

CYTOSKELETON & DISEASE

Janmey PA, Chaponnier C: Medical aspects of the actin cytoskeleton. Curr Opin Cell Biol 1995;7:111.
McLean MHI, Lane EB: Intermediate filaments in disease. Curr Opin Cell Biol 1995;7:118.
Satir P, Dirksen ER: Function-structure correlations in cilia from mammalian respiratory tract. In: Handbook of Physiology. American Physiology Society, 1985.

SUGGESTED READING

Goody RS: Motor proteins: Two-way structure. Nature 1996;380:483.
Kull FJ et al: Crystal structure of the kinesin motor domain reveals a structural similarity to myosin. Nature 1996;380:550.
Moritz M et al: Microtubule nucleation by γ-tubulin-containing rings in the centrosome. Nature 1995;378:638.
Oakley BR: A nice ring to the centrosome. Nature 1995;378:555.
Sablin EP et al: Crystal structure of the motor domain of the kinesin-related motor ncd. Nature 1996;380:555.
Zheng Y et al: Nucleation of microtubule assembly by a γ-tubulin-containing ring complex. Nature 1995;378:578.

8

Cell Junctions, Cell-Cell Adhesion, & the Extracellular Matrix

KEY TERMS

Cell adhesions
Tight junction
Adherens junctions
Cadherins
Catenins
Desmosomes
Hemidesmosomes
Integrins
Cell adhesion molecules
Glycosaminoglycans
Hyaluronan
Proteoglycans
Collagens
Elastin
Fibronectin
Laminin

The organization of cells into groups that form **tissues** is not random. Rather, cells are integrated into units that are attached to each other in a highly organized fashion. The structure of a particular tissue results from the specific adhesion of groups of cells, their connections with the internal cytoskeleton, and cellular interactions with the **extracellular matrix (ECM).**

The ECM is a complex mixture of different macromolecules that form a supporting framework to hold cells and tissues together. This highly organized array of cells and tissues constitutes an **organ.** During tissue formation, individual cells do not simply stick together but rather are organized so that their positions within the tissue and orientation allow for intercellular communication and integration of function. The development and maintenance of specific tissue function result from the complex interactions between the tissue and its physical environment, ie, cell-cell adhesion coupled to a variety of signaling processes that control information transfer between adjacent cells. Cell adhesion should therefore not be thought of as a process whereby groups of cells are simply tethered together by an inert set of molecules, analogous to the nuts and bolts that hold scaffolding together.

Rather, cell adhesion is a dynamic process, and many of the molecules that mediate cellular adhesion and tissue organization also participate in signaling reactions.

CELL-CELL ATTACHMENT & COMMUNICATION

The evolutionary transition from single cell protozoa to multicellular organisms required a mechanism for cell-cell attachment and communication. Indeed, during normal embryogenesis, adhesive interactions function in morphogenetic processes throughout the development of the organism. These interactions involve not only contacts between adjacent cells, but also cell adhesion to and with the ECM. The coordinate interactions of cell-surface receptors and the activity of the cytoskeleton within the cells are necessary to effect a variety of developmental events, including cell proliferation, mobility, and differentiation. These processes of ligand-receptor interaction and cytoskeleton-driven morphogenesis lead to changes in cell behavior and are interdependent (Geiger & Ayalon, 1992). Hence changes in local cell adhesion interactions can produce alterations in the cytoskeleton. Similarly, cell differentiation events can alter the expression of genes that encode adhesion molecules or genes that regulate cytoskeletal proteins. These highly complex events—and the molecules involved in these processes—are addressed in this chapter (Table 8–1).

CELL JUNCTIONS & ADHESION

The various combinations of groups of cells and tissues within an organ are in contact with their adjacent partners and with the ECM. The ECM is a complex secretion composed of protein fibers, collagen,

Table 8–1. Anchoring junctions.[1]

Junction	Transmembrane Linker Protein	Extracellular Ligand	Intracellular Cytoskeletal Attachment	Intracellular Attachment Proteins
Adherens (cell-cell)	Cadherin (E-cadherin)	Cadherin in adjacent cell	Actin filaments	Catenins, vinculin, α-actinin, plakoglobin
Desmosome	Cadherin (desmogleins & desmocollins)	Cadherin in neighboring cell	Intermediate filaments	Desmoplakins, plakoglobin
Adherens (cell-matrix)	Integrin	Extracellular matrix proteins	Actin filaments	Talin, vinculin, α-actinin
Hemidesmosome	Integrin	Extracellular matrix (basal lamina) proteins	Intermediate filaments	Desmoplakin-related

[1]Modified from Alberts B: *Molecular Biology of the Cell.* Garland, 1994, p. 958, with permission.

and a gelatinous material referred to in older histology texts as *ground substance.* This material is now known to consist of glycoproteins and **proteoglycans.** The ECM holds cells together by providing physical support and a matrix in which cells can migrate, signal each other, and interact. Cells frequently adhere to each other by direct connections known collectively as cell-cell **junctions** or **adhesions.**

The major tissue types are nerve, muscle, blood, lymphatic, epithelium, and connective tissue. (See Chapter 1.) Connective tissue has relatively few cells and a large volume of ECM to which the cells are attached. In contrast, epithelial cells—the simplest of which comprise a layer of cells lining body surfaces such as the digestive and respiratory tracts—adhere to each other in sheets that are held together by **tight** interactions. These cells reside on a thin layer of ECM called the **basal lamina.** In epithelia, specialized junctions between adjacent cells (1) facilitate intercellular interaction and communication and (2) enable cells to resist physical stress through the action of filaments attached to the cell membranes (Figure 8–1).

JUNCTIONAL COMPLEXES

Individual epithelial cells are tethered to adjacent neighboring cells and the ECM by cell junctions (Table 8–1), which are grouped into three major categories:

1. **Tight or occluding junctions:** These form an impervious seal between adjacent cells and prevent even small molecules (eg, ions) from penetrating between cells or moving from one side of the epithelial sheet to the other.
2. **Anchoring junctions:** These attach cells to their neighbors or to the ECM.
3. **Communicating junctions:** As their name implies, these junctions allow passage of small molecules and electrical signals between adjacent cells.

TIGHT JUNCTIONS

A common feature of epithelia is that they constitute a highly selective permeability barrier that separates dissolved material on one side of the cell from that on the other. For example, in epithelial cells that line the small intestine, the contents of the lumen are separated from underlying cells and small blood vessels. These epithelial cells selectively transport nutrients, sugars, amino acids, and other materials from the lumen, through the cell, and into the extracellular fluid of the connective tissue—and hence into the blood. This functional asymmetry of the cell is achieved because the cell has a highly differentiated plasma membrane (Figure 8–2).

The surface closest to the lumen is referred to as the **apical membrane;** it actively transports selected molecules into the cell. The other surface consists of two components:

- the **lateral membrane,** or the surface on which adjacent cells are attached at either side
- the **basal membrane,** or the surface that sits on the extracellular fluid and the interface of the ECM.

Together these components are referred to as the **basolateral** surface or membrane.

Basolateral Surface: Selected Clinical Correlates

Molecules transported into the cell by the apical plasma membrane exit at the basolateral surface, thereby delivering molecules into the circulation. In these **polarized** epithelia, therefore, many cellular proteins (eg, sugar or amino acid transporters and ion pumps) are restricted to the apical or basolateral surfaces. Findings from research on the infection of epithelial cells by various viruses—eg, influenza and the vesicular stomatitis virus—suggest that different viral membrane proteins are specifically targeted to either the apical or basolateral plasma membranes. Indeed, new virus particles bud from only one mem-

Apical surface

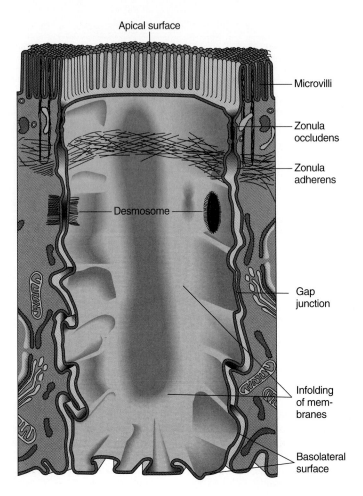

Microvilli

Zonula
occludens

Zonula
adherens

Desmosome

Gap
junction

Infolding
of mem-
branes

Basolateral
surface

Figure 8–1. The cell-cell junction in epithelial tissue. This diagram shows structures that facilitate interaction and adhesion between an intestinal epithelial cell and its neighbors. The gap junction between cells is involved in intercellular interaction. The regions termed the zonula adherens and the desmosome contain numerous filaments that strengthen the connections between cells and enable the tissue to withstand physical stresses. (Modified and reproduced, with permission, from Krstić RV: *Ultrastructure of the Mammalian Cell.* Springer-Verlag, 1979.)

brane of the infected cells; for example, influenza is released from the apical surface, whereas vesicular stomatitis virus buds from the basolateral surface of epithelial cells. To maintain the asymmetry of function—ie, to restrict membrane proteins to their correct surface and prevent molecules from nonspecifically passing from the lumen of the gut between adjacent cells and into the ECM—these cells possess **tight junctions** (Chapter 2). These junctions have two major functions:

1. They prevent apical and basolateral membrane proteins from diffusing between these two surfaces.
2. They seal adjacent cells together, thereby preventing soluble molecules from passing between them.

Although the integrity of the apical and basolateral membrane proteins is always maintained, the permeability barrier to small molecules and ions can vary considerably. The molecular constituents of tight junctions are not well understood. Morphologically they appear as *focal connections* between the outer leaflets of two adjacent plasma membranes (Figure 8–2).

ANCHORING JUNCTIONS

Anchoring junctions also connect adjacent cells to each other. In addition, these junctions tether cells to the ECM. In both cases, this involves connections from the cell membrane to cytoskeletal proteins that impart resistance to physical stress. Consequently,

Table 8–2. Tight junctions and filament proteins.

Junction	Filament Proteins
Adherens junctions	Actin filaments
Desmosomes	Intermediate filaments
Hemidesmosomes	Actin/intermediate filaments

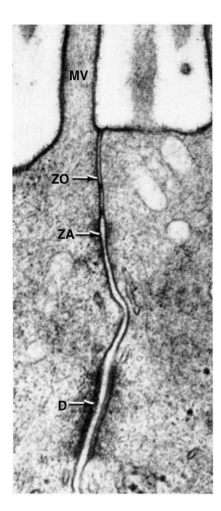

Figure 8–2. Structure and function in an intestinal epithelial cell. This electron micrograph shows the relationship between structure and function of the cell membrane. The apical cell membrane, typified by a microvillus (MV), is selectively permeable to the variety of nutrients within the lumen. The tight adhesion between adjacent epithelial cells ensures that luminal contents do not diffuse between cells and into the underlying tissue. × 80,000. (ZO = zonula occludens; ZA = zonula adherens; D = desmosome.) (From Junqueira LC et al: *Basic Histology,* 8th ed. Appleton & Lange. 1995, p. 65, with permission.)

anchoring junctions are abundant in cells that are exposed to shearing forces, eg, skin epidermis and cardiac muscle. Three types of tight junctions that are structurally and functionally distinct—adherens junctions, desmosomes, and hemidesmosomes—have been characterized. These junctions and their corresponding filament proteins are listed in Table 8–2.

Two types of adherens junctions have been characterized:

1. those that mediate direct cell-cell interactions;
2. those involved in cell-matrix interactions.

Detailed biochemical analysis suggests that adherens junctions possess three structural domains:

- cytoskeletal actin filaments
- a plaque structure that links the filaments to membranes
- membrane components directly involved in mediating adhesive interactions (Geiger, 1992).

Although these junctions have many components in common, each also possesses specialized proteins. Thus, one family of integral membrane proteins, the cadherins, appears to be confined to cell-cell junctions, whereas another family, the integrins, is involved in cell-matrix junctions and cell-cell interactions.

CELL-CELL ADHERENS JUNCTIONS

In various cells, adherens junctions connect **actin filaments** in the cortical cytoplasm of adjacent cells; in epithelial sheets, these junctions form a continuous belt often referred to as the **zonula adherens** in histology texts (Figure 8–2). Bundles of contractile actin filaments run parallel to the plasma membrane in these epithelial sheets and are attached to the adhesion "belt" by a set of intracellular attachment proteins that include:

- alpha α-, beta β-, and gamma γ-catenin
- vinculin
- α-actinin.

Cadherins

Cell-cell adherens junctions are essential in the maintenance of solid tissues; the interacting adjacent membranes are held together by transmembrane Ca^{2+}-dependent adhesion receptors called **cadherins.** These molecules also have important functions in cell recognition and sorting during development. The cadherins comprise a superfamily of cell surface monotypic type I transmembrane glycoproteins that range in size from approximately 120 to 140 kDa. All vertebrate cells express cadherin-type molecules, which were originally named after the tissues from which they were discovered. To date, more than a dozen members of the cadherin family have been identified; some are listed in Table 8–3.

The different cadherin polypeptides share a high degree of amino acid sequence homology:

- Each can be divided into five ectodomains (EC1–EC5) of about 110 amino acids.
- Each shares between 52 and 73% amino acid identity across different species.

In addition, all cadherins have four invariant cysteine residues close to the transmembrane domain, and several motifs in the cytoplasmic tails are also conserved. A similar overall structure of the ectodomain is also present in the transmembrane proteins of desmosomes. These proteins are called **desmogleins** and **desmocollins.**

Role of calcium in cell-cell adhesion. The association of cadherins with the adherens junction requires calcium, as has been demonstrated in vitro by chelation of extracellular Ca^{2+} with the use of ethyleneglycoltetraacetic acid (EGTA). This causes the tissues to dissociate into individual cells, thereby demonstrating that cell-cell adhesion is a calcium-mediated reaction. In addition, cell-cell adhesion is also dependent on **homophilic** interactions between cadherin molecules; ie, cadherin molecules on one cell bind to and interact with the identical molecules on adjacent cells. In contrast, polypeptides that bind different molecules on adjacent cells are said to undergo **heterophilic** interactions.

Cadherin homophilic binding regions have been identified by x-ray crystallographic studies; these findings have also provided significant insight into how cadherins in adjacent cells interact. These studies suggest that in N-cadherin, the extracellular 1 (EC-1) domain from one cell forms a dimer that interacts with two adjacent EC-1 dimers in an antiparallel orientation by the adhesive binding domains, thus forming a continuous **cadherin zipper** at the cell contact zones (Figure 8–3).

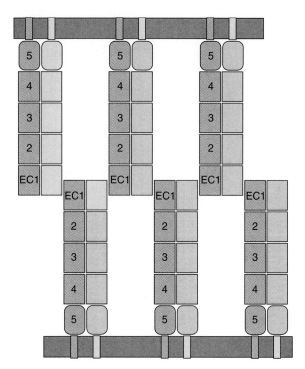

Figure 8–3. Cadherin-mediated cell adhesion. The cell membranes of adjacent cells (dark bands at top and bottom) have cadherin dimers protruding from the cell surfaces. The dimers associate tightly in antiparallel orientation to form a cadherin zipper along the line of cell-cell adhesion. The terminal, EC1 domain of the cadherin protein is thought to contain the adhesive activity in this model based on x-ray crystallographic studies. (Modified and reproduced, with permission, from Gumbiner B: Cell Adhesion. Cell 1996;84:34 copyright © 1993 by Cell Press.)

Table 8–3. Types of cadherins and their primary sites of action.

Type of Cadherin	Location
E-cadherin	Epithelial cells, skin, ovary, placenta, kidney
N-cadherin	Nerve, muscle, lens cells
P-cadherin	Placenta, epidermis
R-cadherin	Retina
Desmogleins and desmocollins	Cardiac skeletal muscle, epithelial cells

Catenins

Cadherins are transmembrane proteins that mediate interaction between the actin cytoskeletons of the cells, which they join together. Cadherins themselves, however, do not bind to the cortical actin cytoskeleton directly; rather, linker proteins called **catenins** attach the carboxyl terminus of cadherins to the actin filaments. At least three catenins—α, β, and γ—are known; the interaction between the cadherin molecule and catenins is essential for cell adhesion.

α-Catenin has been shown to possess actin-binding activity in vitro. Transfection of complementary deoxyribonucleic acid (DNA) encoding α-catenin into tissue culture cells that lack this protein can induce the formation of tightly adherent epithelial cells. α-Catenin is related to **vinculin,** a polypeptide that binds membrane proteins to the actin cortical cytoskeleton at sites of cell-cell and cell-ECM interaction. β-Catenin appears to be less essential for cell adhesion than α-catenin. β-Catenin binds α-catenin to the carboxyl tail of cadherins; α-catenin itself does not interact directly with cadherin molecules.

β-Catenin has recently been shown to

1. be a substrate for several tyrosine kinases that inhibit cell adhesion and
2. interact with the epidermal growth factor receptor.

These findings implicate β-catenin in the regulation of cell adhesion, and this putative regulatory role may influence cadherin-mediated cell-cell interactions during embryonic development. It is well established that embryonic tissue segregation correlates with the expression of different cadherin genes.

Embryonic patterning: *Armadillo* gene. β-Catenin is ~ 70% identical to a *Drosophila* segment polarity gene called *Armadillo.* This gene is one of a family that encodes the proteins required for cell fate determination during early embryonic development. Similarly, β-catenin is involved in regulating embryonic patterning in the frog *Xenopus laevis* and, in part, is responsible for regulating the formation of the dorsal-anterior body axis. These observations—and the demonstration that β-catenin can be phosphorylated on tyrosine residues—has led to the conclusion that β-catenin may regulate cadherin-catenin interaction.

CELL-MATRIX INTERACTIONS

Desmosomal Junctions

In contrast to adherens junctions, **desmosomes** link cytoskeletal **intermediate filaments** to the cell membrane (Chapter 7). By acting in and through adjacent cells, desmosomes and intermediate filaments form a network throughout tissues, and this network imparts high tensile strength on the tissue. In most epithelial cells, **cytokeratin filaments** are attached to desmosomes. In cardiac muscle cells, however, **desmin** filaments are the primary intermediate filament proteins. These proteins link myofibrils in the tubular system of cardiac skeletal muscle.

These cytoplasmic interfilament proteins are attached to a complex of intracellular attachment cytoplasmic **plaque** proteins called **desmoplakins** and **plakoglobin,** which interact with the cytoplasmic tail of transmembrane proteins. The transmembrane linker proteins in desmosomes—called **desmogleins** and **desmocollins**—are also members of the cadherin family. Although the ectodomains of these proteins and the cadherins are homologous, the amino acid sequences of their cytoplasmic tails differ. In part, it is these sequence differences in the carboxy terminal tail region that confer binding specificity toward intermediate filament proteins vs actin.

Desmosomal Junctions: Selected Clinical Correlates

The clinical importance of intermediate filament–desmosome interactions in maintaining tissue integrity—is demonstrated by several forms of the potentially fatal skin disease **pemphigus,** a genetic disease that leads to various forms of skin blistering. Patients who have one form of this disease, pemphigus vulgaris, have autoantibodies to desmoglein-3. These patients have severely blistered skin that results from loss of cell-cell adhesion during the early stages of keratinocyte differentiation into epidermal cells.

Another form of the disease, pemphigus foliaceus, is caused by autoantibodies to desmoglein-1; severe blistering occurs as a result of compromised cell-cell adhesion at a later stage in epidermal cell differentiation. Data from the phenotypes of patients with these diseases have provided genetic evidence that desmosomes—in concert with intermediate filament proteins—give the mechanical and tensile strength to maintain the intactness of the epidermis.

HEMIDESMOSOMES

Morphologically, hemidesmosomes have a similar appearance to desmosomes, but they are biochemically and functionally different. Hemidesmosomes attach epithelial cell basal plasma membranes to the **basal lamina,** a thin strip of ECM on which the cells sit; thus, hemidesmosomes promote cell-matrix interactions. In contrast to desmosomes, the transmembrane proteins that link the cells to the ECM belong to the **integrin** family of receptors rather than to cadherins (see Figure 1–3).

INTEGRINS

Integrins are heterodimeric receptors; ie, they possess two noncovalently associated subunits:

• the α subunit (~ 1000 amino acids)
• the β subunit (~ 750 residues).

Each is a type I **transmembrane glycoprotein.**

The integrins comprise a family of at least 20 different receptors with diverse specificity. Some integrins bind only a single component of the ECM: eg, fibronectin, collagen, or laminin. Other integrins interact with several of these polypeptides (Table 8–1). In contrast to hormone receptors, which have high affinity and low abundance, the integrins exhibit low affinity and high abundance. This means they can bind weakly to several different but related matrix molecules. This property allows the integrins to promote cell-cell interactions as well as cell-matrix binding. Indeed, cellular factors may interact with or modulate integrin binding specificity, because some integrins appear to manifest cell-specific ligand binding.

One essential factor for integrin receptor function is the presence of divalent cations—Ca^{2+} or Mg^{2+}—depending on a particular integrin. In addition, many matrix proteins are ligands for several different integrins; eg, eight isoforms of integrin interact with fibronectin, and presumably only some of these bind to the **RGD (Arg-Gly-Asp)** motif (Figure 8–4).

Integrins: Selected Clinical Correlates

As their name implies, integrins integrate and transduce signals from the ECM to the cytoskeleton by means of their transmembrane orientation. Members of the integrin family are classified according to their β-chains, of which nine separate polypeptides have been described. Because there are at least 14 α-subunits that can bind to more than one of the β-chains, an enormous diversity of ligand specificity is available. Some integrins are present on many cells

(eg, the $\alpha_5\beta_1$ fibronectin receptor and $\alpha_6\beta_4$ integrin that bind to laminin in the basal lamina). Many integrins, however, are cell specific. The $\alpha_L\beta_2$ integrin—also known as the lymphocyte function–associated integrin—is therefore present only on lymphocytes, as the designation implies. Indeed, integrins that possess β_2 subunits are present on white blood cells exclusively. These integrins are thought to function by enabling the cells to attach to and penetrate endothelial cells that line blood vessels at sites of infection.

Blood platelets also express β_2 integrins, which play a role in binding fibrinogen, von Willebrand factor, and fibronectin during blood clotting; such binding helps mediate platelet adhesion and aggregation around a clot. Patients who have a defect in α_2/β_3 subunits have normal numbers of platelets but abnormal clot retraction and bleeding; this condition is known as **Glanzmann's thrombasthenia.** Patients who have the disease **bullous pemphigoid** have autoantibodies that lead to destruction of the hemidesmosome basement membrane and hence loss of cell attachment. Most integrins interact on their cytoplasmic, carboxy terminal tails with actin-binding proteins in the cell cortex. During ligand binding, the β-subunits of integrins interact with both **talin** and **α-actinin,** which in turn initiate assembly of other attachment proteins that link integrins to actin filaments. This transmembrane attachment to the cytoskeleton is essential for cells to bind to the ECM. These interactions are also two-way signaling pathways; eg, the actin filaments can alter the orientation of secreted fibronectin molecules in the ECM. In addition, disruption of the actin cytoskeleton by cytochalasin treatment results in disorganization of secreted fibronectin filaments that normally align with intracellular stress fibers. Conversely, the ECM can profoundly influence the organization of the cytoskeleton in a target cell (Table 8–1). These integrin-mediated signaling events are discussed in more detail in Chapter 10.

GAP JUNCTIONS

Gap junctions, which are the most abundant cell junctions, are present in most tissues in all species (Figure 8–1). The designation stems from the electron microscopic appearance of this junction as a patch between adjacent cells, where the respective plasma membranes are separated by a narrow gap of 2–4 nm.

The gap consists of channel-forming proteins that allow the selective passage of small molecules of up to ~ 1000 daltons, eg, ions and low molecular weight metabolites. Gap junctions can therefore mediate both electrical and metabolic coupling between cells. Such interactions are clearly necessary for cells to respond to local changes in the environment, especially during development. The individual protein subunits

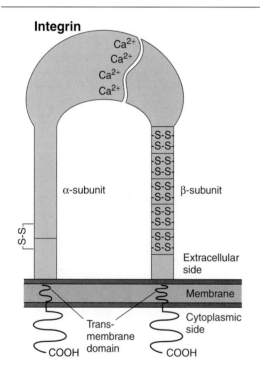

Figure 8–4. Integrin-mediated cell adhesion. In this diagram, integrin protrudes upward from the cell membrane. The binding of a divalent cation, Ca^{2+}, allows the N-terminal regions of the two protein subunits to associate with each other and to bind to the extracellular matrix. (Modified and reproduced, with permission, from Nermut MV et al: Electron microscopy and structural model of human fibronectin receptor. EMBO J 1988;7:4093.)

of each gap junction, called **connexins** (MW 26,000–54,000), are arranged as a ring-like structure of six identical subunits; each subunit is called a **connexon** (Figure 8–5). The alignment of two connexons from two adjacent cells results in the formation of an aqueous channel through which small molecules (< 1000 daltons) can pass. On freeze-fracture electron micrographs, gap junctions characteristically appear as clusters of intramembranous particles. The aqueous pore of the junction—diameter ~ 1.5 nm—does

not open permanently to allow the flux of ions and small metabolites. Similar to voltage-gated channels, however, gap junctions can rapidly oscillate between an open and closed state. Individual connexin polypeptides presumably undergo reversible conformational changes that translate into opening and closing of the channel. Like many cellular components whose electron microscopic appearance might suggest a static structure, gap junctions are actually quite dynamic.

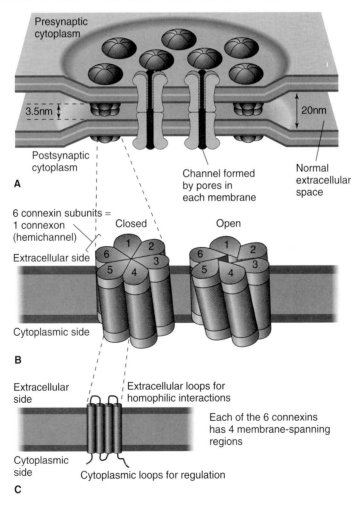

Figure 8–5. Gap junction. This model of a synapse demonstrates intercellular communication through channel-forming proteins. Each of the two cells involved (A) contributes half of the communication channel, a hemichannel. Each hemichannel, or connexon (B), consists of six connexin subunits. Orientation of the subunits determines whether the hemichannel is open or closed. Communication between cells can occur when both hemichannels are open. The placement of each connexin subunit within the cell membrane (C) is also shown. (Modified and reproduced from Kandel ER et al: *Essentials of Neural Science and Behavior.* Appleton & Lange, 1995, p. 190.)

EXTRACELLULAR MATRIX

The ground substance or **ECM** of all cells is not simply an inert mass of packing material that cushions and supports the cells. Although this is certainly one function of the ECM, which comprises a network of intermeshed macromolecules that include collagen, polysaccharides, and glycoproteins, the ECM also participates in such key processes as

- signal transduction
- maintenance of cell shape
- cell development (ie, cell migration and growth).

These processes are mediated by growth factors and hormones, as well as by small molecules. The pancreas, thyroid, and spleen, for example, are encapsulated by a dense, fibrous matrix that anastomoses throughout the organ and divides it into increasingly small functional units. This concentrated ECM constitutes the **connective tissue.** Connective tissue is very important because it provides a supporting matrix for tissues and imparts tensile strength, as well as the ability to resist compression on tissues.

FIBROBLASTS & THEIR CELLULAR PRODUCTS

The ECM is produced locally by **fibroblasts** that secrete

- glycosaminoglycans (GAGs)
- collagen, elastin, fibronectin, laminin and other proteins.

The GAGs are polysaccharide chains that are usually covalently attached to proteins to form **proteoglycans,** which in turn complex with water to form a flexible gel-like substance that can resist compression, much like rubber or sponge packing material. Collagen fibers that run through and are embedded in this gel matrix provide tensile strength, not unlike steel rods embedded in reinforced concrete. Proteins such as **fibronectin** promote attachment of cells to the ECM, whereas **laminin** facilitates cell binding to the basal lamina.

Basal Lamina

The basal lamina is a tough, thin, sheet-like structure that provides a substratum on which cells sit; it is also important for cell differentiation and tissue remodeling. The **basal lamina**—sometimes called basement membrane, which is an older and some-

what misleading term—is composed of proteoglycans, glycoproteins, type IV collagen, and laminin.

In addition to providing a support function, in some tissues the basal lamina acts as a molecular sieve for the selective filtration of small molecules from the blood. This occurs, for example, in the renal glomerulus (Hudson et al, 1993). Each component of the ECM is discussed in the following section, which addresses the key role in signal transduction and cell differentiation played by various ECM molecules and the structures they generate.

EXTRACELLULAR MATRIX IN SIGNAL TRANSDUCTION & CELL DIFFERENTIATION

Major Properties of GAGs

The polysaccharide chains that comprise GAGs consist of repeating unbranched disaccharide units up to 200 sugars long. One sugar is always an amino sugar (N-acetylglucosamine or N-acetylgalactosamine)—hence the name, glycosaminoglycan; frequently GAGs are also sulfated. The other sugar of the disaccharide repeat is glucuronic acid or iduronic acid. The presence of sulfate or carboxyl groups imparts a large net negative charge. Two major properties of GAGs are

1. They can form gels that have a large volume even at a low concentration of GAG
2. Their high distribution of negative charge results in strong cation binding.

Because GAGs are very hydrophilic, they can readily absorb water, which causes the matrix to swell significantly. This ability to swell enables the matrix to withstand huge compression forces; consequently, many joints in the body have a cartilaginous matrix rich in GAGs. When you jump, for example, the shock of landing is partially absorbed by the cushioning that GAGs impart on the knee and ankle joints.

Major GAG Groups

On the basis of their sugar residues, GAGs are divided into four major groups:

1. hyaluronic acid, which is the only GAG that lacks sulfate and is not covalently linked to protein;
2. chondroitin sulfate and dermatan sulfate;
3. heparan sulfate and heparin;
4. keratin sulfate.

Hyaluronan (hyaluronate or hyaluronic acid). Hyaluronan consists of an unbranched chain of up to 12,000 glucuronic acids and N-acetylglucosamine disaccharide repeating units. A diagnostic feature of this GAG is that it lacks sulfate. Unlike other GAGs, hyaluronic acid is not attached to protein. It is distributed in many tissues as a component of loose connective tissue and is also found in the synovial fluid of joints, where it acts as a lubricant. Some cells of the ECM possess hyaluronic acid–binding proteins. Hyaluronic acid is also thought to function during embryonic development, where it acts as filler in intracellular spaces into which cells can migrate; it is also produced in large amounts during wound repair (Figure 8–6; Table 8–4).

Proteoglycans

All GAGs, except hyaluronic acid, are covalently attached to protein backbones to form **proteoglycans.** Because the protein is secreted, it possesses a signal peptide that targets the protein and facilitates translocation across the endoplasmic reticulum (ER). Unlike the synthesis of N-linked glycoproteins, however, where the core carbohydrate is added en bloc during protein translocation, the GAG chains are added later in the secretory pathway, ie, in the Golgi apparatus. The initial linkage present in all proteoglycans is a set of four core sugars, **xylose–galactose–galactose–glucuronic acid,** which is linked to serine residues. Because the serine is linked via oxygen,

such carbohydrates are often referred to as **O-linked** (Figure 8–6B).

After the addition of the tetrasaccharide core, specific glycosyl transferase enzymes add one sugar residue at a time. This process most likely occurs in the cisternae of the late Golgi apparatus and the *trans* Golgi network. In proteoglycans, up to 95% of the mass can be contributed by the carbohydrate side chains—mostly as long unbranched GAG chains. The core protein can also be a glycoprotein and, hence, can also possess N-linked carbohydrates. As a result of the variation in repeating disaccharide units and in the protein backbone, proteoglycans are extremely heterogeneous in size and composition. Given this diversity, it is not surprising that these large complex macromolecules have many different functions and are involved in:

1. Formation of matrices of variable pore size and charge around cells; these matrices can regulate the movement of small molecules through the gelatinous matrix of the ECM.
2. Intercellular signaling by acting as receptors for growth factors and peptides, eg, fibroblast growth factor. The activity of these ligands can be modulated (see below).

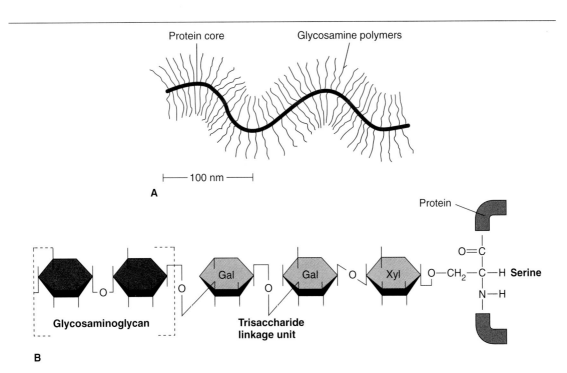

Figure 8–6. Glycosaminoglycans. The basic structure of a proteoglycan—protein core and attached glycosamine polymers—is shown in overview (A). The individual linkage relationship between a glycosaminoglycan (GAG) and the protein core is also shown (B). Note that hyaluronic acid, as discussed in the text, is different from other GAGs: It is not attached to a protein molecule. (Modified and reproduced, with permission, from Zubay G: *Biochemistry,* 3rd ed. Brown, 1993.)

Table 8–4. Composition and distribution of glycosaminoglycans in connective tissue and their interations with collagen fibers.[1]

| Glycosaminoglycan | Repeating Disaccharides | | Distribution | Electrostatic Interaction with Collagen |
	Hexuronic Acid	Hexosamine		
Hyaluronic acid	D-glucuronic acid	D-glucosamine	Umbilical cord, synovial fluid, vitreous humor, cartilage	. . .
Chondroitin 4-sulfate	D-glucuronic acid	D-galactosamine	Cartilage, bone, cornea, skin, notochord, aorta	High levels of interaction, mainly with collagen type II
Chondroitin 6-sulfate	D-glucuronic acid	D-galactosamine	Cartilage, umbilical cord, skin, aorta (media)	High levels of interaction, mainly with collagen type II
Dermatan sulfate	D-iduronic acid or D-glucuronic acid	D-galactosamine	Skin, tendon, aorta (adventitia)	Low levels of interaction, mainly with collagen type I
Heparan sulfate	D-glucuronic acid or D-iduronic acid	D-galactosamine	Aorta, lung, liver, basal laminae	Intermediate levels of interaction, mainly with collagen types III and IV
Keratan sulfate (cornea)	D-galactose	D-galactosamine	Cornea	None
Keratan sulfate (skeleton)	D-galactose	D-glucosamine	Cartilage, nucleus pulposus, annulus fibrosus	None

[1]From Junquiera LC et al: *Basic Histology,* 8th ed. Appleton & Lange, 1995, p. 90, with permission.

3. Binding other secreted proteins: Some secreted proteases and inhibitors interact with proteoglycans, whose function may be to modulate enzyme activity at the site of secretion. This may play a role in the inflammatory response, wound repair, and the regulation of tumor metastasis.

In addition to forming essential components of the ECM, proteoglycans can be present on the plasma membrane of cells, where some, eg, the **syndecans,** function as receptor molecules. These proteoglycan molecules possess a transmembrane domain and function as fibronectin and collagen receptors. The cytoplasmic tails of these proteoglycans can interact with the cortical actin cytoskeleton (cf, cadherins and integrins) and thus provide a link between the ECM and the cytoskeleton (Table 8–5).

COLLAGEN

Collagens are the most abundant protein in mammals and the major component of connective tissue. They comprise a family of fibrous proteins secreted by fibroblasts and connective tissue cells. A characteristic feature of a collagen molecule is its long rigid triple-helical structure: three collagen polypeptide chains—called α-chains—are woven around each other into a right-handed superhelix that forms a rod-like molecule.

Collagens have the following characteristics:

1. They are rich in **proline** and **glycine** residues, both of which facilitate the formation of triple helices. Every third residue of the α-chain is a glycine, the only amino acid that can be accommodated in the central core of the helix.
2. Approximately 25 separate collagen α-chains have been identified; each is encoded by a separate gene, and different combinations of α-chains are expressed in different tissues.
3. To date, approximately 15 types of collagen molecules have been found.
4. Collagens possess **hydroxyproline** and **hydroxylysine** residues that are generated by the post-

Table 8–5. Proteoglycans and their location.

Proteoglycan	Location and Role
Chondroitin sulfate	Major component of cartilage
Dermatan sulfate	Widely distributed
Heparan sulfate	Many cell surfaces; skin fibroblasts
Heparin	Mast cells; anticoagulant (binds antithrombin III)
Keratin sulfate	Cornea, loose connective tissue

translational hydroxylation of proline and lysine residues. The formation of these residues is catalyzed by the enzymes prolyl hydroxylase and lysyl hydroxylase, respectively.

Connective tissue collagen consists of several different collagens; **type I** is the most abundant (Table 8–6). These types of collagen are designated **fibrillar** and have the rope-like triple helix structure.

Collagen Biosynthesis

Collagen biosynthesis involves extensive post-translational modifications. Collagen polypeptides are secreted into the extracellular space and assembled into ordered polymers of collagen **fibrils** that (1) are 10–300 nm in diameter and (2) can be several hundred micrometers long. These fibrils aggregate into bundles of collagen fibers, which are cable-like structures up to 3 mm in diameter. The collagen fibrils are cross-linked to each other and to other ECM components by fibril-associated collagens (types IX and XII); these cross-links are essential for the tensile strength of collagen. Types IV and VII are network-forming collagens, and type IV is a major constituent of the basal lamina (Table 8–7).

Procollagen

Characteristic of secreted proteins, collagens are synthesized as precursors with a signal peptide that targets them to the ER. Collagens also have a **propeptide** at the N- and C-terminus of 20 and 30 kDa, respectively. The propeptides are cleaved after secretion of the collagen triple helices. After translocation into the lumen of the ER, selected proline and lysine residues are hydroxylated by their respective hydroxylases, in reactions that require ascorbic acid—vitamin C—to form hydroxyproline and hydroxylysine. The pro-α-chains then combine in the lumen of the ER to form the hydrogen-bonded triple helix **procollagen.**

It is thought that the hydroxyl groups of hydroxyproline and lysine form interchain hydrogen bonds that stabilize the triple helix. In addition, the N- and C-terminal propeptides form **disulfide bonds** in the oxidizing atmosphere of the ER lumen; these disulfide bonds are also thought to facilitate formation of the triple helix. The secreted forms of fibrillar collagens are proteolytically processed to mature collagen molecules in the extracellular space by removal of the N- and C-terminal propeptides by specific amino- and carboxypeptidases. On removal of the propeptides, the triple helical molecules assemble into fibers (Figure 8–7).

Procollagen is relatively soluble, whereas the mature molecule is insoluble. It is therefore thought that the propeptides serve two functions during collagen biosynthesis:

Table 8–6. Types of collagen and their genes.[1,2]

Type	Genes	Tissue
I	COL1A1, COL1A2,	Most connective tissues, including bone
II	COL2A1	Cartilage, vitreous humor
III	COL3A1	Extensible connective tissue such as skin, lung, and the vascular system
IV	COL4A1–COL4A6	Basement membranes
V	COL5A1–COL5A3	Minor component in tissues containing collagen I
VI	COL6A1–COL6A3	Most connective tissues
VII	COL7A1	Anchoring fibrils
VIII	COL8A1–COL8A2	Endothelium, other tissues
IX	COL9A1–COL9A3	Tissues containing collagen II
X	COL10A1	Hypertrophic cartilage
XI	COL11A1, COL11A2, COL2A1	Tissues containing collagen II
XII	COL12A1	Tissues containing collagen I
XIII	COL13A1	Many tissues
XIV	COL14A1	Tissues containing collagen I
XV	COL15A1	Many tissues
XVI	COL16A1	Many tissues
XVII	COL17A1	Skin hemidesmosomes
XVIII	COL18A1	Many tissues (eg, liver, kidney)
XIX	COL19A1	Rhabdomyosarcoma cells

[1]Adapted, from Prockop DJ, Kivirrikko KI: Collagens: molecular biology, diseases, and potentials for therapy. Annu Rev Biochem 1995;64:403, with permission.
[2]The types of collagen are designated by Roman numerals. Constituent procollagen chains, called proα chains, are numbered using Arabic numerals, followed by the collagen type in parentheses. For instance, type I procollagen is assembled from two proα1(I) chains and one proα2(I) chain and is thus a heterotrimer. Type 2 procollagen is assembled from three proα1(II) chains and is thus a homotrimer. The collagen genes are named according to the collagen type, written in Arabic numerals for the gene symbol, followed by an A and the number of the proα chain that they encode. Thus, the COL1A1 and COL1A2 genes encode the α1 and α2 chains of type I collagen, respectively.

1. to facilitate intracellular formation of triple helices;
2. to prevent intracellular formation of collagen fibrils, which would block the secretory pathway because collagen is insoluble.

In the extracellular space, mature collagen molecules form fibrils close to the cell surface, often

Table 8–7. Main characteristics of the different collagen types.[1]

Collagen Type	Tissue Distribution	Appearance (Light Microscope)	Ultrastructure	Site of Synthesis	Interaction with Glycosaminoglycans	Main Function
I	Dermis, bone, tendon, dentin, fascias, sclera, organ capsules, fibrous cartilage	Closely packed, thick collagen fibers	Densely packed thick fibrils with marked variation in diameter	Fibroblast, osteoblast, odontoblast, chondroblast	Low level of interaction, mainly with dermatan sulfate	Resistance to tension
II	Hyaline and elastic cartilages	Loose, collagenous network	No fibers: very thin fibrils embedded in abundant ground substance	Chondroblast	High level of interaction, mainly with chondroitin sulfates	Resistance to intermittent pressure
III	Smooth muscle, endoneurium, arteries, uterus, liver, spleen, kidney, lung	Loose network of thin fibers; reticular fibers	Loosely packed thin fibrils with more uniform diameters	Smooth muscle, fibroblast, reticular cells, Schwann cells, hepatocyte	Intermediate level of interaction, mainly with heparan sulfate	Structural maintenance in expansible organs
IV	Epithelial and endothelial basal laminae and basement membranes	Thin, amorphous membrane	Neither fibers nor fibrils detected	Endothelial and epithelial cells, muscle cells, and Schwann cells	Interaction with heparan sulfate	Support and filtration
V	Muscle basal laminae	Insufficient data	Insufficient data	Insufficient data	Insufficient data	Insufficient data

[1]Modified from Junquiera LC et al: *Basic Histology,* 8th ed. Appleton & Lange, 1995, p. 94, with permission.

within invaginations of the plasma membrane. Mature collagen fibers have a characteristic morphology when observed at the electron microscopic level: They possess **cross-striations** every 67 nm, which result from the staggered packing of individual collagen polypeptides in the fibril (Figure 8–8).

Collagen Tensile Strength

After the formation of collagen fibrils, cross-linking between lysine residues to form both intra- and interchain cross-links greatly enhances the tensile strength of the collagen fibrils. Depending on the tissue, collagen fibrils have different diameters and orientations that have evolved to perform specialized functions. In skin, for example, the fibrils are arranged in a wickerwork crisscross pattern that enables the tissue to resist shearing stresses in many different directions; in tendons, the fibrils are aligned in parallel bundles along the axis of tension.

This specific orientation of the collagen fibers may be facilitated by fibril-associated collagens (types IX and XII). These collagens bind to the surface of the

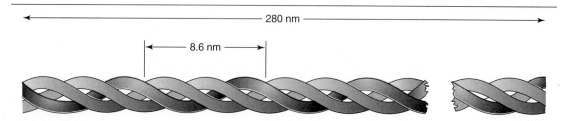

Figure 8–7. Collagen. All types of collagen have the same basic structure of three α chains wrapped around each other to form a right-handed helix. Every third amino acid residue is glycine, which enables the chains to wrap into the tight, rope-like structure. Each complete helical turn is 8.6 nm in length. A collagen fibril may be several hundred micrometers long. (From Junqueira LC et al: *Basic Histology,* 8th ed. Appleton & Lange. 1995, p. 94, with permission.)

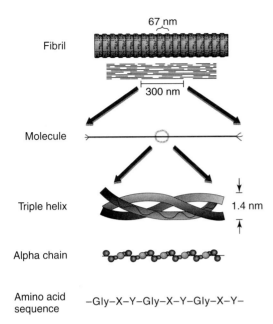

Fibril

67 nm

300 nm

Molecule

Triple helix

1.4 nm

Alpha chain

Amino acid sequence

–Gly–X–Y–Gly–X–Y–Gly–X–Y–

Figure 8–8. Organization of collagen. The amino acid sequence of each α chain is shown at the bottom and the association of molecules into fibrils is depicted at the top. In electron micrographs, collagen fibrils show a characteristic cross striation at intervals of 67 nm. The cross striation is due to the staggered positioning of collagen polypeptides within the fibril. (Modified and reproduced, with permission, from Eyre DR: Collagen: molecular diversity in the body's protein scaffold. Science 1980; 207:1315. Copyright 1980 American Association for the Advancement of Science.)

fibrils with a distinct periodicity and interact with both the fibrils and with other matrix components, thereby regulating the organization of the fibrils.

Type IV Collagen

Basal lamina specific; nonfibrillar. Like fibrillar collagen, the monomeric unit of type IV collagen is also a triple helical molecule composed of three α-chains (Tables 8–6 and 8–7); each chain has a long collagenous domain of ~ 1400 Gly-X-Y repeats. At the N-terminus, type IV collagen has an ~ 15–amino acid noncollagenous sequence, and the carboxyl terminus possesses a long noncollagenous domain (~ 200 residues). Each chain is highly glycosylated with ~ 50 hydroxylysine-linked disaccharides, as well as an asparagine-linked oligosaccharide near the N-terminus (Hudson et al, 1993).

The triple helices self-associate to form a superstructure, and this involves several different interactions. Monomeric triple helices therefore associate at the carboxy termini to form dimers and at the amino terminus to form tetramers. The N-terminal 15-residue noncollagenous sequence has four cysteine residues that are thought to participate in forming intra- and interchain disulfide bonds that stabilize these macromolecules. In addition to end-to-end interactions, the triple helices can intertwine to form supercoiled structures. Furthermore, Type IV collagen is a family of six genetically distinct α-chains. This genetic diversity is reflected in the existence of several different triple helices of different chain composition (Tables 8–6 and 8–7).

Clinical Correlates:
Collagen Diseases

Several genetic diseases involve defective collagen biosynthesis. Various genetic defects result in incomplete assembly, destabilized triple helices, defective cross-linking of collagen, or other lesions. Mutations can result in defective post-translation modifications that involve, for example, lysine hydroxylase, or in the absence of procollagen biosynthesis (Table 8–8).

Menkes disease. Menkes disease is associated with a defect in the metabolism of copper. Because lysine oxidase, which mediates collagen cross-linking, is a copper-requiring enzyme, the activity level of lysine oxidase is diminished in patients who have

Table 8–8. Examples of clinical disorders resulting from defects in collagen synthesis.[1]

Gene or Enzyme	Disorder	Defect	Symptoms
COL3A1	Ehlers-Danlos type IV	Faulty transcription or translation of type III	Aortic and/or intestinal rupture
Lysyl hydroxylase	Ehlers-Danlos type VI	Faulty lysine hydroxylation	Augmented skin elasticity, rupture of eyeball
Procollagen N-proteinase	Ehlers-Danlos type VII	Decrease in procollagen peptidase activity	Increased articular mobility, frequent luxation
—	Scurvy	Lack of vitamin C (cofactor for proline hydroxylase)	Ulceration of gums, hemorrhages
COL1A1, COL1A2	Osteogenesis imperfecta	Change of one nucleotide in genes for collagen type I	Spontaneous fractures, cardiac insufficiency

[1]Modified from Junquiera LC et al: *Basic Histology,* 8th ed. Appleton & Lange, 1995, p. 98, with permission.

Table 8–9. Major differences between collagen and elastin.[1]

Collagen	Elastin
Many different genetic types	One genetic type
Triple helix	No triple helix; random coil conformations permitting stretching
(Gly-X-Y)$_n$ repeating structure	No (Gly-X-Y)$_n$ repeating structure
Presence of hydroxylysine	No hydroxylysine
Carbohydrate-containing	No carbohydrate
Intramolecular aldol cross-links	Intramolecular desmosine cross-links
Presence of extension peptides during biosynthesis	No extension peptides present during biosynthesis

[1]From Murray RK et al: *Harper's Biochemistry*, 24th ed. Appleton & Lange, 1996, p. 671, with permission.

this disease. The result is incompletely cross-linked collagen molecules.

Goodpasture syndrome. Goodpasture syndrome, which is an autoimmune disease characterized by glomerulonephritis and pulmonary hemorrhage, is caused by autoantibodies that bind to the basal laminae of renal glomerular and pulmonary alveolar cells. The α_3 (IV) chain of collagen is the component of the basal lamina that is recognized by—and binds to—the autoantibodies. These antibodies presumably prevent collagen dimers from forming efficiently, thereby leading to defects in suprastructure assembly.

Alport syndrome. Another genetic disease, **Alport syndrome,** affects approximately 1 in 5000 individuals and leads to renal failure in males; females are less severely affected. This inherited kidney disease causes defects in the glomerular basal lamina and is associated with mutations in the gene encoding the α_5 (IV) collagen chain (Table 8–9) (Hudson et al, 1993).

FIBRONECTIN

Fibronectin is a major, ubiquitous, insoluble glycoprotein component of the ECM and is also present in body fluids as a soluble molecule (Figure 8–9A). Fibronectin is secreted as a dimer. The monomers have a molecular weight of 220,000–250,000 and are linked by two disulfide bonds located near their carboxy termini. The fibronectins are multidomain proteins (Figure 8–9A) and possess binding sites for sev-

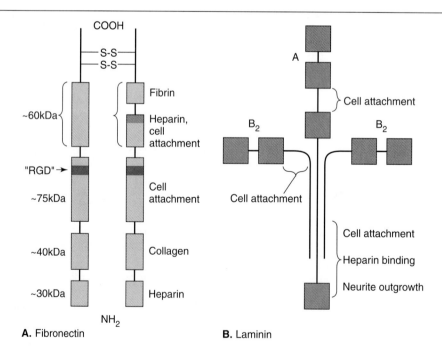

Figure 8–9. Fibronectin and laminin, constituents of the extracellular matrix (ECM). Fibronectin (A) is a glycoprotein dimer joined by disulfide bridges near the carboxyl terminals of each monomer. It has multiple domains that can bind to cells or other components of the ECM. Fibronectin facilitates cell adhesion to the ECM through binding of integrin (see Figure 8–4). Laminin (B) is a glycoprotein found in large quantities in the basal lamina. It consists of three chains held together by disulfide bonds. Laminin has binding domains for type IV collagen and for integrin, thus acting as an intermediate in cell adhesion to the basal lamina. (Modified and reproduced, with permission, from Kandel ER et al: *Principles of Neural Science,* 3rd ed. Appleton & Lange, 1991, p. 920.)

eral other ECM components, including collagen, heparins A and B, fibrin, and chondroitin sulfate. Much information on the structure of these different domains has been obtained because their tertiary structure has been determined with the use of high-resolution nuclear magnetic resonance techniques (see Gumbiner, 1996).

Integrin-Fibronectin Receptor: Clinical Implications for Some Metastases

Fibronectins have rod-like domains that are separated by flexible regions; these domains consist of a series of repeating amino acids encoded by separate exons. One of the best understood motifs in fibronectin is the RGD tripeptide sequence—the one letter code for these amino acids. This sequence motif is recognized by special cell surface receptors: integrins that bind to fibronectin. Moreover, the RGD motif is present in several proteins of the ECM in addition to fibronectin, eg, collagen and laminin. Fibronectin is encoded by a single gene with more than 50 kilobases and 50 exons. Alternate splicing gives rise to approximately 20 different fibronectin isomers that are expressed in cells in a tissue-specific and de-

velopmentally regulated fashion. The protein assembles in the ECM as insoluble filaments in which the dimers are cross-linked by disulfide bonds; the assembly process occurs on the cell surface and probably requires assembly factors released from the cell.

The function of fibronectin is to facilitate adhesion of cells to the ECM through binding to its integrin receptor. This allows the cellular exterior to communicate with the interior. Fibronectin also plays an important function in mediating cell migration by binding cells and facilitating their movement through the ECM. Indeed, the level of fibronectin is reduced in transformed cells, thereby leading to the speculation that decreased cell binding to the ECM allows greater mobility and thus may contribute to some metastases.

LAMININ

Like type IV collagen, **laminin** is an extremely abundant component of the basal lamina (Figure 8–9B). It is a large elongated glycoprotein—MW 850,000 and ~ 70 nm long—that is composed of three distinct chains designated A, B1, and B2. These

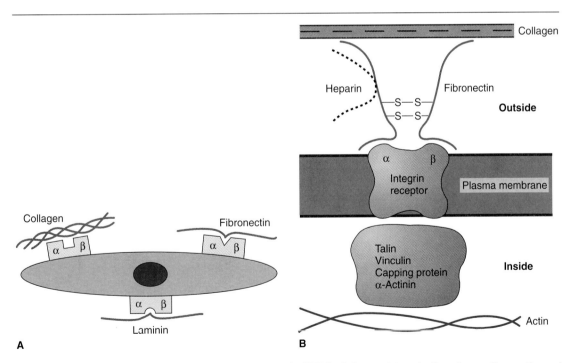

Figure 8–10. Cellular interaction with the extracellular matrix (ECM). Cells can interact with collagen, fibronectin, and laminin through the binding of these ECM components to integrin (A). The integrin binding site is shown diagrammatically as a block in the cell membrane containing α and β subunits. The fibronectin-mediated interaction between a cell and collagen (B) is also shown. Additional external interaction is represented by heparin binding to fibronectin; internal interaction by actin binding to integrin. (A, redrawn after Yamada KM: Adhesive recognition sequences. J Biol Chem 1991;266:12809. B, modified and reproduced, with permission, from Murray RK: *Harper's Biochemistry,* 24th ed. Appleton & Lange, 1996, p. 672.)

polypeptides are arranged in the form of an **elongated cross,** and the individual chains are held together by disulfide bonds. Like fibronectin, laminin has a distinct domain structure; different regions of the molecule bind to type IV collagen, heparin sulfate, entactin (a short protein that cross-links each laminin to type IV collagen), and cell surface **integrins.** The interaction between type IV collagen and laminin is thought to anchor the basal lamina to cells because collagen does not bind integrins directly; this attachment occurs through its interaction with laminin (Figure 8–10).

ENTACTIN

Entactin is a cell attachment glycoprotein of major importance. It contains an RGD motif and binds tightly to both laminin molecules and type IV collagen. Entactin is thought to function as a cross-linker between type IV collagen and laminin, thereby facilitating interactions between the cell and the basal lamina.

CELL ADHESION MOLECULES

Cell adhesion molecules (CAMs) facilitate **calcium-independent cell-cell adhesion.** These molecules are related structurally to immunoglobulin polypeptides because they possess domains similar to those present in immunoglobulin molecules. The **neural CAM (N-CAM)** is expressed in nerve and other cells and is one of the best characterized members of this complex family of polypeptides. N-CAMs bind cells together by **homophilic interac-**

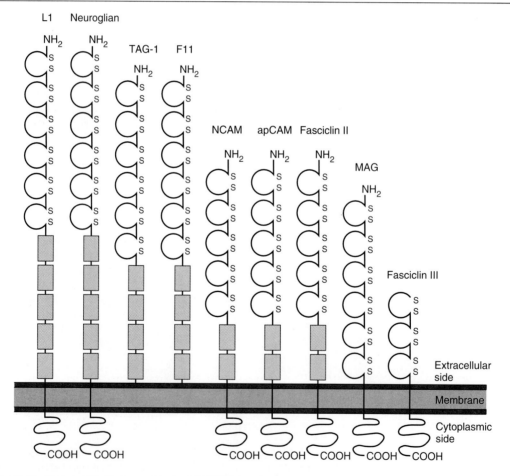

Figure 8–11. Neural cell adhesion molecules (N-CAMs). In this diagram, an N-CAM is shown at the center of a family of structurally related molecules. All of the adhesion molecules share the characteristic of immunoglobulin loops within the extracellular portion of the protein. N-CAMs bind cells to each other through homophilic interactions. Studies have indicated N-CAMs play a significant role during neural development. (Modified and reproduced, with permission, from Kandel ER et al: *Principles of Neural Science,* 3rd ed. Appleton & Lange, 1991, p. 919.)

tions between N-CAM polypeptides on adjacent cells. In addition, another class of CAMs—**I-CAMs**—promote intercellular adhesion by **heterophilic** binding; ie, I-CAMs bind to their cell surface proteins rather than to other I-CAMs.

N-CAMs

N-CAMs are a heterogenous family of approximately 20 related molecules that are derived by alternate splicing of a ribonucleic acid (RNA) transcript from a single N-CAM gene. These molecules are a somewhat heterogeneous family of high molecular monotypic type I transmembrane proteins and are thought to be involved in signaling and binding to cytoskeletal proteins. Alternate splicing gives rise to isoforms of N-CAMs that have the same extracellular sequence, containing five immunoglobulin repeats but a different carboxyl terminus. At least three forms of N-CAM have been described:

- type I transmembrane N-CAMs
- N-CAMs attached to the membrane via a glycosylphosphatidyl inositol anchor
- secreted forms of N-CAM.

Several N-CAMs are highly glycosylated and possess multiple repeating sialic acid residues that impart a net negative charge on the molecule (Figure 8–11). The function of these highly charged N-CAMs is unclear; it is thought that very negatively charged sialic residues promote an outgrowth of nerve processes during development. Indeed, N-CAMs have been implicated in several developmental processes:

1. binding of cells together, although cell-cell interactions by cadherins are much stronger;
2. promotion of nerve outgrowth, ie, nerve processes growing from the retina to the brain;
3. transient expression during development of non-neural tissues;
4. regulation of cell-cell adhesion interactions during development.

SIGNAL TRANSDUCTION & CELL ADHESION

When macromolecules present in the ECM are extracted and added to cells grown in tissue culture, they have a profound effect on the shape, movement, polarity, and differentiation of those cells. Many of these phenotypic changes are mediated by integrins that cluster at sites of contact with matrix components and active intracellular signaling pathways, for example, pathways that involve inositol phospholipid metabolism and tyrosine kinase cascades.

The activation of these integrin-mediated signal transduction events is analogous to that of hormone-receptor signaling at the plasma membrane of target cells. Interestingly, the response of many cells—including epithelial cells—to certain polypeptide growth factors also requires the involvement of integrins. For example, cells grown in tissue culture are

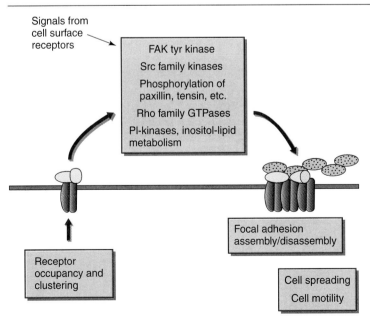

Figure 8–12. Regulation of integrin-mediated cell adhesion. Cell surface signaling events mediated by ligand-receptor binding cause integrin polypeptides to cluster together. Clustering leads to focal adhesion assembly and disassembly, both of which are essential for cell mobility and spreading. Analogous signaling events occur when surface growth-factor receptors are stimulated by ligand binding. Subsequent events due to receptor activation may also be involved in regulation of focal adhesion assembly and disassembly. (Modified and reproduced, with permission, from Gumbiner B: Cell adhesion. Cell 1996;84:345. Copyright © 1993 by Cell Press.) See also Figures 10–16 and 10–17.

refractory to growth factors unless they are attached to the ECM by integrins; when the latter occurs, the growth factor can cause cell differentiation (Figure 8–12).

Phosphorylation of the cytoplasmic tail of integrins plays an important role in their signaling function. In some cancer cells grown in tissue culture, phosphorylation of a tyrosine residue on the cytoplasmic tail reduces the affinity of the integrin-talin interaction, which is thought to lead to diminished adhesion of some cancer cells to fibronectin.

REFERENCES

Geiger B, Ayalon O: Cadherins. Annu Rev Cell Biol 1992;8:307.

Gumbiner B: Cell adhesion: The molecular basis of tissue architecture and morphogenesis. Cell 1996;84:345.

Hudson BG, Reeders ST, Tryggvason K: Type IV collagen: Structure, gene organization, and role in human diseases. J Biol Chem 1993;268:26033.

Mecham RP: Laminin receptors. Annu Rev Cell Biol 1991;7:71.

Schwartz MA, Schaller MD, Ginsberg MH: Integrins: Emerging paradigms of signal transduction. Annu Rev Cell Dev Biol 1995;11:549.

Stanley JR: Autoantibodies against adhesion molecules and structures in blistering skin diseases. J Exp Med 1995; 181:1.

Molecular Mechanisms in Signal Transduction: Basic Cell Signaling Pathways

9

KEY TERMS

Phosphorylation
Second messengers
Signaling molecules
Signaling pathways
Nitric oxide
Lipophilic-nuclear receptors
Ion-channel receptors
Eicosanoids
G protein–coupled receptors
G protein activation cascade
cAMP pathway
Calcium pathway
IP$_3$-pathway

This chapter focuses on the ways cells receive, process, and respond to biomolecular signals that arrive from extracellular origins. Mechanisms used by a cell in response to a particular signal typically involve a cascade of molecules that form an **integrated pathway** of chemical reactions. The eukaryotic cell can react to many types of information-carrying molecules. Fortunately, a number of common features among different pathways make it possible to understand and predict a cellular response to signaling molecules. Hormones—both steroid and polypeptide—are among the most familiar **exogenous signaling molecules;** however, the cell also responds to many other biomolecular signals.

Although subtle variations exist in signaling pathways, it appears that most cells follow similar intracellular pathways and often use the same **enzyme cascades,** regardless of the type of signaling molecule.

When a signal arrives at the cell surface to alert the cell to follow a certain course of action—eg, to begin cell proliferation—an integrated complex of pathways is initiated. An incoming signal usually leads to different responses in the different cells. The specificity of the cellular response is largely determined by the type of **receptor** that the cell expresses. Each cell type has a complement of receptors on its surface, cytosol, or nucleus. These receptors are designed to receive a specific signal and initiate an enzymatic cascade that leads to a cellular response.

The overall scheme of the signaling process is simple and involves five fundamental steps (Figure 9–1). Each stage in the signaling pathway corresponds to a point at which signal variations can occur; defects in the signaling process can lead to physiologic abnormalities and, possibly, human disease, as discussed in this chapter.

PHOSPHORYLATION & CELL SIGNALING

The reversible formation and hydrolysis of phosphate ester bonds are among the most crucial chemical reactions carried out by living organisms. Phosphate ester chemistry is central to the determination of genetic material, protein translation, biological membranes, and many other reactions in the cell. Phosphorylation and dephosphorylation are the key underlying events in signal transduction pathways; therefore, the two classes of enzymes that play a major role in these processes—kinases and phosphatases—also play a crucial role in cell signaling.

KINASES & PHOSPHATASES

The enzymes responsible for forming phosphate esters on proteins are called **kinases.** The two general types of kinases are the **tyrosine (Tyr)** and **serine-threonine (Ser-Thr)** kinases, and the Tyr kinases generate phosphate esters on selected Tyr residues of specific substrates. The **Ser-Thr kinases** form phosphate esters on selected Ser or Thr residues. It is estimated that the cell has more than a thousand different kinase enzymes, which suggests that these enzymes

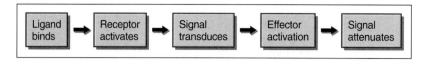

Figure 9–1. The five major steps in cellular signal transduction.

are major participants in cellular function. For example, the processing of hundreds of different messages by cells occurs largely through the action of kinases.

Role of Phosphorylation

Phosphorylation serves two basic purposes in signal transduction. First, in nearly every instance, the addition of a phosphate changes the conformation of proteins and activates enzymatic functions, which in turn usually involves more kinase activity. The transmission of the signal therefore represents a wave of **protein activation.** Second, phosphorylation, especially of Tyr, creates **docking sites** on the affected proteins. The appearance of these docking sites recruits other target proteins, with which newly activated elements of the signaling pathway may interact. Signal transduction is therefore not only a linear progression of activation but also the transient assembly of intracellular messengers.

Proteins accumulate at appropriate sites in the cell, eg, the inner surface of the plasma membrane. *Often it is the phosphorylation of a kinase by a specific kinase that drives the signaling pathway.* Various signaling events repeatedly use phosphorylation-dephosphorylation. Some receptors are themselves kinases, and some are substrates of kinases. The phosphorylation of these proteins most often initiates a cell signaling event. Other crucial loci for cell signaling are found in the cytoskeleton, where proteins are activated by upstream components of the particular pathway.

Role of Dephosphorylation

Equally important to the phosphorylation of a substrate (on either its Ser-Thr or Tyr residues) is the removal of these phosphates. In some instances, the removal of a phosphate occurs by simply turning off the signal events. In other instances, however, the removal of phosphate is the activation event. These processes are described later in this chapter. Just as there are two types of kinase, there are two general types of phosphatases: Ser-Thr phosphatases and Tyr phosphatases. Like the kinases, the phosphatases must be specific, ie, they must remove the phosphates from only specified substrates. The implication is that for every kinase there is a phosphatase; however, this is not exactly the case. Some Ser-Thr phosphatases are more generic and remove phosphates from various substrates. Tyr phosphatases, however, appear to

maintain substrate specificity, and these enzymes are about as numerous as the Tyr kinases.

GTPase FAMILIES

A second general theme of *information processing* within a cell that involves phosphate ester chemistry is carried out by two types of guanine nucleotide triphosphatases (GTPases). Most intracellular communication—eg, vesicle trafficking, endocytosis, import into the nucleus, reformation of the nuclear envelope, and elongation of polypeptide chains during translation—occurs by the small proteins that bind GTP in their activated state. These proteins, however, can rapidly hydrolyze bound GTP to guanosine diphosphate (GDP), which in turn inactivates the molecule. As pointed out in Chapter 4, these monomeric proteins are intracellular **molecular switches** that are key components to most regulated events in the cell.

Another member of the GTPase family that is particularly important in cell signaling by surface receptors is a trimeric protein called the **G protein.** The three subunits of the G protein—alpha α, beta β, and gamma γ—are noncovalently associated. The α-subunit is a GTPase; like the monomeric GTPase, this subunit can bind GTP and hydrolyze it to the GDP form. The core GTPase domains bear a striking family resemblance in three dimensions: their β-sheet and α-helices are arranged identically to the α-subunit of the G protein. Of interest, the α-subunit has several forms, each of which performs different functions in signal transduction. These functions are discussed in more detail later in the chapter.

SECOND MESSENGER MOLECULES

Second messengers are small molecules that are rapidly formed, often in large quantities. These molecules amplify a molecular signal that is initiated through receptor activation. Second messengers are usually active for a brief time and then are inactivated by specific mechanisms. Five common small intracellular molecules are now recognized as second messengers. These substances, which play a central role in cell signaling and information exchange, are found in numerous settings:

1. cyclic adenosine monophosphate (cAMP)
2. cyclic guanosine monophosphate (cGMP)
3. diacylglycerol (DAG)
4. inositol 1,4, 5-trisphosphate (IP_3)
5. calcium.

cAMP

cAMP is formed from adenosine triphosphate (ATP) by the membrane-bound enzyme adenylate cyclase. cAMP is rapidly produced by the activated enzyme, and intracellular levels of cAMP are rapidly increased. These levels are also quickly diminished, however, by the intracellular enzyme cAMP phosphodiesterase. cAMP is a central participant in the cell signaling pathway, and its formation is regulated both positively and negatively by actions of cell surface receptors (Figure 9–2A).

cGMP

cGMP is rapidly formed by guanylyl cyclase and degraded by cGMP phosphodiesterase (Figure 9–2B). cGMP is involved in signal transduction in vertebrate vision. This signal pathway is explained in more detail in the section that addresses mechanisms of sensory transduction.

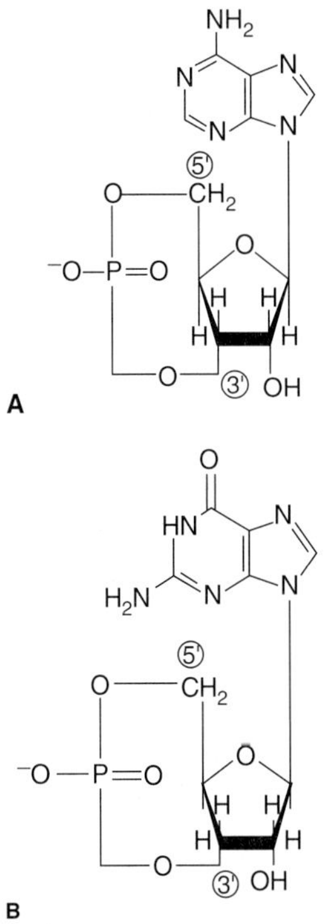

DAG

DAG and IP_3 are both formed from the same parent molecule. DAG is the membrane-bound moiety of the specialized membrane lipid **inositolphospholipid.** DAG is formed after cleavage of the phosphoinositol head group by members of the phospholipase C family of enzymes (Figure 9–3). It associates with the major cellular Ser-Thr kinase, **protein kinase C (PKC),** and aids in its activation. In addition, one of the acyl-chains of DAG is often arachadonic acid— a C-20 unsaturated fatty acid that serves as the parent structure in the formation of prostaglandins.

IP_3

IP_3 is the water-soluble head group component of the phosphoinositol lipid; after IP_3 is cleaved from the lipid, it is distributed into the cytosol, where it binds to intracellular membrane Ca^{2+} channel proteins and initiates their opening. This allows Ca^{2+} to flow from sequestered sites into the cytosol (Figure 9–4).

Calcium

Calcium plays an important role in cellular signaling and therefore has been classified as one of the major second messenger molecules (Figure 9–5). Calcium exerts its role primarily by binding to specific sites on kinases or on specialized calcium-binding proteins (eg, calmodulin) that serve as activators of a number of crucial kinases. The role of calcium is explored in more detail later in the chapter.

EXTRACELLULAR ROUTES OF SIGNALING MOLECULES

The classic definition of a hormone is that it is synthesized by cells of an endocrine gland and is translocated to its target cell by the circulatory system. This **endocrine pathway** was the first signaling route to be recognized. It has recently become evident that cells use various extracellular routes to bring a signaling molecule to a responsive cell. These routes are called the **paracrine, autocrine,** and **juxtacrine** pathways. Together with the endocrine pathway, they constitute the extracellular communicating system (Figure 9–6).

Paracrine Pathway

In a **paracrine pathway,** one cell type in a tissue secretes a signaling molecule that activates the immediately adjacent cell. For example, when a neuron secretes a neurotransmitter at a cell synapse, such as acetylcholine, a second cell that possesses an acetylcholine receptor on its surface binds the neurotransmitter and responds by propagating a bioelectrical signal. In paracrine signaling, the signal molecule is not usually picked up and carried in the circulation. The paracrine signaling system is prominent during

A

B

Figure 9–2. The structure of second messenger molecules. (A) Cyclic 3′,5′ adenosine monophosphate, cAMP. (B) Cyclic guanosine monophosphate, cGMP.

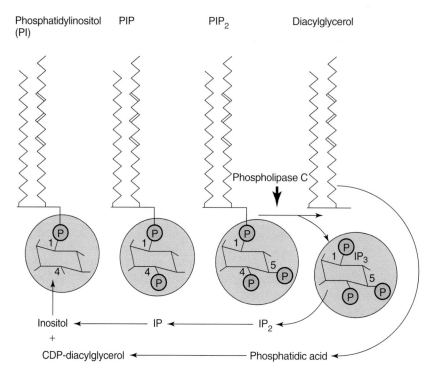

Figure 9–3. Generation of diacylglycerol (DAG) during the metabolism of phosphatidylinositol in cell membranes. Successive phosphorylation of phosphatidylinositol (PI) yields first phosphatidylinositol 4-phosphate (PIP) and then phosphatidylinositol 4,5-bisphosphate (PIP_2). The breakdown of PIP_2 to inositol 1,4,5-trisphosphate (IP_3) and DAG is catalyzed by phospholipase C; both of these interactions initiate signaling events. The metabolism of DAG and IP_3 proceeds along the illustrated pathways until these compounds combine to make phophatidylinositol, and the cycle begins again.

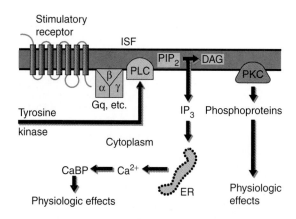

Figure 9–4. Ligand-receptor binding results in hydrolysis of phosphatidylinositol 4,5-bisphosphate (PIP_2) and formation of second messengers inositol trisphosphate (IP_3) and diacylglycerol (DAG), which subsequently move through a Ca^{2+} signaling pathway. (PKC = protein kinase C; ER = endoplasmic reticulum; CaBP = calcium binding proteins.) (Modified and reproduced, with permission, from Ganong WF: *Review of Medical Physiology,* 17th ed. Appleton & Lange, 1995, p. 38.)

wound healing, tissue repair, and embryonic development.

Autocrine Pathway

Local communication is a widely used mechanism for cells to respond to limited signals. In the **autocrine loop or pathway,** *a cell responds to its own signal:* The cell produces a signaling molecule and, at the same time, has the appropriate receptor on its surface to respond to a secreted signaling ligand. A cell typically cannot respond to a signaling molecule that it produces unless it receives the message through a receptor; therefore, the signal must first be secreted before a cell can respond. Cells of the immune system often rely on autocrine stimulation, and autocrine and paracrine stimulation often occur simultaneously.

Juxtacrine Pathway

The **juxtacrine** signaling system involves the **adhesion** of cells, eg, the adhesion of blood cells to one another or to cells of the vascular wall during hemostasis or inflammation. Signaling between juxtacrine cells is also crucial, and one or both cells may be

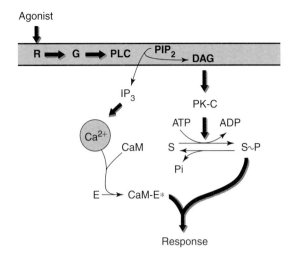

Figure 9–5. Calcium also acts as a second messenger in signaling pathways. The release of Ca^{2+} from internal storage sites is accomplished via the phosphoinositide pathway. IP_3 activates calcium channel proteins in the internal membranes that open the channels, and Ca^{2+} flows down a concentration gradient. The major calcium-binding protein, calmodulin, is activated after it binds Ca^{2+}. Calmodulin (CaM) binds to specific kinases (S) and initiates a phosphorylation signaling cascade. (S~P = phosphorylated kinase.) (Modified and reproduced, with permission, from Katzung BG: *Basic & Clinical Pharmacology,* 7th ed. Appleton & Lange, 1995, p. 25.)

stimulated when signals are passed during adhesion. Intercellular adhesion and signaling are tightly coupled; for example, aggregation of platelets at the site of initial injury and adhesion of neutrophils and monocytes at the endothelial site of injury or infection indicate that the processes of signaling and adhesion—ie, **cell-cell binding**—are spatially and temporally regulated. The juxtacrine pathway not only links cells together but also links cells to molecules of the extracellular matrix.

CELLULAR RESPONSES TO SIGNALING MOLECULES BY RECEPTORS

Gain & Loss of Function

Cells within tissues and organs are continuously bombarded with potentially significant signaling information. To distinguish between all the possible signaling molecules available, the cell has programmed the expression of its specific complement of **receptors.** It therefore responds only to the signal for which it has a receptor. The corollary to this principle is that the complement of receptors may change during development and differentiation. A signal that tells a cell to make more of a particular differentiated protein is unheeded by a cell that has not yet achieved its differentiated phenotype and has not yet expressed the receptor to respond to the signal for increased production of that specific molecule. The capacity of a cell to gain or lose a function is often based on whether the receptor is expressed or lost. Both events are part of the programmed events of **cell differentiation.**

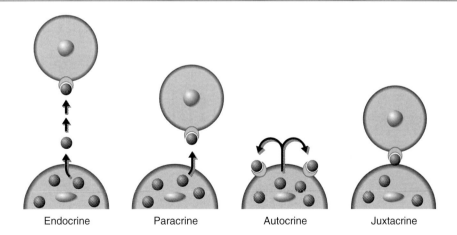

Figure 9–6. Intercellular signaling. Four mechanisms are shown: endocrine, paracrine, autocrine, and juxtacrine. The biologically active mediators, or ligands, are depicted as round and the receptors as crescent-shaped. Note that in juxtacrine signaling the ligand molecule is not released from the signaling cell into extracellular fluid. Instead, it remains part of the external surface of the cell membrane. (Modified and reproduced from Zimmerman GA et al: Juxtacrine intercellular signaling and the way to do it. Am J Resp Cell Mol Biol 1993;9:573.)

Some Cells Require a Signaling Ligand to Survive Programmed Cell Death

Certain cells must receive a specific signal to survive. The failure of the signaling molecule to reach its receptor or the failure of a receptor to respond to an essential ligand sets in motion a program that leads to cell death (see Chapter 6). Certain incoming signals are therefore required for cell survival. A number of programmed cell death models have been devised. During embryonic development, for example, many more neurons are produced than are eventually retained—approximately one half die soon after reaching their targeted location in the body. This **programmed cell death** likely occurs as a result of competition for the available neurotrophic factor—called nerve growth factor (NGF)—that is secreted by the target cell. NGF is produced in small quantities, and cells that do not receive it die. Through this loss of cells and cellular energy, organisms can tailor the appropriate number of cells for efficient neuronal transmission of bioelectrical signals.

Different Cells Respond Differently to the Same Signal

One hallmark of the signaling system is the specificity of the receptor for a ligand. It is therefore somewhat confusing to see different cells respond differently to the same ligand. For example, after acetylcholine binds to its receptor on skeletal muscles, the cell contracts; however, acetylcholine causes cardiac muscles to relax, and binding of acetylcholine to secretory cells initiates massive secretion. These observations indicate that although the receptor ligands are similar, proteins that are downstream of the activated receptor interpret the signal differently.

Downregulating the Signal

The ability to turn off a signal is as important as the ability to turn it on. A cell that cannot turn off a signal will eventually die. Various mechanisms are used in normal cell growth and differentiation to deactivate cell signaling. The cell may do the following:

1. Internalize the signaling complex—the ligand and receptor—by endocytosis. This is the mechanism used most frequently.
2. Desensitize the receptor. **Desensitization** most often occurs by phosphorylation; in addition to activating a downstream substrate, a receptor **autophosphorylates** at another site in the protein, thereby reducing its response to a bound ligand. This is referred to as **homologous desensitization.** A variation occurs when another molecule phosphorylates the receptor and attenuates its capacity to activate downstream substrates. This is called **heterologous desensitization.**

3. Degrade an effector molecule or sequester pools of activating molecules.

COMMUNICATING PARADIGMS IN MAMMALIAN CELLS

Mammalian cells have developed a number of ways to receive and process information, and each will be discussed in detail. The different pathways, which are listed below, are grouped on the basis of the location and characteristics of the receptor.

Group 1: Lipophilic Receptor Family

Ligands for this family include

- steroids, eg, the glucocorticoids, mineralocorticoids, and sex steroids
- the thyroid hormone, thyroxine
- retinoids, a large group of molecules related structurally to vitamin A and the vitamin D family.

These ligands are sufficiently lipophilic to pass through the lipid bilayer and enter the cytosol. The ligands are most often transported by carrier proteins, which have hydrophobic binding pockets that hold the ligand. The empty receptors of this family often reside in the cytosol and are complexed with another protein. Once the ligand enters the cell and binds to a receptor, the complex translocates to the nucleus where it binds to specific DNA sequences in the central regions of genes.

Group 2: Hydrophilic Receptor Family

The hallmark of this family is that the receptor is an **integral membrane protein.** This large group of receptors is subdivided according to the biochemistry of the receptor. The numerous ligands for this group are mostly hydrophilic. They are described by group, and there is a specific receptor for each ligand.

Receptors Coupled to G Proteins. The ligand leads to activation of the specific G protein. Activated G protein subunits modulate activity of molecular targets, in particular, adenylate cyclase, phospholipases, ion channels, and cGMP phosphodiesterase.

Receptors as Ion Channels. The ligand binds to the receptor—the channel protein—thereby causing the channel to open, leading to the influx or efflux of respective ions.

Atrial Natriuretic Factor (ANF)–Receptor. The ligand binds and causes the activation of a guanylyl cyclase catalytic domain. Activation of the receptor leads to Na^+ influx.

Receptors That Have Kinase Domains. Ligand binding leads to activation of an intrinsic protein Tyr kinase catalytic domain; this in turn phosphorylates cytoplasmic substrates. Receptors can be either protein Tyr kinases or Ser-Thr kinases.

Receptors Activated by Cytosolic Tyrosine Kinases. Protein Tyr kinases that are noncovalently associated with the surface receptor are activated by binding of the ligand to the receptor.

Receptors That Are Phosphatases. The ligand binds and activates a phosphatase domain.

Cytokine Receptors. These receptors are related in structure; they often share **signal-transducing** subunits and exhibit redundancy and pleiotropy.

SIGNALING PATHWAYS WITH RECEPTORS NOT EXPOSED TO THE CELL SURFACE

COMMUNICATION THROUGH GAP JUNCTIONS

Role of Secretin & Calcium

The gap junction signaling system is a highly efficient mechanism for the modulation of **cell-cell communication** between cells that are very closely linked, eg, epithelial cells (see Chapter 8). Gap junctions are located along the lateral surfaces of adjacent cells, which allows for the direct exchange of small molecules. For example, the second messenger cAMP can pass through pores created by the molecules that comprise a gap junction (see Figure 8–5). Stimulation of a one or a few cells in such tissue can typically initiate a response in all cells of that tissue; this delivery of cAMP throughout connected cells occurs through gap junctions. Such stimulation can occur by **secretin,** a hormone that induces release of enzymatic proteases from pancreatic acinar cells. Secretin binds to receptors on one or a few cells, thereby causing an increase in cAMP; this in turn releases intracellular calcium ions (Ca^{2+}), which triggers release of secretory enzymes from **storage vesicles** in all cells of the respective gland.

Ca^{2+} is a key signaling molecule that is often involved in movement through gap junctions of adjacent cells. For example, calcium waves in adjacent smooth muscle cells induce **coordinated peristalsis** and **uterine contraction,** respectively. This type of controlled release of calcium is integrated over many cells, which implies that calcium flows through adjacent cells. High concentrations of Ca^{2+}, however, cause gap junctions to close rapidly. When a cell is ruptured, for example, the sudden increase of Ca^{2+} from 10^{-7} to 10^{-3} mol/L causes proteins in the gap junction of the cell—the connexins—to contract and close their pores (see Figure 8–5). This closure leads

to the retention of essential small molecules that could otherwise be lost through the junction.

CELL SIGNALING BY NITRIC OXIDE

For more than a century, nitroglycerin has been recognized as an effective medication for angina; yet the mechanism of action of this drug for easing cardiac pain was elucidated only in the early 1990s. Nitroglycerin is a substrate that is rapidly converted into nitric oxide (NO). It causes endothelial and smooth muscle cells of the coronary vessels to relax, thereby enabling a larger flow of blood to the cardiac muscle. It has long been thought that human cells synthesize oxides of nitrogen; however, the full effect of NO in biological systems has been recognized only recently. In the context of cell biology, the realization that a carbonless gas can perform so many different functions suggests new ways to think of cellular controls and novel signaling processes. NO molecular signaling occurs through changes in the subhydroxyl (SH; thiol) groups of proteins and through alterations in redox reactions on metal ions that are positioned as coordinate complexes. For more on the biochemistry of NO, the reader is referred to several excellent reviews in the reference section of this chapter and to *Harper's Biochemistry,* 24th edition, by RK Murray et al (Appleton & Lange, 1996).

Nitric Oxide: Selected Clinical Correlates

Although most cells can produce NO, this signaling molecule appears to function primarily in three broad categories:

1. at the endothelial cell to cause endothelial relaxation
2. during neurotransmission to facilitate central nervous system function
3. in cell-mediated immune responses to facilitate immunologic function

Production of NO is the result of the enzymatic reaction of a very large enzyme complex, **NO synthetase (NOS),** which deaminates arginine to citrulline. NO is produced through oxidation that involves five electron equivalents of one of the guanidine N atoms of L-arginine to yield citrulline and NO. Figure 9–7 represents the formation of NO in an endothelial cell from arginine, with NO synthase as the catalyst.

Role of NOS in Production of NO. There are two main classes of **NOS:**

1. The constitutive enzymes produce short-lasting and small quantities of NO at a basal level, which allows NO to serve the regulatory role of

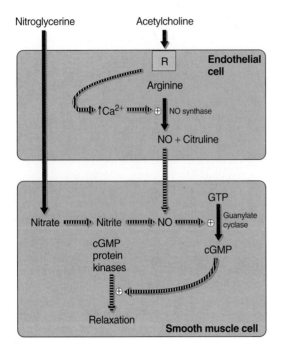

Figure 9–7. Nitric oxide and intercellular signaling. The role of nitric oxide in communication between an endothelial cell and a smooth muscle cell is shown. Nitric oxide (NO) is formed in the endothelial cell (top) after activation of the acetylcholine receptor binding causes an increase in intracellular Ca^{2+} and activation of nitric oxide synthase. In the smooth muscle cell (bottom), nitric oxide stimulates formation of cyclic guanosine monophosphate (cGMP), which in turn activates cGMP-dependent protein kinases. The end result of the intercellular signaling is relaxation of the smooth muscle cell. (Modified and reproduced, with permission, from Murray RK: *Harper's Biochemistry,* 24th ed. Appleton & Lange, 1996, p. 700.)

controlling vascular tone by acting as an endothelium-derived relaxing factor.
2. NO regulates **platelet aggregation** and participates as a **neuromediator** by acting primarily through its molecular target, guanylate cyclase. The activation of guanylate cyclase leads to increased levels of **cGMP** and to a cascade of molecular events within the target cells, eg, smooth muscle cells.

Another form of NOS—the inducible form Ca^{2+}-independent calmodulin-containing enzyme—is induced by endotoxins. Cytokines, such as γ interferons, tumor necrosis factor, and interleukin-1, can stimulate production of larger quantities of NO over a longer period of time, eg, many hours or even days. The production of larger amounts of NO at first shows powerful positive physiologic effects on the immune system, hormone release, cellular secretion,

and reproduction; however, the continuous production of large amounts of NO can become a serious problem because it leads to overstimulation of guanylate cyclase and hence unregulated cell signaling.

The complex versatility of NO in part results from its reliance on covalent modification—**phosphorylation**—which is how kinases act to transfer biomolecular signals. Specifically, NO exerts its effects by its reaction with the SH (thiol) groups of proteins and with proteins that contain metal ions. Essential components of the NO response therefore include ion channel proteins, enzymes, surface receptors, and transcription factors—all of which contain either transition metals or thiol strategically located at allosteric or reactive sites (Table 9–1).

NO in Neurons. The actions of NO are not confined to anatomical structures or to the circulation; rather, the generation of NO can easily move into cells by **transcellular diffusion.** NO is not stored; rather, it is synthesized on demand. Its actions are mediated by diffusion to intracellular targets rather than by binding to specific plasma membrane receptors, and there is no known inactivation or uptake mechanism. NO is considered a neurotransmitter; its neural functions include the facilitation of (1) peripheral nonadrenergic-noncholinergic neurotransmission in contractile and secretory tissue, (2) synaptogenesis, (3) sensory input processing, and (4) synaptic plasticity and learning.

LIPOPHILIC LIGANDS & NUCLEAR RECEPTORS

A surprisingly large number of ligands are sufficiently lipophilic to cross the cell membrane and bind to their receptors, which are located either in the cytosol or in the nucleus. As indicated earlier, hormones that belong to this group include the steroids, vitamin D_3, thyroid hormone, and the retinoids. These ligands are potent regulators of development, cell differentiation, and organ physiology. Unlike the water-soluble peptide hormones and the growth factors and cytokines that bind to surface receptors, the fat-soluble steroid hormones pass through the bilayer and interact with their cognate receptors (Figure 9–8).

Steroid hormone receptors are located in the cytoplasm and exist as a large multiprotein complex of **chaperones,** including heat shock protein 90 (hsp90) and the immunophilin molecule hsp56. These cytoplasmic complexes maintain the receptors in an inactive but "ligand-friendly" conformation. When the ligand—ie, the hormone—binds to its receptor, the Hsp is released. The receptor-ligand complex is then transported to the nucleus, where it binds to specific DNA sequences in the promoter regions of specific genes. The DNA binding motif of the target gene is known as the **hormone response element (HRE).** Of

Table 9–1. Cellular activation and inhibition functions of nitric oxide synthatase.

	Tissue Messenger	Toxic Effects
Blood vessel	Endothelium-derived relaxing factor, antithrombic ischemic protection, anti-atherosclerotic inhibition of smooth muscle proliferation, antiadhesive	Septic shock, inflammation, reperfusion injury, microvascular leakage, atherosclerosis
Heart shock	Cornary perfusion, ischemia	Myocardial "stunning," sepsis
Lung	Ventilation-perfusion matching, bronchiociliar motility, mucus secretion, immune defense	Immune complex–induced aveolitis, silo filler's disease, asthma, adult respiratory distress syndrome
Kidney	Tubuloglomerular feedback, glomerular perfusion, renin secretion	Acute kidney failure, glomerulonephritis
Central nervous system	Synaptogenesis, synaptic plasticity, memory formation, cerebral blood flow and ischemia, neuroendocrine secretion, visual transduction, olfaction	Neurotoxic proconvulsive, migrane, hyperalgesia, reperfusion
Pancreas	Endocrine/exocrine secretion	B cell destruction
Gut	Blood flow, peristalsis, exocrine secretion, mucosal protection	Mutagenesis, mucosal damage
Immune system	Antimicrobiol, antitumor	Anti-allograph, graft-vs-host disease, inflammation, septic shock, tissue damage

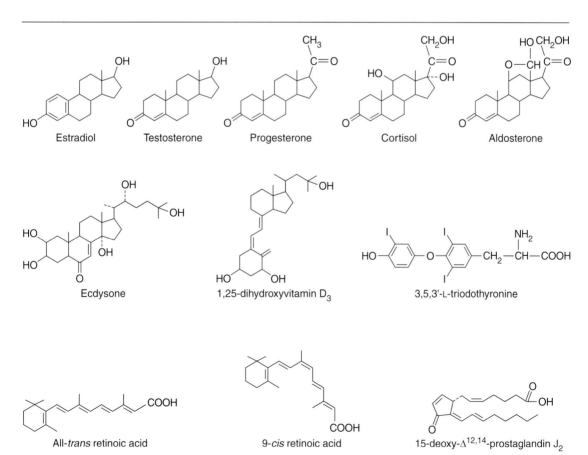

Figure 9–8. Steroid hormones and other ligands that bind to receptors in the nucleus. (Reproduced, with permission, from Mangelsdorf DJ et al: The nuclear receptor superfamily: the second decade. Cell 1995;83:835. © 1995 Cell Press.)

interest, the nucleotide sequence of the HRE is identical for all steroid-binding receptors.

This finding raises an intriguing question concerning gene specificity. Some receptors of this group reside in the nucleus and are already associated with their HREs, albeit in an inactive configuration to stimulate transcription of the downstream gene. In fact, the unoccupied receptor often acts as a repressor of the particular gene. When the hormone binds to the ligand-binding domain on this receptor, it causes an **allosteric rearrangement,** which leads to the activation of the gene. Thyroid hormone and estrogen receptors are examples of this type of repressor-inducer control system.

Nuclear receptors are grouped into four classes depending on their ligand binding, DNA binding, and dimerization properties. Figure 9–9 is a schematic representation of a nuclear receptor that contains a DNA-binding domain, a ligand-binding domain, a variable amino acid region, a variable hinge region, and a variable C-terminal region.

STEROID SIGNALING SYSTEM

In contrast to surface receptor signaling pathways, hormones in the steroid signaling system produce their effects after a characteristic **lag period** that lasts several hours. This means that the lipophilic hormone signaling system does not activate genes that must respond within a rapid time frame, ie, second or minutes. In fact, the steroid cellular response can persist for hours or days after the concentration of hormones has been reduced to baseline levels. This persistence is caused by the relatively slow turnover of most enzymes and proteins that are controlled by the steroid hormone signaling system. Lipophilic hormones and their receptors often bind to promoters of genes that encode other DNA binding proteins—ie, **transcription factors**—which themselves control the expression of genes. Genes responsive to lipophilic hormones are therefore involved in regulating genes that, in turn, modulate differential expression.

Clinical Correlate: Obesity

Adipocytes are formed from fibroblast cells during normal development and in various pathologic circumstances. **Obesity** is an excessive accumulation of adipose tissue that is characterized by an increase in the number or size of adipocytes. The adipocyte normally serves as a site for storage and release of fatty acids and contributes to the regulation of food and energy balance through the production of **leptin,** the product of the obese gene. The adipocyte may also influence glucose homeostasis through other regulatory molecules.

One of the earliest events in the differentiation of adipocytes is the expression of the γ isoform of the **peroxisomal proliferator activated receptor (PPARγ),** which is located in the nucleus. The PPARγ is a member of the nuclear receptor subfamily that includes receptors for thyroid steroids and

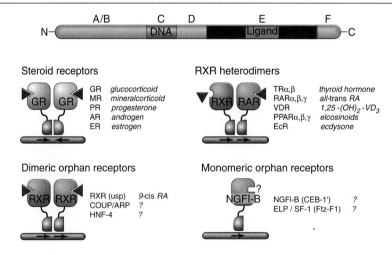

Figure 9–9. Common domains among nuclear receptors. The protein structure of a nuclear receptor is shown at the top of the figure with the amino terminal on the left (N-) and the carboxyl terminal on the right (-C). The sequences of the DNA binding domain (C) and the ligand binding domain (E) are the same. The N-terminal region, the region between the binding domains, and the C-terminal region vary in sequence. Nuclear receptors can be divided into four types based on DNA binding, ligand binding, and dimerization characteristics. Representatives of each type are shown at the bottom of the figure. (Reproduced, with permission, from Mangelsdorf DJ et al: The nuclear receptor superfamily: the second decade. Cell 1995;83:835. © 1995 Cell Press.)

retinoid hormones. Like other members of this super-family, PPARγ contains a central DNA binding domain that binds to *cis*-acting elements, ie, HREs, in the promoter of the PPAR gene. The nucleotide sequence of the **PPAR response elements (PPRE)** have been determined. To recognize a PPRE, PPARγ must form a heterodimer with the retinoic acid receptor.

When the PPARγ is overexpressed in fibroblasts, it initiates a cascade of events that leads to the differentiation of the fibroblast into an adipocyte. This finding implies that signals that modulate the PPARγ may serve a primary regulatory role in energy and fat metabolism. During the search for the ligand of the PPARγ, it was discovered that a metabolite of arachidonic acid in the prostanoid pathway, prostanoid PGJ_2, is the natural PPARγ ligand. This prostanoid activates PPARγ-dependent adipogenesis and thus represents a primary adipogenic signal. The search for the natural ligand of the PPAR receptor has therefore produced insights into prostaglandin synthesis and nuclear receptor signaling. PGJ_2 derivatives appear to be unique among the prostaglandins because they can act through a nuclear receptor without requiring second messenger pathways.

PATHWAYS THAT INCLUDE RECEPTORS EXPOSED TO THE CELL SURFACE

Ion Channel Receptors

Found in all cells, ion channels are **integral membrane proteins** that traverse the cell membrane and are involved in regulating the passage of specific ions into and out of the cell. The size of the pore of the various ion channels is narrow; for ions to pass through, they must shed their water of hydration. The size of the pore of the ion channel therefore behaves like a **molecular sieve.** As the water of hydration is removed, the ion forms a weak **electrostatic interaction** with polar amino acids that line the wall of the channel. Because loss of water from the ion is energetically unfavorable, the ion traverses the channel only if the electrostatic interaction compensates for the loss of water. The loss of the water of hydration and electrostatic interactions with the pore last only briefly (microseconds) during the passage of the ion. Only ions of a certain size can pass through the narrow channel formed in the bilayer by the channel receptor. Ion channels for Na^+, Ca^{2+} (Figure 9–10), K^+, and Cl^- are the most common in eukaryotic cells.

Conformational States of Ion Channels: Regulatory Mechanisms

All known ion channels exist in one of two conformational states:

1. the channel is **open,** thereby allowing the movement of ions down their **concentration gradient;**
2. the channel is **closed,** thereby inhibiting the passage of ions.

The transition of a channel between these different states is called **gating.** The molecular events of gating likely involve significant changes in the overall conformation of the channel protein. This process creates a channel through which ions of different sizes can move into and out of the cell.

Several mechanisms have evolved to regulate the conformational state of the ion receptor. Some channels are regulated by the binding of chemical ligands to specific domains on the channel—eg, neurotransmitters and hormones that bind to extracellular sites of the channel—or they may be second messengers within the cell that are activated by transmitters, which in turn act on the cytoplasmic side of the channel. Some ion channels are activated by changes in membrane potential, whereas others are activated by the mechanical stretch of the membrane (Figure 9–11).

The activity of the different channels can be modified by a number of events including (1) metabolic reactions and phosphorylation and (2) the effects of toxins and drugs. Certain autoimmune diseases, such as **myasthenia gravis,** result from the actions of specific antibodies that interfere with channel function. As more molecular details are elucidated on the structure and function of the different ion channel proteins, it may be possible to devise therapeutic approaches to treat certain neurologic and psychiatric disorders that are caused by different ion channel proteins.

G PROTEIN–COUPLED RECEPTORS & THEIR SIGNALING PATHWAYS

The G Protein–linked Receptor Family

The basic molecular design of **G protein–linked receptors** is described in Chapter 2. Recall that the amino terminus is located extracellularly, the polypeptide stitches through the membrane seven times, and the cytoplasmic domain contains the sites for G protein binding. Hundreds of different forms of the G protein receptors exist, and the chemical diversity of the ligands that bind to this family of receptors is extraordinary (Table 9–2). Members of the family of highly specific seven-membrane–pass receptors include

- small molecules, such as catecholamines, peptides, and chemokines
- larger molecules, such as glycoprotein hormones
- thrombin

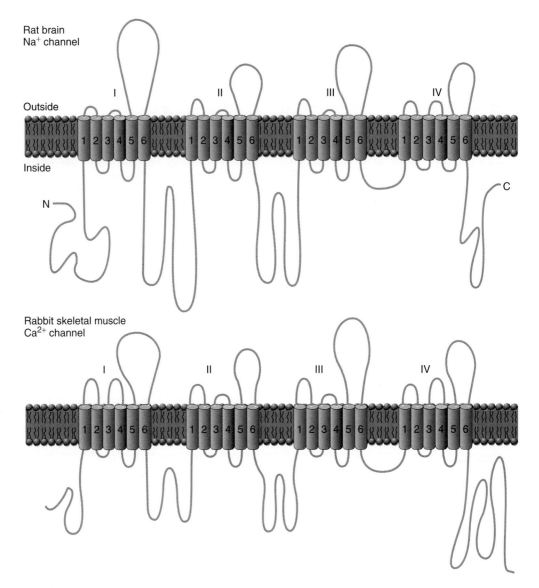

Figure 9–10. Similarities of ion channels. The structures of two mammalian ion channels are shown (Na$^+$ channel from rat brain and Ca^{2+} channel from rabbit skeletal muscle). Note that both membrane proteins have four major subunits (I–IV), and that each major subunit includes six α-helical domains that span the cell membrane. In addition, the amino and carboxyl terminals of both channels are located within the cytoplasm. (After WK Catterall. Modified and reproduced from Hall ZW: *An Introduction to Molecular Neurobiology.* Sinauer, 1992.)

- light-activated signals
- volatile odorant molecules.

Although the same basic design is used, important variations exist among G proteins, notably,

1. the way these proteins are inserted into the lipid bilayer
2. the three-dimensional variations of the receptor that account for the diverse binding sites and the specificity of these molecules.

Figure 9–12 illustrates some of the subtle differences in the structure of G protein–coupled receptors and suggests how these proteins can account for the wide range in ligand structure.

G Proteins: Selected Clinical Correlates

A loss of function or an activating mutation in G protein–linked receptors is the underlying cause of various human diseases (Table 9–3). The loss-of-function mutations behave as **recessive traits,** and

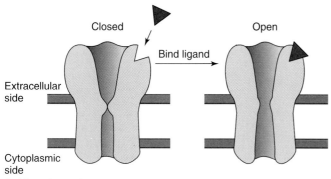

Closed   Open

Bind ligand

Extracellular side

Cytoplasmic side

A. Ligand-gated

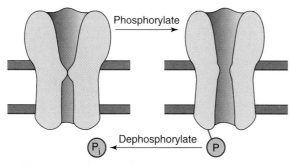

Phosphorylate

Dephosphorylate

B. Phosphorylation-gated

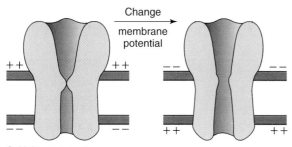

Change membrane potential

C. Voltage-gated

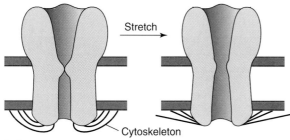

Stretch

Cytoskeleton

D. Stretch or pressure-gated

Figure 9–11. Ion channels. Four different types can be distinguished based on the stimulus regulating the opening and closing of the channel. (A) Calcium-gated channels fall within the ligand-gated type. The ion channel opens because of energy from ligand binding. (B) For phosphorylation-gated channels, the energy to open the channel is derived from the transfer of a high-energy phosphate group to the channel protein. (C) The energy responsible for opening voltage-gated channels comes from changes in the electrical potential across the cell membrane. (D) Pressure-gated channels open in response to stretching or pressure on the cell membrane and adjacent cytoskeleton. (Reproduced, with permission, from Kandel ER et al: *Essentials of Neural Science and Behavior.* Appleton & Lange, 1995, p. 127.)

Table 9–2. A sampling of G proteins and their physiologic effects.[1]

Stimulus	Affected Cell Type	G Protein	Effector	Effect
Epinephrine, glucagon	Liver cells	G_S	Adenylate cyclase	Breakdown of glycogen
Epinephrine, glucagon	Fat cells	G_S	Adenylate cyclase	Breakdown of fat
Luteinizing hormone	Ovarian follicles	G_S	Adenylate cyclase	Increased synthesis of estrogen and progesterone
Antidiuretic hormone	Kidney cells	G_S	Adenylate cyclase	Conservation of water by kidney
Acetylcholine	Heart muscle cells	G_i	Potassium channel	Slowed heart rate and decreased pumping force
Enkephalins, endorphins, opioids	Brain neurons	G_i/G_o	Calcium and potassium channels, adenylate cyclase	Changed electrical activity of neurons
Angiotensin	Smooth muscle cells in blood vessels	G_q	Phospholipase C	Muscle contraction; elevation of blood pressure
Odorants	Neuroepithelial cells in nose	G_{olf}	Adenylate cyclase	Detection of odorants
Light	Rod and cone cells in retina	G_t	cGMP phosphodiesterase	Detection of visual signals
Pheromone	Baker's yeast	GPA1	Unknown	Mating of cells

[1]Reprinted, with permission, from Linder M, Gilman AG: G Proteins. Sci Am 1992;267:56.
cGMP = cyclic guanosine monophosphate.

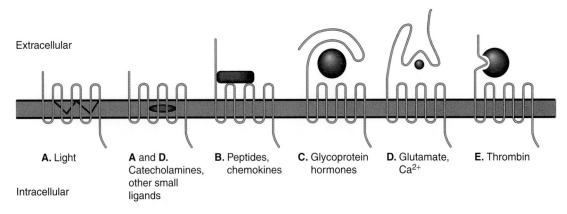

Figure 9–12. Different ways in which ligands are recognized by receptors coupled to G proteins. Examples of each group of ligands are given beneath the six recognition models. Rhodopsin, the receptor whose informational changes are associated with light stimulation, is shown at the far left. From near left to right, five other models show ligands binding to regions of the receptor—to membrane-spanning domains (A, D); to the external surface (B); to the large, external amino-terminal domain (C); to a small region within the large, external amino-terminal domain (D); and to a new amino-terminal domain determined by ligand cleavage of the original sequence (E). (Modified and reproduced, with permission, from Coughlin SR: Expanding horizons for receptors coupled to G proteins: diversity and disease. Curr Opin Cell Biol 1994;6:195.)

Table 9–3. Examples of G protein pathway–linked diseases in humans.[1]

Disease	Defective G Protein Receptor	Defective G Protein
Familial hypocalciuric hypercalcemia	Human analogue of BoPCaR1	
Neonatal severe hyperparathyroidism	Human analogue of BoPCaR1 (homozygous)	
Hyperthyroidism (thyroid adenomas)	Thyrotropin receptor	
Precocious puberty	Luteinizing hormone receptor	
X-linked nephrogenic diabetes insipidus	V2 vasopressin receptor	
Retinitis pigmentosa	Rhodopsin receptor	
Color blindness, spectral sensitivity variations	Cone opsin (iodopsin) receptor	
Familial glucocorticoid deficiency, isolated glucocorticoid deficiency	Adrenocorticotropic hormone receptor	
Albright's hereditary osteodystrophy and pseudohypoparathyroidisms		$G_{\alpha s}$
McCune–Albright syndrome		$G_{\alpha s}$
Pituitary tumors (*gsp* oncogene)		$G_{\alpha s}$
Pituitary, thyroid, adrenal cortical, ovarian tumors (*gip* oncogene)		$G_{\alpha i}$

[1]Modified and reproduced, with permission, from Clapham DE: Mutations in G protein–linked receptors: novel insights on disease. Cell 1993;75:1237. © 1993 Cell Press.

the phenotypes of individuals homozygous for these mutations demonstrate the relative importance of each affected receptor in normal biology. In addition, several naturally occurring mutations that cause constitutive activation of the seven-membrane domain receptors have been identified; for example, **hyperfunctioning thyroid adenomas** caused by somatic mutations in the thyrotropin receptor are an important recent finding.

Basic Signaling Pathway of the G Protein. G proteins are made up of three polypeptides: an α subunit, which binds and hydrolyzes GTP, and β and γ subunits, which form a dimer that is tightly linked by noncovalent forces. When GDP is bound to the α subunit, it associates with the βγ subunits to form an inactive trimer that associates with the C-terminal portion of the receptor. When a ligand binds to the receptor, the cytoplasmic domain of the receptor changes its conformation. The GDP-ligand α subunit also responds with a conformational change of its own that decreases GDP affinity so that GDP leaves the active site on the α subunit.

GTP quickly binds to the active site because it is approximately 10-fold greater in concentration in the cell than GDP. Once GTP is bound, the α subunit assumes an active conformation and dissociates from both the receptor and the βγ subunits. The GTP-bound α subunit activates other effector molecules (eg, adenylate cyclase, which produces cAMP). The activated state of the α subunit lasts until GTP is hydrolyzed to GDP by the intrinsic GTPase activity within the α subunit. Once GTP is hydrolyzed to GDP, the α and βγ subunits reassociate and return to the receptor. Figure 9–13 illustrates the steps in this process.

It was once believed that only the α subunit of the G protein was involved in activating the effector molecule and that the βγ subunits either were not in-

volved or acted as a negative regulator. It is now recognized that the βγ subunit can also activate downstream effector molecules (eg, muscarinic K$^+$ channels). Thus, both α and βγ subunits, therefore, are involved in the regulation of cellular responses.

G Protein Effector Molecules. G proteins play a pivotal role in activating downstream effector molecules. The major downstream effector molecules controlled by G proteins include

- adenylate cyclase
- phospholipase C (PLC)
- phospholipase A$_2$ (PLA$_2$)
- phosphoinositide 3-kinase (PI$_3$-kinase)
- β–adrenergic receptor kinase (βARK).

Both the α and βγ subunits are involved with many of these downstream effectors, but the pattern of regulation is specific. For example, there are several different forms of adenylate cyclase, and each form of the effector molecule apparently uses a different activator subunit: one type uses the α subunit, another uses the βγ subunit, and still others require both.

1. THE α-SUBUNIT FAMILY OF THE G PROTEIN

Thus far, we have implied that the α subunit is the same for all G proteins. This is not the case; in fact, there are as many as 20 different forms of the α subunit. These forms have been grouped into four classes on the basis of their amino acid sequence similarity. Most forms of the α subunits are found in all cells associated with the G proteins; however, unique α subunits are found in cells of the sensory system, including vision, taste, and smell. We also know that

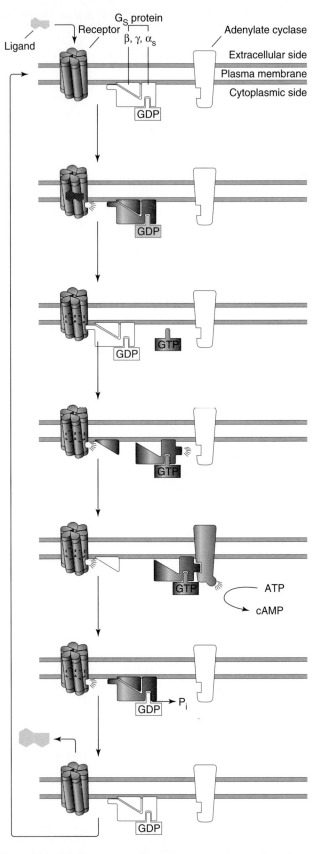

Ligand binding alters conformation of receptor, exposing binding site for G_S protein.

Diffusion in the bilayer leads to association of ligand-receptor complex with G_S protein, thereby activating it for GTP-GDP exchange

Displacement of GDP by GTP causes the α subunit to dissociate from the G_S complex, exposing a binding site for adenylate cyclase on the α subunit

α subunit binds to and activates cyclase to produce many molecules of cAMP

Hydrolysis of the GTP by the α subunit returns the subunit to its original conformation, causing it to dissociate from the cyclase (which becomes inactive) and reassociate with a $\beta\gamma$ complex

The activation of cyclase is repeated until the dissociation of ligand returns the receptor to its original conformation

Figure 9–13. G protein signaling pathway. (See text for details.) (Adapted from Alberts B et al: *Molecular Biology of the Cell,* 2nd ed. Garland, 1989. Modified and reproduced, with permission, from Kandel ER et al: *Essentials of Neural Science and Behavior.* Appleton & Lange, 1995, p. 248.)

there are different isoforms of the β and γ subunits that perform different regulatory functions and are effector molecules:

1. $G\alpha_s$: This subunit acts as a stimulatory molecule of adenylate cyclase.
2. $G\alpha_i$: This subunit inhibits the activity of adenylate cyclase.
3. $G\alpha_o$: This subunit primarily mediates Ca^{2+} channel closure and inhibits phosphoinositol (PI) turnover.
4. $G\alpha_T$: This subunit is located in the outer segments of photoreceptor rods and mediates stimulation of phosphodiesterase. Other specialized α subunits of the sensory system are designated α-olf, for olfactory (smell), and α-gust, for gustation (taste).

The βγ complex plays three functional roles:

1. facilitator of the α subunit (the complex increases the affinity of the α subunit for GDP)
2. activator of the β family of PLC enzymes
3. modulator of the role of the α subunits in regulating the adenylate cyclase enzyme.

In addition, a few α subunits are located in neural cells.

Not surprisingly, the various forms of α subunits function differently on downstream effector molecules. Moreover, certain bacterial toxins appear to exert their effects on mammalian cells by modifying the α subunit of the G protein.

How G Proteins Are Tethered to the Cell Membrane

G proteins are not classic membrane-bound proteins; rather, they are tethered into the cytoplasmic face of the membrane by one of four types of lipid linkages, as shown in Table 9–4.

The γ subunit of the trimeric G-protein contains both a myristate acid linked through an amide bond to the N-terminus, as well as a thioester-linked palmitoyl group. The α subunit contains a thioether-linked geranylgeranyl isoprenoid, as well as a methylated carboxyl terminus. These linkages to the inner surface of the membrane provide a way to target these reactive molecules to sites in close proximity to their activating receptors—and, in many instances, to membrane-bound effector molecules (Table 9–4).

2. G PROTEIN EFFECTOR PATHWAYS

At least *four* major signaling pathways originate from an activated seven-membrane–pass G protein system, and each is discussed below. There is much crossover among these pathways within the cell, however, because a signaling molecule often elicits a number of metabolic responses.

Role of Adenylate Cyclase in Pathway Involving cAMP and Ca^{2+}

The enzyme adenylate cyclase catalyzes formation of the second messenger molecule cAMP. Adenylate cyclase is a large (MW ~ 120,000) protein that has two clusters of six transmembrane-spanning domains (Figure 9–14). The eight isoforms of the enzyme are divided into two groups: those that require the calcium-binding protein **calmodulin** for activation and those that do not. All cells contain adenylate cyclase, but there are substantial differences in the patterns of expression of the enzyme; these differences reflect the specific activity of the particular cell.

The $G\alpha_s$ protein causes activation of adenylate cyclase, $G\alpha_s$, which leads to the formation of cAMP. It

Table 9–4. Lipid linkages.[1]

Lipid	Structure	Representative Proteins Modified	Position of Modification
N-Myristoyl	(O) N-Gly / H	Trimeric G proteins (α) NRTKs	NH_2-terminus
S-Palmitoyl (*S*-acyl)	(O) S-Cys	Trimeric G proteins (α) GPCRs Ras	Internal; no defined consensus
S-Prenyl	S-Cys Geranylgeranyl / S-Cys Farnesyl	Trimeric G proteins (γ) Small G proteins Retinal GRK	COOH-terminus
GPI	Complex structure containing ethanolamine, sugars, and phosphatidylinositol	Many cell-surface proteins	COOH-terminus

[1]Reproduced, with permission, from Casey PJ: Lipid modifications of G proteins. Curr Opin Cell Biol 1994;6:219.

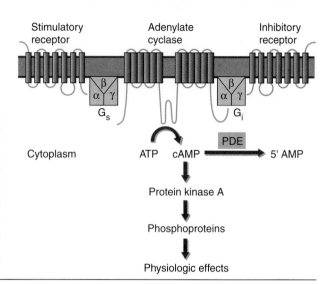

Figure 9–14. Structure of adenylyl cyclase and stimulation and inhibition through the cAMP system. Interaction of adenylyl cyclase with a stimulatory receptor–G$_s$ protein complex leads to formation of cAMP and its subsequent physiologic effects. Interaction of the same enzyme with an inhibitory receptor–G$_i$ protein complex leads instead to production of 5′ AMP. In the latter case, the cAMP-dependent physiologic effects do not occur. (ISF = interstitial fluid.) (Modified and reproduced, with permission, from Ganong WF: *Review of Medical Physiology,* 17th ed. Appleton & Lange, 1995, p. 39.)

is believed that the βγ subunits can augment the stimulatory action of the Gα$_s$ subunit in certain isoforms of adenylate cyclase. The signal transducer effect of the Gα$_s$ subunit occurs because the protein interprets the conformational state of the receptor after ligand binding by altering its association with both GDP and its other subunits. When the Gα$_s$ subunit associates with adenylate cyclase, the original signal is amplified 1000-fold by forming the second messenger molecule cAMP. The signal is turned off during three events:

1. when the GTPase of the Gα$_s$ subunit converts GTP to GDP, which causes dissociation from the enzyme (adenylate cyclase)
2. when newly generated cAMP activates a phosphodiesterase enzyme that hydrolyzes cAMP to 5′AMP, thereby diminishing the intracellular concentration of the second messenger
3. once the activated G α subunit dissociates from the βγ subunit; the receptor loses its affinity for the ligand and is no longer in the active configuration.

In this type of signaling system, therefore, a mechanism for on-off signaling is necessary, and agonists must be available to stimulate the response (Figure 9–15).

Different isoforms of the α subunit exert different physiologic effects. For example, in adipocytes, epinephrine and glucagon activate adenylate cyclase by Gα$_s$, whereas prostaglandin E$_1$ inhibits adenylate cyclase. Prostaglandin E$_1$ binds to its receptor (a seven-membrane–pass receptor) and activates a G protein that has the Gα$_i$ isoform of the α subunit. This isoform also binds GTP and associates with the adeny-

late cyclase enzyme; however, the isoform inhibits the enzyme instead of activating it to produce cAMP.

Two bacterial toxins affect cells by their interaction with G proteins. The toxin secreted by the bacterium *Vibrio cholerae* catalyzes the modification—ie, the adenosine 5′-diphosphate (ADP)-ribosylation—of the Gα$_s$ subunit. This modification inhibits the GTPase activity of the subunit. Consequently, the Gα$_s$ does not hydrolyze its bound GTP; thus, it continuously stimulates adenylate cyclase to produce cAMP. The huge quantity of cAMP exceeds the capacity of cAMP's inhibitor, phosphodiesterase, to bring the level of cAMP into the normal range. The most prominent target cells of cholera toxin are the epithelial cells that line the intestine. The high levels of cAMP generated by cholera toxin alters the electrolyte balance of these cells, resulting in extensive loss via diarrhea.

Pertussis toxin, the toxin derived from the bacterium that causes whooping cough, also affects the G protein; however, this process occurs through the ADP-ribosylation of a Gα$_i$ subunit, which inhibits the function of the subunit. GDP therefore remains bound to the subunit, and adenylate cyclase is not appropriately inhibited. Because Gα$_i$ is also important for activating K$^+$ ion channels, this gating system is also inhibited.

Many human diseases have been linked to the G protein signaling family (see Table 9–3).

cAMP & PROTEIN KINASE A

cAMP regulates numerous cellular functions by activating or inhibiting specific cellular proteins. cAMP can also affect the expression of various genes by modifying the activities of a specific group of pro-

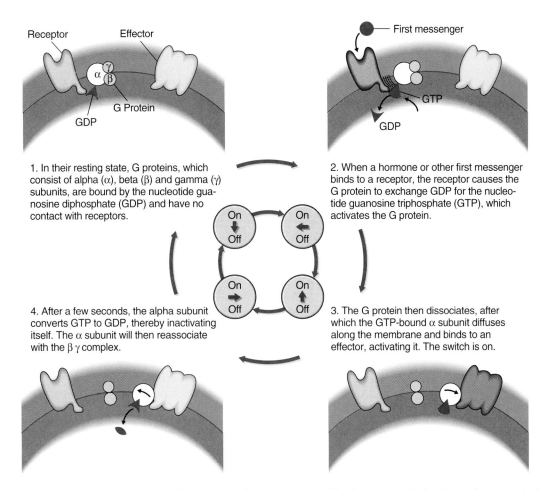

Figure 9–15. G proteins as the on-off switch for effector molecules. The four-step cycle is shown diagrammatically: (1) binding of first messenger, (2) transduction through the G protein, (3) activating the effector, (4) resetting of the G protein complex and inactivating the effector. (Reprinted, with permission, from Linder M, Gilman AG: G Proteins. Sci Am 1992:56. © 1992 Scientific American. All rights reserved.)

teins through the action of cAMP-dependent protein kinase A (PKA, or A-kinase). Several features of this pivotal enzyme (PKA) are worth noting. It is composed of four polypeptides—two regulatory peptides and two catalytic peptides that are held together by noncovalent forces; the complex is inactive in this conformation. When the cytoplasmic levels of cAMP increase, two cAMP molecules bind to each regulatory subunit, thereby altering the conformation of the complex. The two catalytic subunits dissociate from the complex and are then free to phosphorylate available substrates.

The catalytic subunits have an ATP binding site located at the amino terminus, and the subunits transfer the terminal ATP phosphate group to specific Ser and Thr residues of acceptor proteins. Phosphorylation of these substrate proteins regulates their activity. The catalytic domains share extensive sequence homology with all eukaryotic protein kinases.

PKA

Activation of PKA by cAMP is a major starting point for a large number of downstream signaling pathways. Activated PKA initiates the following:

1. a metabolic event
2. a transcription event
3. activation of the enzyme system that removes the phosphates from PKA to downregulate its action.

PKA Metabolic Event

Glycogen, the major storage form of glucose, is found in relatively high concentrations in muscle cells and hepatocytes. Glycogen is formed by three enzymatic reactions:

1. hexokinase, which places a phosphate into position 6 on the glucose

2. phosphoglucomutase, which rearranges the glucose, moving it to position 1
3. pyrophosphorylase plus uridine triphosphate, which forms uridine diphosphoglucose (UDP-glucose), the required unit for the formation of a glycogen polymer

In the final step, **glycogen synthetase** uses UDP-glucose to build the glycogen polymer.

Muscle cells continuously form glycogen within each cell in order to have a rapid source of energy when required. Epinephrine (adrenalin) stimulates the activation of PKA through the G protein pathway discussed above. PKA activates the breakdown of glycogen by phosphorylating the enzyme **glycogen phosphorylase kinase,** which activates glycogen phosphorylase:

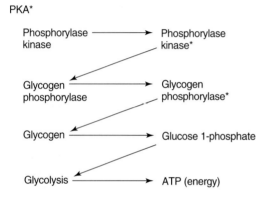

Although this metabolic scheme has been known for several decades, the connection between adrenalin and the G protein activation of PKA has only recently been explained. We emphasize here that PKA also plays a regulatory role in many other metabolic pathways.

PKA Transcription Event: cAMP Controls Transcription of Various Genes

Nearly all genes have a region upstream from the transcription start site called the **regulatory** or **promoter region.** This region contains DNA sequences to which specific DNA binding proteins bind and aid in the transcription of that gene. The specific nucleotide sequence to which the protein binds is called the **responsive element (RE).** When PKA is activated by increased cAMP, some of the activated catalytic subunits are transported to the nucleus, where they phosphorylate specific proteins—the cAMP responsive element binding protein (CREB). The activated PKA in the nucleus phosphorylates a Ser residue (Ser133) on CREB, thereby allowing it to activate genes that contain the response element in their promoters. CREB can also be activated through pathways that involve increased levels of Ca^{2+}. Increased

cytosolic levels of calcium activate a calcium-calmodulin (CaM) kinase, which will also phosphorylate Ser133.

PKA Event: Role of Protein Phosphatases in Cell Signaling

Protein phosphatases remove the phosphates that have been put on substrates by protein kinases. The level of phosphorylation in a cell depends on a balance between the activating kinases and phosphatases. Phosphatases usually have a broader range of specificity than do kinases. There are two major types of phosphatases:

1. those that remove phosphates from Ser-Thr residues **(Ser-Thr phosphatase)**
2. those that remove phosphates from Tyr residues **(Tyr phosphatases).**

Four types of Ser-Thr phosphoprotein phosphatases have been identified: I, IIA, IIB, and IIC. Each type has homologous catalytic subunits that are linked to different regulatory subunits:

- **Phosphatase I** inactivates many enzymes stimulated by PKA, including CREB.
- **Phosphatase IIA** is thought to remove phosphorylations catalyzed by Ser-Thr kinases; it is important in regulating events of the cell cycle.
- **Phosphatase IIB,** also called **calcineurin,** is abundant in the brain and is activated by free calcium.
- **Phosphatase IIC** is structurally different from the other types; it has high specificity for the enzymes that regulate cholesterol metabolism.

Phosphatases have been shown to be among the proteins most highly conserved throughout evolution, which suggests that these enzymes perform functions that are essential for all eukaryotic cells. For example, phosphorylation on Ser and Thr residues accounts for more than 97% of the protein-bound phosphate in stimulated cells.

A second type of phosphorylation event that occurs in cell signaling uses certain Tyr residues in target proteins. Details of these signaling cascades are discussed in Chapter 10. Here, it is sufficient to note that the Tyr phosphatases comprise a more diverse family of enzymes than do the Ser-Thr phosphatases.

MOBILIZATION OF THE SECOND MESSENGER MOLECULE, CALCIUM

The concentration of calcium in the cytoplasm is maintained at a low level, 10^{-7} mol/L; when this concentration increases, a number of enzymatic events are initiated. Sudden regulated increases of intracellular calcium—with a concomitant activation of different signaling pathways—demonstrate that free calcium serves as a second messenger molecule. For calcium to serve in this capacity, its steady-state concentration must be rigorously maintained.

The cell has developed several mechanisms to maintain a low intracellular concentration of calcium in the face of a much higher concentration on its extracellular surface. The plasma membrane, as well as the endoplasmic reticular membrane and mitochondrial membranes, has ATP-driven Ca^{2+} channels that actively remove free calcium from the cytosol to the outside or into the lumen of these organelles. Any leakage of calcium from outside the cell or from intracellular reservoirs is usually removed quickly. Within the endoplasmic reticulum (ER) are high-capacity, low-affinity, calcium-binding proteins that hold free calcium to a loosely bound substrate.

Two pathways of calcium signaling have been identified and extensively studied. One pathway occurs in nerve cells. Depolarization of the nerve causes an influx of Ca^{2+} into the nerve terminal, thereby initiating the secretion of neurotransmitter substances. The Ca^{2+} enters through voltage-gated channels that open when the plasma membrane depolarizes. The second pathway is found in all cells and occurs through a signal generated at the cell surface through membrane-bound receptors. Increases in cytosolic levels of Ca^{2+} occur from the release of sequestered Ca^{2+} in the ER and involve yet another second messenger molecule, IP_3.

PKC & CELL SIGNALING

Role of Plasma Membrane–associated Phosphoinositol

Phosphatidylinositol is the low-abundance lipid found primarily in the inner leaflet of the plasma membrane (see Chapter 2). This phospholipid is an important part of the receptor-initiated signaling cascade and is the substrate for PLC, which is an important subclass of membrane lipases. The PLC family has a number of isotypes. As discussed below, PLC-β is the major player in the cleavage of the phosphoinositide head group from its acyl chains.

Most cellular responses to the occupancy of membrane receptors include the hydrolysis of phosphoinositol lipids. Two well-studied second messengers—IP_3 and DAG—are produced from phosphoinositide lipids, and a number of different molecules are involved in their generation (see Figure 9–3). Generation of the derivatives of plasma membrane–associated phosphoinositols is shown in Figure 9–3. Each enzyme substitutes a phosphate group in place of a hydroxyl group located on specific carbon atoms of the inositol ring. *This phosphorylated product is an important component in several signaling pathways.* The inositol phosphate pathway is complex and in-

volves a number of newly discovered enzymes. The three major types of myoinositol-containing lipids are

1. phosphatidylinositol (PI) 80%
2. phosphatidylinositol-4-phosphate (PIP) 15%
3. phosphatidylinositol-4, 5-bisphosphate (PIP_2) 5%.

The enzymes responsible for hydrolyzing the inositol lipids are C-type phospholipases. Three families of PLC have been identified: β, γ, δ. Within each family are subtypes designated by the addition of the Arabic number, eg, PLC-$β_1$ and PLC-$β_2$.

Two distinct regulatory pathways are involved in the activation of PLC-β and PLC-γ. PLC-β is regulated by G proteins, whereas PLC-γ is regulated by Tyr kinases. In the case of PLC-β, the Gα subtypes known as G_q ($Gα_q$) are primarily involved in activating this phospholipase. When agonists (ie, ligands), such as acetylcholine, histamine, epinephrine, 5-OH-tryptamine, thromboxane, and glutamate, bind to their seven-membrane–pass receptor and elicit G protein activation, one form of the G protein that contains the G_q subtype will activate PLC-β, which cleaves PIP_2 from the membrane, thereby forming IP_3 and DAG. Although most cells have the $Gα_q$ subtype, this molecule is most abundantly located in the brain.

Likewise, receptors that are activated by growth factor ligands—eg, epidermal growth factor—involve phosphorylation of Tyr residues on the receptor cytoplasmic domains that participate in the activation of PLC-γ. This process also leads to the production of IP_3, DAG, and other important intracellular messengers. PI-3 kinase and the γ isoform of PLC bind to the cytoplasmic domain of many receptors of the Tyr kinase family, thereby bringing the enzyme close to their substrates and stimulating their catalytic activity. Figures 9–3 and 9–4 summarize the two major receptor-mediated pathways for stimulating the formation of IP_3 and DAG.

Cell Signaling Functions of IP_3. IP_3 functions as the ligand to activate calcium-release channels located in the ER. In muscle cells, the smooth ER is called the **sarcoplasmic reticulum,** and the calcium-release channels are identified as **ryanodine channels.** The channels appear to be identical regardless of cell type; IP_3 operates as the ligand that binds to the channel protein, thereby causing it to open and allowing Ca^{2+} to flow down a concentration gradient and into the cytosol. There are also calcium-binding domains on the channels, and one of the first augmentation events that Ca^{2+} exerts is to facilitate additional channel openings. These occur within 1–2 seconds and are followed by the introduction of a calcium wave into the cytosol.

The basic paradigm for this phenomenon is as follows:

- A ligand stimulates G protein activation.
- Gα_q activates PLC-β which cleaves IP$_3$ from PIP$_2$, thereby generating IP$_3$.
- IP$_3$ binds to Ca^{2+} and opens membrane channels.
- Ca^{2+} flows from the smooth ER into the cytosol.
- IP$_3$ is dephosphorylated by cytoplasmic phosphatases and is released from the ion channel.
- The channel closes.
- Ca^{2+} is removed from the cytosol by ATP activity and by Ca^{2+} pumps.

PIP$_2$ and Actin-binding G Proteins. The receptor-mediated hydrolysis of PIP$_2$ is frequently accompanied by increased cell motility and by changes in cell structure, both of which are attributable to changes in the physical properties of **actin networks.** The properties of these networks depend on the length and concentration of actin filaments and on the number and geometry of the cross-links between them. Actin-binding G proteins regulate and promote or prevent filament formation. In many cases, the interactions between the network proteins and actin are altered by molecules implicated in cell signaling, including Ca^{2+} and PIP$_2$. The actin-binding G proteins that interact with PIP$_2$ include

- the actin monomer–sequestering protein profilin
- the actin filament–severing G proteins gelsolin, villin, severin, adseverin, destrin, and cofilin
- protein gCap39, which blocks the ends of actin filaments
- the actin filament–cross-linking protein α-actinin.

The interactions between actin-binding proteins and PIP$_2$ usually promote actin **polymerization,** whereas the interaction between these proteins and Ca^{2+} usually promote **depolymerization.** The decreased levels of PIP$_2$, coupled with increased levels of Ca^{2+}, therefore favor the depolymerization of filaments. Changes in cell migration and shape are controlled in part by the concentration of PIP$_2$ and Ca^{2+}. Additional functions of Ca^{2+} as a second messenger molecule are addressed later in the chapter.

Cell Signaling Functions of DAG. The lipid moiety of phosphatidylinositol is DAG, and examination of the acyl chains reveals that one group is the polyunsaturated C-20 fatty acid **arachidonate,** which is esterified to the glycerol backbone. Arachidonate is often cleaved from diacylglycerol by PLA$_2$ and serves as the substrate for the various prostaglandins and **eicosanoids** discussed earlier. Intact DAG also serves a second crucial second messenger role by activating PKC. The association between DAG and this pivotal protein kinase enhances their activity.

Intact DAG plays a crucial role in activating another membrane-bound protein kinase, PKC. Because the half-life of DAG is brief (a few seconds), it cannot serve as a sustained activator of PKC. Other agonist-induced lipases are required to help maintain the activity of this kinase for longer periods. DAG, however, is considered the major inhibitor of PKC activation.

Role of PKC in Cell Signaling

PKC, also known as C-kinase, is a protein with a molecular mass between 65 and 78 kDa. There is an extended family of PKC isoforms, which accounts for the range in size of the molecule. Within the protein are regulatory domains located in the amino half of the molecule. The catalytic (kinase) domain is found in the latter half of the protein, and an ATP-binding site is located near the catalytic domain.

The full activation of PKC requires Ca^{2+}, DAG, and association with phospholipids on the inner surface of the plasma membrane, primarily phosphatidylserine. In its inactive state, PKC is a cytosolic soluble protein. The cytosolic concentration of free calcium increases after IP$_3$ stimulation of the calcium channel opening. Cytosolic translocation of PKCs to the membrane occurs as the Ca^{2+} concentration increases. The enzyme "docks" to the membrane and is held in place—in part by ionic interactions of the negatively charged phospholipid phosphatidylserine. At such sites, association with the membrane facilitates the activity of PKC. PKC itself has calcium-binding domains that are important in altering its conformation and enhancing its catalytic activity. PKC phosphorylates target proteins on specific Ser and Thr residues. PKC is inactivated when DAG is hydrolyzed or when the intracellular level of Ca^{2+} decreases.

Physiologic Roles of PKC

There are at least 10 subtypes of PKC, and each has a different range of characteristics in terms of calcium requirements, substrate preference, intracellular localization, tissue distribution, and rate of inactivation. In addition, there is more than one type of PKC within the same cell. The PKCγ isoform, for example, is found only in the brain and spinal cord and is thought to be involved in specialized neuronal processes. PKC is also involved in a number of key cellular responses including cell division, secretion, exocytosis, ion conductance, smooth muscle contraction, and gene expression. From this list, one can readily see that PKC is an important regulatory kinase.

Of particular interest is the role that PKC plays in controlling **gene expression.** In one pathway, PKC activates a pivotal cytosolic kinase, **mitogen-activated protein (MAP) kinase.** This kinase initiates a cascade that leads to the phosphorylation of nuclear transcription factor Elk-1, whose response component—called the serum response element—increases transcription of genes that encode proteins involved in **cell replication.** PKC initiates a second gene regulatory pathway that involves the release of NFkB, an inactive cytosolic transcription factor that is activated after its release from the inactivating complex IkB (see Chapter 10).

INTRACELLULAR CA^{2+} RELEASE CHANNELS

As the previous discussion suggests, Ca^{2+} is a key regulatory ion in intracellular signaling pathways. The use of specific binding dyes to examine release of Ca^{2+} demonstrates that the ion is released in a **pulsatile** manner, with so-called Ca^{2+} spikes that occur in discrete regions then spread in a wave-like motion throughout the cell. Cells use two sources of Ca^{2+} to generate signals:

1. Ca^{2+} released from internal stores
2. Ca^{2+} entry from across the plasma membrane.

Release of Ca^{2+} from internal stores is controlled by two families of channels: ryanodine receptors and IP$_3$ responsive receptors. Although multiple isoforms of each type exist, all types are somewhat similar in determining channel opening. Findings from several studies suggest that channels demonstrate a bell-shaped sensitivity curve to Ca^{2+}. At low extracellular concentrations, Ca^{2+} promotes release of calcium from intracellular stores. At high extracellular concentrations, however, Ca^{2+} inhibits the intracellular flow of calcium by shutting down the receptor channel. These stimulatory effects mean that Ca^{2+} contributes to a rapid sudden movement—called **a Ca^{2+} spike**—followed by a wave-like flow of the ion throughout the cytosol. The release and re-uptake of Ca^{2+} is complex, and understanding the release mechanism provides additional information on the spatiotemporal property of calcium signaling.

Calcium acts as a second messenger molecule in two ways:

1. It can bind directly to a number of effector molecules, eg, PKC.
2. It binds to an inactive cytosolic protein, which then becomes the effective modulator of effector molecules.

CALMODULIN: A UBIQUITOUS CALCIUM-BINDING PROTEIN

Calmodulin, a small protein (16 kDa) with four binding sites for calcium, is an abundant protein in all cells. It mediates a number of effector functions. A unique characteristic of this calcium receptor is the dramatic conformational change it undergoes after Ca^{2+} binding. The calmodulin-calcium complex is involved in regulating a number of enzymes, including the Ca^{2+}-activated pump that removes free calcium from the cytosol. Calcium and calmodulin are also in-

volved in phosphorylation events; these molecules are a necessary cofactor for activation of a family of kinases called **calcium-calmodulin–dependent kinases (CaM kinases)** (see Figure 9–5), which phosphorylate Ser and Thr residues on specific protein substrates.

CaM-kinase II is among the best characterized kinases. It comprises approximately 2% of the total protein mass in mammalian brain cells and is thought to reside in all animal cells. CaM-kinase is concentrated at synapses and is believed to function as a memory molecule that switches on when stimulated by Ca^{2+} and calmodulin, then maintains its biomolecular signal *even after the stimulation of calcium ceases*. When activated by calcium and calmodulin, CaM-kinase phosphorylates itself as well as other proteins. This autophosphorylation continues to activate the enzyme after levels of calcium decrease, thereby extending the signaling effects. When the autophosphorylation is inhibited by other kinases, the signal turns off.

MOLECULAR BASIS OF SIGNALING PATHWAYS OF SENSORY CELLS

The mammalian sensory system involves specialized cells for

- vision—photoreceptors
- smell—olfactory neurons
- taste—receptors on the tongue for salt, sweet, sour, and bitter
- touch—mechanoreceptors.

Most sensory cells are specialized epithelial cells that connect to neurons, which in turn transmit signals to the brain. For olfactory cells, the receptor is a modified neuron. In the case of mechanoreceptors, stretch receptors, touch receptors, and taste receptors located on the tongue, the receptor molecule is the **sodium (Na$^+$) channel protein** located in the cell membrane. The molecular signal is transduced when the channel protein opens, thereby allowing the influx of sodium ions, which in turn leads to depolarization of the cell.

In at least two types of sensory cell—the photoreceptor cell and the olfactory neuron—the sensory receptor is a seven-membrane–pass receptor that relies on a specialized G protein signaling system.

MOLECULAR BASIS OF VISION

Photoreceptor Signaling System: Rod Cells

The human retina contains two types of photoreceptors: rods and cones. Rods are stimulated by low levels of light, and cones are activated in bright light. It is important to understand the intracellular membrane arrangement of the rod cell and its proximity to the plasma membrane (Figure 9–16).

The outer segment of the photoreceptor contains a series of membrane stacks, or disks, that are studded with multiple copies of the seven-pass–membrane receptor protein **rhodopsin.** The extracellular domain of the opsin protein has a hydrophobic binding pocket for the light sensitive pigment, 11-*cis* retinal. The 11-*cis* isomer is a stereoisomer of vitamin A and is the only form that binds to the opsin protein. As soon as binding occurs, the receptor is primed to be activated by a photon of light. The light energy of the **photon** is absorbed by the pigment (11-*cis* retinal), which causes a conformational change to all-*trans* retinal; this results in its release from the receptor, opsin (see Figure 9–18, below). This process leads to the activation of the G protein that contains the unique subunit. Thousands of opsins are in the membrane stack of the outer segment in close proximity with the Na⁺ channel proteins.

The resting dark-adapted rod cell is in a state of **depolarization** with respect to neurons or other electrically excitable cells. The low resting potential occurs because the Na⁺ channel proteins are continuously in the open configuration, and sodium has relatively free access to the inside of the cell. Under these conditions, the photoreceptor is also secreting neurotransmitters, and the interfacing bipolar neuron is continually firing (Figure 9–17).

Rhodopsin Complex. When a photon of light in the range of 400–600 nm strikes a **rhodopsin complex,** it causes an atomic rearrangement of the 11-*cis* isomer to the all-*trans* form, which causes the isomer to be released from the opsin protein (Figure 9–18). This conformational rearrangement of the pigment is sufficient to activate the opsin protein, which translates this photon energy into a signal sufficient to activate a trimeric G protein that is associated with the inner surface of the receptor. In this case, the removal of the ligand—the light-absorbing pigment—activates the receptor. This differs significantly from all other known G protein–linked receptors, which are activated by binding of an agonist.

The Gα subunit of the photoreceptor was the first to be identified. This subunit has retained its original name, **transducin** (also called Gα_T). As in other G protein signaling systems, Gα_T dissociates from the $\beta\gamma$ subunit and activates its membrane-associated effector molecule.

In the photoreceptor rod cell, the Na⁺ channels are activated by cGMP, a product of guanylate cyclase. In the resting state, the Na⁺ channels are in the open

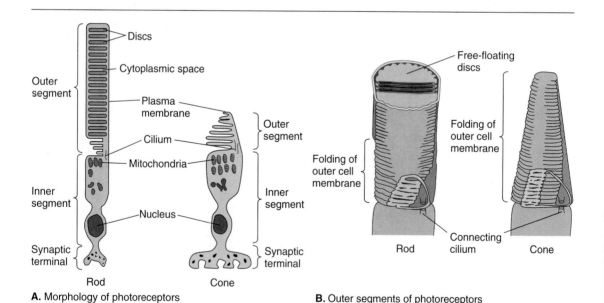

A. Morphology of photoreceptors

B. Outer segments of photoreceptors

Figure 9–16. The structure of photoreceptor cells. (A) Rods and cones are named for their overall shape. They have a similar structural organization, with both consisting of an outer and inner segment distal to the synaptic terminal. The outer segments contain the photoreceptor apparatus, the membranous discs. (B) Membranous discs are formed from infoldings of the plasma membrane. In rods, however, the folds separate from the membrane into free-floating discs. In cones, the discs remain part of the plasma membrane. (Adapted from O'Brien DF: The chemistry of vision. Science 1982;218:961 and Young RW: Visual cells. Sci Am 1970 (October); 223:80. Modified and reproduced, with permission, from Kandel ER et al: *Essentials of Neural Science and Behavior.* Appleton & Lange, 1995, p. 411.)

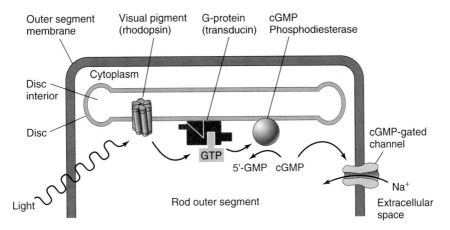

Figure 9–17. Signal transduction in rod cells. Phototransduction involves closing of ion channels. Without light stimulation, the channels are maintained in an open position by the presence of intracellular cGMP and an inward current carried largely through Na⁺ ions. The stimulus of light is transduced into the closing of ion channels in a three-step process. First, light is absorbed by the retinal portion of the rhodopsin molecule. Second, the activated form of rhodopsin interacts with the G protein transducin to activate the enzyme cGMP phosphodiesterase. The intracellular concentration of cGMP decreases owing to enzymatic metabolism to 5′-GMP. In the third step, the lowered concentration of cGMP causes the closing of the cGMP-gated channel, which reduces the inward current and causes the receptor to hyperpolarize, generating the neural response to light. (Modified and reproduced, with permission, from Kandel ER et al: *Essentials of Neural Science and Behavior.* Appleton & Lange, 1995, p. 412.)

position. To maintain these proteins in the open configuration, high concentrations of cGMP—three molecules per receptor—are required. On light activation of the signaling receptor, $G\alpha_T$ is released; it binds to and activates a cGMP phosphodiesterase that rapidly hydrolyzes cGMP to GMP, and this process leads to the closing of the Na⁺ channels.

The cellular form of cGMP phosphodiesterase is inactive as long as an inhibitor subunit is bound to the enzyme. The $G\alpha_T$ (in its GTP-bound state) associates with the phosphodiesterase then dissociates the inhibitor subunit from the enzyme, thereby allowing it to hydrolyze cGMP rapidly. As with other $G\alpha$ subunits, bound GTP is rapidly hydrolyzed to GDP, which causes dissociation from the diesterase and reassociation with the membrane bound $\beta\gamma$ subunit. In the dark-adapted rod cell, the cGMP-phosphodiesterase is inactive, levels of cGMP increase, the Na⁺ channels open, and the 11-*cis* isomer reassociates with the opsin molecule.

Photoreceptor Signaling System: Cone Cells

Rod cells are inhibited by bright light, and **cone cells** are insensitive to low levels of light. When an individual moves from bright light to dim light, a brief period of adaptation is needed to see. The dissection of the molecular signaling events involved in the conversion of light energy to chemical energy is one of the remarkable discoveries in the past decade.

The biochemistry of adaptation to a light source occurs through a **negative feedback mechanism.** The enzymatic activity of guanylate cyclase is stimulated by Ca²⁺; in the resting cell, levels of Ca²⁺ are high enough to maintain levels of the cyclase-producing cGMP because this cyclic nucleotide controls the Na⁺ and Ca²⁺ channels, both of which open in the presence of high levels of cGMP. The decrease in levels of Ca²⁺ in the cell activates a Ca²⁺ sensing protein, which binds and activates guanylate cyclase. This process is followed by a second modulating process that controls the sensitivity of rod cells to light: An opsin-kinase present in the cytoplasm of rod cells phosphorylates the cytoplasmic face of the opsin receptor at several sites.

Seven potential Ser-Thr residues can be phosphorylated, and the more they undergo phosphorylation, the less able the receptor is to activate the $G\alpha_T$ subunit. Under conditions of intense light, opsin is extensively phosphorylated: the greater the level of light, the more opsin is generated. When an individual moves into a dim light, opsin becomes dephosphorylated, and the lower light signals can be translated into a visual response.

MOLECULAR BASIS OF OLFACTION

It has been estimated that a human being can recognize as many as 10,000 distinct odorant molecules.

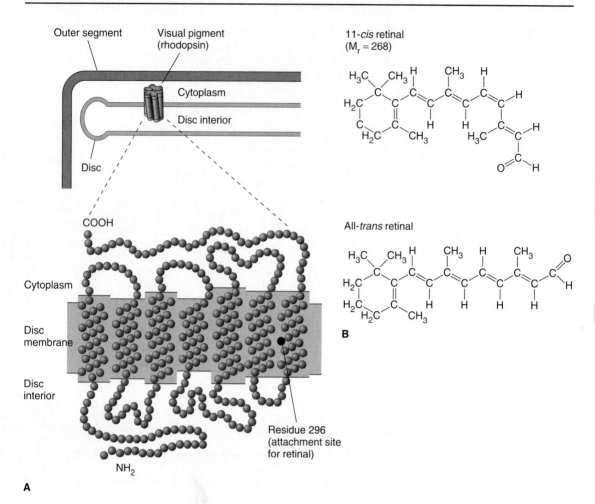

Figure 9–18. Rhodopsin and retinal. (A) Rhodopsin, which consists of the protein opsin and the photoreceptor molecule retinal, is located in the disc membrane of rods. (B) When stimulated by light, the retinal molecule changes from the 11-*cis* configuration to the all-*trans* configuration. This change in retinal configuration is the first step in signal transduction. (A: adapted from Nathans J, Hogness DS: Isolation and nucleotide sequence of the gene encoding human rhodopsin. Proc Natl Acad Sci USA 1984;81:4851. A, B: Modified and reproduced, with permission, from Kandel ER et al: *Essentials of Neural Science and Behavior.* Appleton & Lange, 1995, p. 413.)

Nasal cells that can recognize these molecules are genuine neurons, not specialized epithelial cells. It is thought that a separate neuron exists for each odorant.

Olfactory neurons have specialized cilia that contain the olfactory receptor, which is a seven-membrane–pass protein coupled to a G protein. A specific receptor is thought to exist for each odorant, although this has not been fully established. Signaling events for olfaction involve the solubilization of the odorant molecule into secretions that cover the surface of the olfactory epithelium. Novel cloning strategies have led to the identification of several hundred different odorant receptor genes, and it is expected that more will be identified. Olfactory neurons usually survive for about a month before they are replaced by replicas; these cells are one of the very few types of neurons that undergo replication.

REFERENCES

Baldwin JM: Structure and function of receptors coupled to G proteins. Curr Opin Cell Biol 1994;6:180.

Beato M et al: Steroid hormone receptors: many actors in search of a plot. Cell 1995;83:851.

Bootman MD, Berridge MJ: The elemental principles of calcium signaling. Cell 1995;83:675.

Bourne HR: GTPases: a turn-on and a surprise. Nature 1993;366:628.

Clapham DE: Calcium signaling. Cell 1995;80:259.

Divecha N, Irvine RF: Phospholipid signaling. Cell 1995; 80:269.

Felder CG: Muscarinic acetylcholine receptors: signal transduction through multiple effectors. FASEB J 1995; 9:619.

Forman BM et al: 15-Deoxy-12-14-prostaglandin J2 is a ligand for the adipocyte determination factor PPAR gamma. Cell 1995;83:803.

Goetzl EJ et al: Specificity of expression and effects of eicosanoid mediators in normal physiology and human diseases. FASEB J 1995;9:1051.

Henry Y et al: EPR characterization of molecular targets for NO in mammalian cells and organelles. FASEB J 1993;7:1124.

Lambright DG et al: The 2.0 Å crystal structure of a heterotrimeric G protein. Nature 1996;379:311.

Mangelsdorf DJ, Evans RM: The RXR heterodimers and orphan receptors. Cell 1995;83:841.

Mangelsdorf DJ et al: The nuclear receptor superfamily: the second decade. Cell 1995;83:835.

Marletta MA: Nitric oxide synthase: aspects concerning structure and catalysis. Cell 1994;78:927.

Neer EJ: Heterotrimeric G proteins: organizers of transmembrane signals. Cell 1995;80:249.

Schmidt H, Walter U: NO at work. Cell 1994;78:919.

Strader CD et al: Structure and function of G protein–coupled receptors. Annu Rev Biochem 1994;63:101.

Taussig R, Gilman AG: Mammalian membrane-bound adenylyl cyclases. J Biol Chem 1995;270:1.

Waterman MR: Biochemical diversity of cAMP-dependent transcription of steroid hydroxylase genes in the adrenal cortex. J Biol Chem 1994;269:27783.

10

Cell Signaling Pathways: Communication Via Enzyme-Linked & Enzyme-Associated Receptors

KEY TERMS

Tyrosine kinase domain
Extracellular domain
Transmembrane domain
Cytoplasmic domain
Receptor protein–tyrosine kinases (RPTKs)
RPTK receptors
RPTK ligands
RPTK signaling
Adapter proteins
Ras pathway
Mitogen-activated protein (MAP) pathway
Src family
Protein tyrosine phosphatases (PTPs)
Kinase-associated receptors
Non–tyrosine kinase receptors
Pleiotropy
Redundancy
Cytokine signal pathway
Interferons
Interleukins
Transforming growth factor–β (TGF-β)
Tyrosine kinase cascade

In the previous chapter we discussed mechanisms of cell signaling that involved nuclear receptors, ion channel receptors, and a large family of seven-membrane–pass receptors that transmit signals into the cell via activation of the trimeric G protein family. In this chapter, we consider four additional types of cell surface receptors and their signaling pathways:

1. receptors that are themselves tyrosine kinases, that is, those that have a kinase domain as part of their polypeptide structure (eg, the growth factor receptors)
2. receptors that utilize specific cytoplasmic tyrosine kinases to activate them (eg, interleukin receptors)
3. receptors that have a serine-threonine kinase do-

main as a part of their structure (eg, the transforming growth factor–β [TGF-β] family)
4. integrin receptors.

The receptors in categories 1 and 2 have many more members than those in categories 3 or 4, and their signaling pathways are considered in more detail in the discussion that follows. Both of these types of receptors are activated by phosphorylation of selected tyrosine residues located within the cytoplasmic domain of the receptor.

In general, information signals that operate through the phosphorylation of tyrosine residues are involved in pathways that initiate cell proliferation or cell differentiation. These ligands and their receptors have been classified historically as **growth factors** and **growth factor receptors,** because these signaling molecules often promote cell growth. However, they also can inhibit growth under certain conditions, and in some cases, they regulate crucial cellular functions that have very little to do with cell proliferation. A more useful term—**cytokine**—encompasses a broader spectrum of molecules, not just those that function as growth factors.

Of the two types of signaling pathways discussed in this chapter, the receptors of the larger group contain a kinase domain in the cytoplasmic portion of the molecule. This group is referred to as the **receptor protein–tyrosine kinases (RPTKs).** Receptors of the second group, discussed later in the chapter, do not contain kinase domains. An important point to remember about all signaling pathways is that the ligand (growth factor, hormone, interleukin, etc) is simply the "bearer of the message" and has no additional function after binding to its receptor. It is the receptor where the cellular action, and our discussion, begins.

THE RECEPTOR PROTEIN–TYROSINE KINASES

BASIC STRUCTURE OF RPTK RECEPTORS

Unlike the seven-membrane–pass receptors the polypeptide of the RPTK receptors passes through the membrane only once. Furthermore, they are classed as type I receptors because the amino-terminal portion of the protein is oriented on the exterior of the cell.

The External Domain

Receptors in this class typically have an extensive length of their polypeptide structure on the external surface of the cell. Also the external domains have structural features that are homologous to other types of proteins. For example, many RPTK receptors have regions of amino acid sequences that resemble those of other molecules. These sequences include:

- immunoglobulin-like sequences (Ig-like domains)
- fibronectin type III domains, cysteine-rich domains
- leucine-rich domains
- epidermal growth factor (EGF)–like domains.

The functional significance of these regions is unknown, but they probably participate in the binding of the ligand to its specific receptor. In addition to these different "recognizable" motifs, most of the external domains of these receptors have both *N*- and *O*-linked carbohydrate clusters (Figure 10–1).

The Transmembrane Domain

This portion of the receptor is typical of all single transmembrane-spanning regions. It is composed of approximately 20–24 amino acids with the usual block of basic residues that function as the stop-transfer signal that locks the protein into the lipid bilayer.

The Cytoplasmic Domain

The cytoplasmic domain of most of the RPTKs contains between 250 and 400 amino acid residues. The kinase domain contains approximately 250 residues and is located near the middle of the cytoplasmic domain. Residues on either side of the catalytic domain may function as "spacers" or in other noncatalytic events. A high degree of amino acid homology exists among the catalytic domains of these receptors.

The RPTK Family

Members of this family of receptors share a strong evolutionary relationship, as shown in Figure 10–2, which illustrates the molecular phylogeny of 52 different RPTKs. The map is based on the amino acid homologies within the catalytic domains and demonstrates that different receptor families can be clustered into similar groups.

THE RPTK LIGANDS

The RPTKs were first identified as receptors responding to polypeptide ligands that had been shown to specifically cause cell growth (proliferation) in different types of cells grown in tissue culture. For example, **epidermal growth factor (EGF),** one of the first growth factors identified, was named and characterized because of its effect on cells isolated from murine salivary epithelial cells. **Platelet-derived growth factors (PDGFs)** were identified as special components found in serum but absent in unclotted blood, and later studies showed that when platelets are activated during clotting, they release cellular growth factors. **Nerve growth factor (NGF)** and **fibroblast growth factor (FGF)** were isolated from cell culture media that, when added to certain types of cells, stimulated their growth. Once a specific growth factor had been isolated and purified, it becomes of great interest to determine the "molecular language of the factor" and define how the polypeptide information was transmitted into the cell. This interest led to the identification of the large group of growth factor receptors. We now recognize that there are many different types of ligands, or signaling molecules, and based on their amino acid sequence, they can be grouped into families (Table 10–1).

PRINCIPLES OF RPTK SIGNALING

In Chapter 9 we discussed the paradigm of signaling through the seven-membrane–pass receptors as it involved the activation of the trimeric G proteins. In that signaling system, the initial signal cascade followed a common pathway involving activation of the $G\alpha$ subunit and its subsequent activation of the effector molecules (such as adenylate cyclase, phospholipase C, or protein kinase C [PKC], see Figure 9–4). The initial signaling of the RPTKs also follows a well-defined sequence of molecular events, outlined in the following steps:

1. The kinase domain of the receptor is activated.
2. Docking sites for other substrates form on the cytoplasmic tail of the receptor. This occurs as a result of tyrosine phosphorylation.
3. Docked proteins may be phosphorylated by the receptor.
4. Mechanisms for turning off, or down-regulating, the activated receptor are initiated.

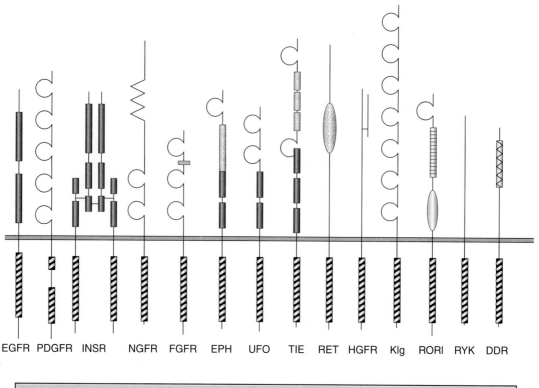

EGFR PDGFR INSR NGFR FGFR EPH UFO TIE RET HGFR Klg RORI RYK DDR

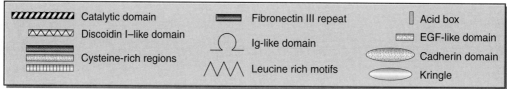

///////// Catalytic domain	▬▬▬ Fibronectin III repeat	▯ Acid box
XXXXX Discoidin I–like domain	⋂ Ig-like domain	⬚ EGF-like domain
▤ Cysteine-rich regions	⋀⋀⋀ Leucine rich motifs	⬭ Cadherin domain
▤		⬯ Kringle

Figure 10–1. Examples of different receptor protein tyrosine kinases (RPTKs). All receptors of this class of proteins have a kinase domain within their cytoplasmic tail. The extracellular domains have amino acid sequence motifs that are also found in nonreceptor proteins. The functional role of these signature motifs is unknown. (Modified from van der Geer P et al: Receptor protein tyrosine kinases and their signal transduction pathways. Annu Rev Cell Biol 1994;10:254. Reproduced, with permission, from the *Annual Review of Cell Biology,* Volume 10, © 1994, by Annual Reviews Inc.)

This is the typical process for RPTK activation. Transmission of the molecular signal from the ligand to the cytoplasmic domain of the receptor occurs by a dimerization (or in some cases, oligomerization) of the receptor complex. This intermolecular event brings together the kinase domains of two (or more) receptor subunits, resulting in autophosphorylation and often cross-phosphorylation of key tyrosine residues. Phosphorylation of key tyrosines in the receptor changes the receptor's conformation, which allows cytoplasmic proteins with special domains to "dock" onto the phosphorylated tyrosine of the receptor. In many instances after the cytoplasmic protein docks, it also is phosphorylated by the receptor's kinase or the special cytoplasmic tyrosine kinase. The

proteins that dock and are themselves phosphorylated generate subsequent signaling events that occur in the first stage of the signaling process. Figure 10–3 illustrates interactions between an RPTK receptor and ligands containing an SH2 domain (see below).

Mutations in the receptor's cytoplasmic domain that affect its kinase activity, the formation of docking sites, or receptor down-regulation lead to abnormal cell responses and consequently human disease. Alterations in a single codon have been shown to constitutively activate the kinase domain, and the protein loses its capacity to be inactivated. The result is uncontrolled growth of the cells containing the mutation. Many of the so-called **oncogenes** (cancer genes) are the result of mutated growth factor receptors.

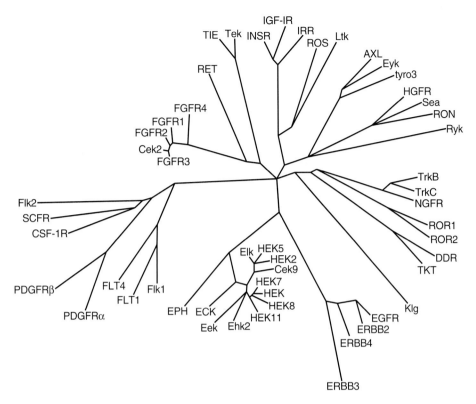

Figure 10–2. Molecular phylogeny of the family of RPTKs. Amino acid sequence analyses of the kinase domain show strong homology among 52 RPTKs. Stronger homologies can be seen within receptors that have similar ligands. (Noteworthy abbreviations: EGFR = epidermal growth factor receptor; FGFR = fibroblast growth factor; PDGF = platelet derived growth factor; INSR = insulin receptor.) (Modified from van der Geer P et al: Receptor protein tyrosine kinases and their signal transduction pathways. Annu Rev Cell Biol 1994;10:258. Reproduced, with permission, from the *Annual Review of Cell Biology,* Volume 10, © 1994, by Annual Reviews Inc.)

Downstream Signaling Events of Activated RPTKs

A major intracellular pathway used in RPTK signaling involves a membrane-associated protein called Ras (discussed below). In addition to activating Ras, RPTKs also activate a variety of other target protein (see Table 10.2) including other enzymes, adapter proteins, and structural proteins.

SH2 & SH3 Domains. To understand the chemical significance of phosphorylation on tyrosine residues, we must understand how this event physically attracts other molecules to interact with the receptor. The unraveling of this process has been a remarkable achievement and reinforces the importance of understanding the three-dimensional structure of protein molecules.

The three-dimensional structure of a soluble cytoplasmic tyrosine kinase called **Src** indicated that a specialized region of this protein was involved in its association with its substrates. This domain of the Src molecule consisted of an approximately 100–amino

acid stretch and appeared to be essential for the kinase to bind its substrate. A very similar amino acid stretch was noted in many proteins that interfaced with the cytoplasmic region of the RPTK. These domains, called **SH2 domains** (Src-homology 2), and another stretch known as **SH3** (about 60 amino acids) were examined at the crystallographic level and shown to have a pocket into which a phosphorylated tyrosine residue would fit. This type of binding motif has been shown in nearly all proteins that bind phosphorylated tyrosines. Both SH2 and SH3 domains are prominent in cytoplasmic proteins that are part of the tyrosine-kinase signaling system.

Adapter Proteins. One of the first cytoplasmic events after RPTK activation is the binding of a special type of protein, called an **adapter protein,** to the receptor. Adapter molecules usually contain one or more SH2 domains and associate with phosphotyrosines on the cytoplasmic surface of the receptor. There, the adapter proteins link other cytoplasmic proteins to the activated receptor. One of the first

Table 10–1. Families of signaling cytokines

Growth factors
  Platelet-derived growth factor family (PDGF)
    PDGF A
    PDGF B
    VEGF
    PLGF
    CSF-1
    SCF (steel factor)
  Fibroblast growth factor family (FGF)
    αFGF
    βFGF
    int 2
    K-FGF
    FGF-5
    GFG-6
    KGF
    FGF-8
    FGF-9
  Insulin family
    Insulin
    IGF-1
    IGF-2
  Epidermal growth factor family (EGF)
  Tumor-derived growth factor α
  Nerve Growth Factor Family (NGF)
    NGF
    BDNF
    NT-3,4,5
  Hepatocyte Growth Factor Family (HGF)
Interferons
  Interferon α
  Interferon β
  Interferon γ
Interleukins
  Interleukin 1–17
Tumor Necrosis Factor (TNF)
  TNFα
  TNFβ
Colony-stimulating factors (CSF)
  G-CSF
  M-CSF
  GM-CSF
Tumor growth Factor-β (TGFβ)

adapter proteins to be identified, **Grb2,** is a 24-kDa protein that contains one SH2 and two SH3 domains. Grb2 links a nucleotide-exchange protein to the activated receptor. Ultimately this complex stimulates a third member of this signaling pathway, called **Ras** (see Figure 10–4), which initiates additional signaling events that will be discussed in more detail below.

A somewhat different type of adapter protein is **insulin growth factor–1 (IGF-1).** This adapter contains no SH2 or SH3 domains but does have several "reactive" tyrosine residues that are phosphorylated during insulin activation of its receptor. The phosphorylated tyrosines then bind to the SH2 domain of Grb2, and this complex acts as an adapter and activates Ras. Another adapter protein, **NCK,** is found in most cells during tissue formation, organ development, and organ differentiation. NCK associates with sites on the PDGF receptor as well as on the EGF receptor.

Figure 10–5 shows an expanded cartoon of the PDGF receptor's cytoplasmic domain and the different locations where adapter molecules bind, as well as where other cytoplasmic proteins link to the activated receptor.

The Ras Pathway. A key protein in the tyrosine signaling cascade is a small (21 kDa) membrane-associated GTPase called Ras. Ras belongs to a family of monomeric GTPases that behave as **molecular switches.** Ras is particularly notable for its activation of downstream molecules involved in cell proliferation. (See Figure 10–4.)

Ras alternates between an active state with bound GTP and an inactive state with bound GDP. The activation-inactivation pathway for Ras involves two other proteins. First, a guanine-nucleotide exchange factor (GEF) binds and causes inactive Ras to exchange its GDP for GTP, which leads to the Ras-GTP, the active form. Then Ras-GTP is inactivated by the binding of GTPase-accelerating protein (GAP), which enhances the intrinsic GTPase activity of Ras.

Interestingly, there are some similarities between Ras and the Gα subunit of the G protein signaling molecule, which indicates that these two proteins are likely related. They share similar amino acid sequences near the GTP binding pockets, and both require the association of other proteins to activate and release GTP.

The GEF that activates Ras in the RPTK signaling cascade is a protein called **SOS.** The name SOS is derived from a study of *Drosophila* eye development, in which a nucleotide-exchange protein was shown to be essential for neuroretinal cell formation. A mutation that resulted in the lack of this protein was called *son of sevenless,* abbreviated SOS. This protein is activated when it binds to the adapter protein Grb2, and in its active form, SOS causes the GDP-GTP exchange on Ras. Activated Ras triggers a protein kinase cascade that leads to changes in gene expression, often involving genes that cause cells to divide.

In summary, the steps of the signaling cascade leading to Ras activation are:

1. Growth factor binds to RPTK.
2. Dimerization of the receptor and autophosphorylation of the receptor's tyrosine residues occur.
3. Grb2 binds to a specific phosphorylated tyrosine through its SH2 domain.
4. Binding results in a conformational change in Grb2, and its SH3 domains bind to SOS.
5. SOS associates with membrane-bound Ras, causing it to exchange GDP for GTP, thereby activating Ras.

What happens downstream of activated Ras involves several other intracellular kinases, as discussed in the next section.

The MAP Pathway. Several lines of evidence have revealed that activated Ras initiates a series of

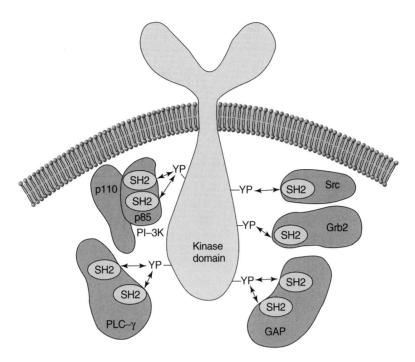

Figure 10–3. Binding of cytoplasmic effector molecules to activated growth factor receptor. Cartoon depicts the association of several cytoplasmic effector molecules with the phosphorylated tyrosines of the receptor cytoplasmic tail. The SH2 domains of effector molecules provide the docking motifs for the phosphotyrosines (YP) on the receptor. (Modified and reproduced, with permission, from Balcavage WX, King MW: *Biochemistry: Examination & Board Review.* Appleton & Lange, 1995, p. 361.)

reactions that stimulate other kinase molecules in the cell, leading to cell division. This pathway, known as the **MAP (mitogen-activated protein) kinase pathway** is conserved in all organisms studied so far and is an important pathway in all cells. It is activated during development, when there is the need to produce new cells as tissues and organs grow, and it is quiescent in fully differentiated, nondividing cells. However, if new cells are needed (ie, for the repair or remodeling of tissues), then this kinase cascade is activated. In addition, many types of cancer result from an unregulated MAP kinase pathway.

The first protein that activated Ras targets is an intracellular serine-threonine kinase called **Raf-1.** Different experiments have shown that activated Ras binds and activates Raf-1 as the first member of the downstream activation pathway. Activated Raf-1 recruits and activates another intracellular kinase that has the unique property of possessing both a catalytic domain for tyrosine phosphorylation and a domain for phosphorylating substrates on Ser-Thr residues. This remarkable kinase, called **MEK (M**AP kinase/ **e**xtracellular signal–regulated **k**inase) or **MAP2K (MAP kinase kinase),** has the ability to divert the RPTK signal down more than one pathway. One such pathway is activation of kinases that control the cy

clins as well as the cyclin-dependent kinases (CDKs; see Chapter 6) leading to cell division.

One of the hurdles to understanding the complex relationships of the signaling cascades in the MAP pathway arises from the confusing and inconsistent nomenclature that is used in the literature. We have attempted to simplify the names whenever possible; however, no universal nomenclature has yet been adopted. Raf-1 is also known as mitogen-activated protein kinase kinase kinase, MAP kinase kinase kinase, or more simply MAP3K.

The NH2-domain of Raf-1 binds to the activated Ras protein. This binding activates Raf-1 to phosphorylate the third member of this pathway, MAP2K. *The MAP2K protein is unique in that it can, by itself, phosphorylate regulatory threonine and tyrosine residues on its substrate, MAP kinase (MAPK), the central member in the MAP pathway.* Other possible substrates have been looked for but only members of the MAPK family can serve as substrates for MAP2K. MAP2K phosphorylates its two residues on MAPK in sequence, first tyrosine-185 (Tyr185), then threonine-183 (Thr183). Once the Tyr and Thr residues have received their phosphate, MAP2K is inactivated by a specific phosphatase.

The MAPK family consists of three isoforms

Table 10–2. Selected substrates and targets of receptor protein–tyrosine kinases.

Enzymes
 PLCγ
 RAS
 Src family of kinases
 SH-PTPs (tyrosine-phosphatases)
 PI3 kinase
Adapter Proteins
 IRS-1
 NCK
 CRK
 GRB-2
 SHC
Structural Proteins
 Annexins
 Ezrin
 Clathrin
 Vinculin
 Talin
 Tensin
 Paxilin
 AFAP (F-actin binding protein)

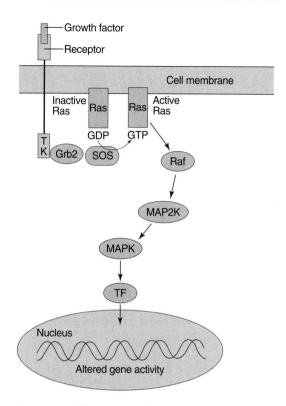

Figure 10–4. The Ras signaling pathway. The simplified model shows how an activated receptor's kinase domain associates with an adapter molecule, Grb2, which then binds and activates a nucleotide exchange protein, SOS, which forces the Ras protein to exchange its bound GDP for GTP. This exchange then activates a kinase cascade that activates several proteins on the way to cell division. (Reproduced and modified, with permission, from Ganong WF: *Review of Medical Physiology,* 17th ed. Appleton & Lange, 1995, p. 41.)

(MAPK, Erk-1, and Erk-2), which can be activated in response to numerous growth factors and mitogens. In all of these molecules, both the tyrosine and threonine residues must be phosphorylated to achieve a fully activated enzyme. Because of the broad nature of its substrate recognition, MAPK can phosphorylate many proteins after they are activated. These proteins are usually regulatory and function in both the nucleus and cytoplasm. They include transcription factors, cytoskeletal regulatory proteins, and even substrates that are part of the initial signaling cascade (SOS, Raf-1, and even the RPTK receptor itself, creating a positive feedback loop for continued signaling events).

The growth factor–stimulated signaling cascade has proven to be a central pathway for the cell. Most of the 50 or more oncogenes that are currently known encode proteins that participate in the various cascade events by which growth factors stimulate normal cell division. These oncogene homologues of the normal proteins involved in the signal cascade are subdivided into four major groups:

- growth factors
- growth factor receptors
- transducers of growth factor responses
- transcription factors.

The transducers of growth factor response are of special interest here because some include members of the MAPK cascade.

Summary of the MAP Pathway. The events of this pathway are as follows:

1. Growth factor binds to its receptor—this leads to dimerization of the receptor and autophosphorylation.
2. Grb2 binds to phosphorylated tyrosines via SH2 domains.
3. SH3 domains provide a binding site for SOS.
4. The Ras-Grb2-SOS complex associates with Ras-GDP, and SOS catalyzes the exchange of GDP to GTP on Ras, thereby activating Ras.
5. Activated Ras-GTP associates with the Raf-1 at its NH2 domain, and Raf-1 is activated.
6. Activated Raf-1 recruits and binds MAP2K to its C-terminal domain, activating MAP2K.
7. Activated MAP2K in turn activates MAP and the kinases for other pathways.
8. Activated MAP phosphorylates transcription factors to activate other genes.

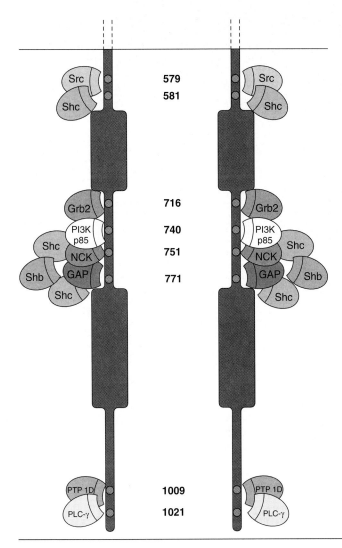

579
581

716

740

751

771

1009

1021

Figure 10–5. Binding of various signal-transducing molecules to different phosphorylated tyrosines in the PDGF receptor. The PDGF receptor has a split kinase domain. The locations of phosphotyrosines to which various effector molecules bind are shown. The binding of Src to its phosphotyrosine is near the membrane. Binding and activation of phospholipase C–γ (PLC-γ) is very near the C terminus of the receptor. The outlined area in each signal-transduction molecule represents the SH2 domain. (Reproduced and modified, with permission, from Claesson-Welsh LJ: Platelet derived growth receptor signals. J Biol Chem 1994;269:32023.)

THE Src FAMILY OF INTRACELLULAR TYROSINE KINASES

Approximately 85 years ago Francis Peyton Rous identified a virus, called **Rous sarcoma virus,** that causes cancer in chickens. The virus was purified and shown to infect and transform chicken tissue culture cells in vitro. A related virus was also isolated that could also infect and replicate in chicken cells without transforming them into tumor cells. This observation suggested that the Rous sarcoma virus carried an oncogene that is missing in the benign virus. When molecular techniques became available to examine the genomes of the two virus strains, it was found that the transforming virus contained an extra gene that was named *v-src* (viral-sarcoma). Additional experiments showed that when the *v-src* gene was transfected into normal cells they became transformed (tumor cells), indicating that *v-src* was an **oncogene.**

Analysis of the genomes of normal cells showed that they contain a very similar gene, called **c-src,** which encodes a protein tyrosine kinase. Because mutations in this gene lead to tumor cells, it is known as a **proto-oncogene.** The appearance of *v-src* is believed to be the result of the virus capturing a copy of the *c-src* DNA from its host. Through many viral generations, the copy of the *src* gene was mutated and its normal control region was lost.

This was the first tyrosine kinase to be identified and was called the **Src kinase** after the type of tumor (sarcoma) that it caused. It is now recognized that Src represents a family of specialized intracellular tyrosine kinases (Figure 10–6). There are currently nine recognized members of the family (Src, Fyn, Yes,

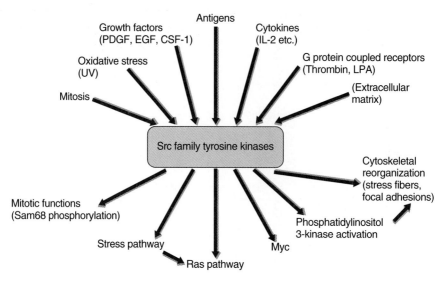

Figure 10–6. Multiple actions of the Src kinases in cell signaling. A variety in external signals will activate the various members of the Src family of kinases. In the lower half of the diagram, the arrows indicate the various pathways or specific substrates that these kinases will activate. (Modified and reproduced, with permission, from Erpel T; Courtneidge SA: Src family protein tyrosine kinases and cellular signal transduction pathways. Curr Opin Cell Biol 1995;7:176.)

Fgr, Lck, Yrk, Hck, Lyn, and Blk). Most of these proteins show restricted tissue distribution with expression in specific hematopoietic cells; however, a few members, such as Src, Yes, and Fyn, are expressed in a wide variety of cell types. Members of the Src family show a high degree of structural homology with common domains and regulatory mechanism.

Interestingly, Src (and members of its family) can be activated through the growth factor–signaling pathways. For example, when PDGF activates its receptor, one of the phosphorylated tyrosines provides a docking site for the SH2 domain of Src. (Recall that the tyrosine-binding domain was first recognized in the Src kinase and was named the Src-homology, or SH2, motif). Src kinases are also activated by receptors that are coupled to G proteins. For example, thrombin, which has a role in coagulation and acts as a growth factor, having its own special receptor coupled through a G protein, also activates Src kinases in several cell types.

Src family members are involved in several signal-transducing pathways, including those that result in cell division, cytoskeletal rearrangements, and responses of cells recovering from oxidative and other forms of cell stress. This family of intracellular kinases have been systematically shown to be major participants in many pathways and cellular behavioral responses and must be considered major regulators of cell function. It is already well known that when these kinases lose their capacity to be carefully

regulated, then dire consequences occur, such as unregulated cell proliferation and hence cancer.

PROTEIN PHOSPHATASES & SIGNAL TRANSDUCTION

The protein phosphatases are divided into two major groups, **protein serine-threonine phosphatases (PSPs)** and **protein tyrosine phosphatases (PTPs).** A given species might have as many as 1000 different phosphatase genes (of course, not all are expressed in the same cell). The activities of the PSP and PTP are carefully regulated in the cell. As indicated in Chapter 6, the PSPs are subdivided into four major types, PP1, PP2A, PP2B, and PP2C; all are essential for the cell and many of them have multiple copies of their catalytic subunit in the same polypeptide. The importance of the PSPs and PTPs to cell function is exemplified by the fact that they are often the targets for microbial or viral products that interfere with cell function. A number of bacterial toxins are specific inhibitors of phosphatase activity. (Purification of several of these toxins has been useful in tracking down the specific function of the phosphatase in the cell.)

Cell signaling pathways require that the action between tyrosine kinases and tyrosine phosphatases be precisely coordinated. When an RPTK is activated in a given cell, the tyrosine phosphorylated event lasts only briefly. If the same cell is treated with a PTP inhibitor (such as sodium vanadate), the duration of the signal is greatly extended. The first PTP to be purified and sequenced from human tissue was found to have a strong homology to a common leukocyte surface antigen called **CD45,** a transmembrane protein with a catalytic phosphatase domain essential for T-cell activation by the T-cell receptor.

Two PTPs that have SH2 domains have been identified and cloned. SH-PTP1 associates with tyrosine residues on the cytoplasmic tail of several growth factor receptors (PDGF, EGF, IGF-1) and is involved in removing phosphates from the tyrosine residues, thereby attenuating the growth factor signal. SH-PTP2, in contrast, binds to phosphotyrosine on substrates farther downstream in the signal cascade. Clearly, a balance between phosphorylation and dephosphorylation is strictly maintained in the growth factor signaling cascade. Figure 10–7 illustrates how several different PTPs and CD45 can function as receptors.

SIGNAL PATHWAY FROM TYROSINE KINASE–ASSOCIATED RECEPTORS

A surprisingly large number of protein signaling molecules that are not specifically recognized as growth factors have been identified in the past few years. For the most part, these small soluble proteins (10–30 kDa) are mainly involved in signaling between cells of the immune and hematopoietic systems and signaling from cells near a site of inflammation. As more has been learned about their function, many have been shown to be involved in other signaling events, particularly those in neural and embryonic development.

The receptors of this large group of molecules initiate the second major signaling pathway that in-

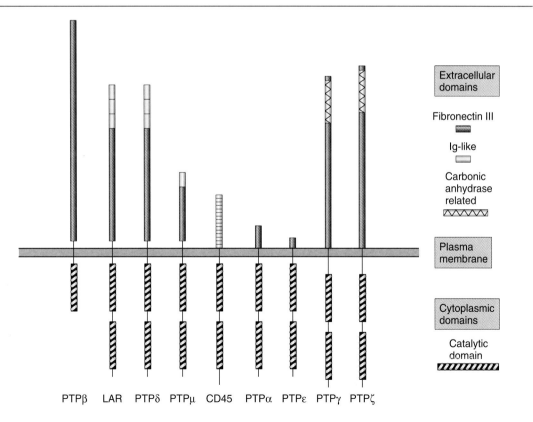

Figure 10–7. Phosphatases also function as receptors in many cell types. Many cells have single-pass membrane proteins that have phosphatase domains as part of their cytoplasmic structure. In almost all receptors of this type, there are two catalytic phosphatase units in the cytoplasmic tail. (Modified and reproduced, with permission, from Hunter T et al: Receptor protein tyrosine kinases and phosphatases. Cold Spring Harbor Symp Quant Biol 1992;57:25.)

volves tyrosine phosphorylation. Like the RPTK receptors, these are single membrane–pass proteins and they are activated after ligand binding by phosphorylation on tyrosine residues located in the cytoplasmic tail of the receptor. However, *unlike* the RPTKs (which have a kinase domain in the receptor itself), these receptors are phosphorylated by a special family of cytoplasmic tyrosine kinases called the **Janus kinases (JAKs),** of which there are four members: **JAK1, JAK2, JAK3,** and **TYK2.** It is believed that these kinases reside in close proximity to receptors on the inner surface of the membrane. The JAKs phosphorylate selected tyrosine residues on both the receptor and signaling proteins that dock on the receptor.

As described in the introduction, these molecules are recognized as cytokines and can be further subdivided into the following categories:

1. **Interferons (IFNs),** of which there are three types—IFNα, IFNβ, and IFNγ. Each type is derived from a different cell type and performs independent but overlapping functions.
2. **Interleukins (IL),** of which as many as 17 different polypeptides (IL-1 to IL-17) are known. The name of this group was chosen as a way to describe molecules that were involved in signaling among cells of the immune system (T-cells, B-cells, NK-cells, dendritic cells, and various types of macrophages).
3. **Tumor necrosis factor (TNF),** which is involved in important cellular functions that occur during acute inflammatory crisis. TNF received its name from one of its early defined functions, that of killing certain kinds of tumor cells.
4. **Colony stimulating factors (CSFs),** named for their individual ability to stimulate the differentiation and maturation of white blood cells in vitro. These cells include granulocyte-colony stimulating factor (G-CSF), monocyte-colony stimulating factor (M-CSF), and granulocyte-monocyte–stimulating factor (GM-CSF).

It is beyond the scope of our discussion to explore the function of each of these molecules. However, many cytokines share important characteristics.

PROPERTIES OF THE NON–TYROSINE KINASE RECEPTORS

Redundancy

Many members of the cytokine family can stimulate the same response in a cell. That is, one cytokine can perform the function of another in signal initiation. In certain instances, the initiation of a cell response is so crucial that having a backup signaling system may provide a survival advantage. It is be-

lieved that the molecular basis of this redundancy involves the cytokine receptor. Molecules that initiate the same response in a cell are said to have redundant signaling signals.

Sharing of Receptor Transducing Subunits

The cell-surface receptors of cytokines that exhibit redundant signaling are composed of two polypeptide chains. One of the subunits is the cytokine-binding or recognition subunit; the other is a subunit used for generating the signal that is transduced into the cell. Because a number of cytokines share the same signal transducing protein, overlapping signal information

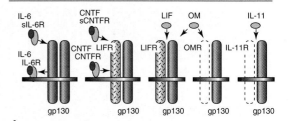

A

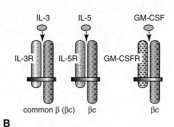

B

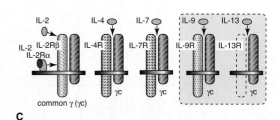

C

Figure 10–8. Sharing of receptor subunits helps explain redundancy in hematopoietic cytokine signaling systems. (A) Five members of the IL-6 subfamily (IL-6, CNTF, LIF, OM, IL-11) all share a common signal-transducing subunit, gp130. Each has its own "cognate" receptor that recognizes the specific cytokine. (B) These three cytokines, IL-3, IL-5, and GM-CSF, share a common subunit, β. (C) This system utilizes a common subunit, the IL-2 γ subunit, but the system also has a common cognate receptor. In the case of IL-2 three different polypeptides are required for signaling. (Modified and reproduced, with permission, from Kishimoto T et al: Cytokine signal transduction. Cell 1994;76:259. © 1994 Cell Press.)

is often generated by two or more cytokines. For example, the following cytokines all share a subunit (see also Figure 10–8):

- IL-6, IL-11, ciliary neurotrophic factor (CNTF), and leukemia inhibitory factor (LIF)
- IL-3, IL-5, and GM-CSF
- IL-2, IL-4, and IL-7.

Pleiotropy

It was expected that each cytokine would exert a specific effect on its particular target cell; however, this turned out not to be entirely true. Instead, many cytokines can affect target cells in more than one way, a feature known as pleiotropy. For example, IL-6 causes activated B lymphocytes to differentiate into plasma cells (antibody-producing cells); it also stimulates hepatocytes to increase production of certain plasma proteins. Moreover, IL-6 is involved in fever production during inflammation and in neural cell development. Thus IL-6 is multifunctional and induces different responses in different cells. This same pleiotropic action is seen in other members of the cytokine family.

Cytokines of the hematopoietic and immune system control an amazing number cellular responses (Table 10–3). In most instances the cytokines in this category carry out their signaling function via a paracrine pathway, although a few are found in the general circulation under pathologic conditions. In general, one may consider that these types of cytokines are of two main functional groups: (1) those involved in a **proinflammatory response** and (2) those serving as general **alarm signals** and are involved in mobilizing the immune system. The proinflammatory cytokine group includes TNF, IL-1, and IL-6. The anti-inflammatory cytokines include IL-2, IL-4, (and often IL-6 as well), and IL-10. The other hematopoietic cytokines regulate specific gene expression in hematopoietic cells.

The classic definition of a hormone is a molecule produced by a cell, secreted into the circulation, and delivered to target cells at some distance from its origin. Some cytokines could be considered hormones under special circumstances. For example, IL-1, TNF, and IL-6 are detectable in the blood in certain pathologic situations (inflammatory crisis, sepsis) and perform their signaling function far from their source. Normally, however, these proteins function in a paracrine fashion. It is obvious there is some overlap in definition among these types of proteins.

Table 10–3. Major sources and activities of selected cytokines.[1]

Cytokine	Primary Cellular Source	Primary Biologic Activity
IL-1	Macrophages	Immunologic and inflammatory mediator; acute phase reactant; augments immune responses
IL-2	T lymphocytes	Promotes T lymphocyte activation, growth
IL-3	T lymphocytes	Hematopoietic growth factor, "multicolony stimulating factor"
IL-4	T lymphocytes	T and B lymphocyte, mast cell growth factor; promotes IgE isotype switching
IL-5	T lymphocytes	B cell growth factor; promotes IgA production; promotes eosinophil growth and differentiation
IL-6	Macrophages, T lymphocytes	B cell differentiation factors; acute phase reactant
IL-7	Stromal cells of the spleen and thymus	Growth factor for very early B and T lymphocytes
TNF	Macrophages, T cells, mast cells, NK cells	Overlaps activity with IL-1 but has more antitumor activity
IFN-α IFN-β IFN-γ	B lymphocytes, macrophages Fibroblasts, epithelial cells T lymphocytes	Antiviral and antitumor activities; activates macrophages; enhances cytotoxic lymphocyte and NK activity
GM-CSF	T lymphocytes, fibroblasts, endothelial cells	Growth factor for granulocytes, macrophage and eosinophil colonies; activates neutrophil phagocytosis; enhances eosinophil-mediated cytotoxicity; promotes basophil histamine release

[1]Reproduced, with permission, from Tierney LM Jr et al: *Current Medical Diagnosis & Treatment,* 33rd ed. Appleton & Lange, 1994, p. 645.
IL = interleukin; TNF = tumor necrosis factor; IFN = interferon; GM-CSF = granulocyte-macrophage colony-stimulating factor; NK = natural killer cells.

HEMATOPOIETIC CYTOKINE RECEPTORS

As previously indicated, the receptors of this large group of molecules initiate signaling cascades in a similar fashion to the RPTK receptors. In general the signaling cascades from these receptors often involve the activation of genes for differentiation and for increased expression of genes. To be certain, signals arising from these cytokines often also activate the Ras pathway to activate genes involved in cell proliferation. Several special features of the hematopoietic receptors are described below. They share several similarities:

- They are all single-pass transmembrane proteins.
- Their extracellular regions possess different types of tandem repeat motifs.
- Their cytoplasmic domains, although variable in length, possess tyrosine residues that when phosphorylated serve as docking sites for substrates involved in downstream signaling.
- *None have an intrinsic kinase domain as a part of their amino acid sequence.*

The last feature is universal among hematopoietic cytokines. In addition as indicated above, many cytokine receptors are composed of at least two subunits, but some are single polypeptides. Of these, **erythropoietin (EpoR), growth hormone (GHR),** and **prolactin (PRLR)** receptors are the most prominent.

Receptors for the various hematopoietic cytokines are diverse and belong to four main families of receptors (Figure 10–9): (1) **class I,** (2) **class II,** (3) **TNF,** (4) **IL-1.** Most of the cytokine binding receptors belong to the class I type of receptor. Members of this group have conserved amino acid sequence motifs in their extracellular domain. These consist of four cysteine residues located in the same relative positions of the receptor as well as the highly conserved sequence Trp-Ser-X-Trp-Ser (W-S-X-W-S), where X is any nonconserved amino acid. The ligands for class II receptors also have the four positionally conserved cysteines but lack the W-S-X-W-S motif.

A fifth group of inflammatory cytokines known as **chemokines** are known for their chemoattractive properties; these cytokines recruit macrophages and neutrophils into areas of inflammation. The receptors for the chemokine molecules are seven membrane–pass receptors and invoke signal cascades utilizing the G protein signal pathways described in Chapter 9.

THE HEMATOPOIETIC CYTOKINE SIGNALING PATHWAYS

Many cytokine receptors are capable of transmitting two types of signals: (1) the signal similar to RPTK receptors and involving the activation of the Ras signaling pathway as described above, and (2) a more specific signal that activates particular cytokine-responsive genes. Experiments in which portions of a receptor's cytoplasmic domain were deleted revealed that sites located in a membrane-proximal region are generally required for stimulation of the Ras pathway (Figure 10–10). In contrast, the carboxy-terminal regions of the receptors appear to have the domains for activating molecules that affect cytokine-specific genes. Rapid, transient phosphorylation of tyrosine residues occurs on the receptor when the cytokine binds to the external domain of the receptor and causes its dimerization. Phosphorylation of tyrosines on cytokine receptors is carried out by a special family of cytoplasmic tyrosine kinases known as the JAKs (see above). These kinases reside close to the inner face of the cell membrane, next to the cytokine receptor. When the receptor dimerizes after ligand (cytokine) binding, the JAK is activated and rapidly phosphorylates the receptor and molecules that will "dock" on the phosphotyrosines of the receptor.

Many types of cytokines utilize "latent" transcription factor proteins that are located in the cytoplasm. After their activation, these transcription factors move to the nucleus and bind to regulatory regions of specific genes. One group of these factors consists of proteins called **STATs** (**S**ignal **t**ransducers and **a**ctivators of **t**ranscription). To date, six different STATs have been identified.

The basic events of STAT activation occur as follows (Figure 10–11):

1. After cytokine receptor activation by JAKs, the STAT associates with the receptor through its SH2 domain.
2. JAK phosphorylates the STAT.
3. STAT is released from receptor and dimerizes with another activated STAT.
4. The STAT dimer quickly moves into the nucleus.

RECEPTORS WITH A SERINE-THREONINE KINASE DOMAIN

TRANSFORMING GROWTH FACTOR–β

Transforming Growth Factor–β (TGF-β) is the "parent member" of a superfamily of related polypeptides that perform a number of important functions in the cell. Members of this family have been shown to be involved in several functions crucial to

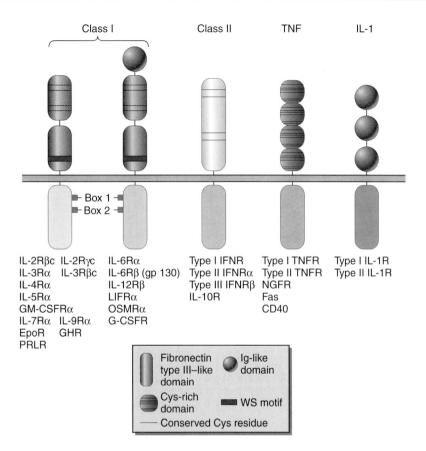

Figure 10–9. Receptor classes and motifs for hematopoietic signaling system. This cartoon depicts the structural motifs that help characterize receptors for the hematopoietic signaling cytokines. The identifying structural motifs contained in the largest family of hematopoietic cytokine receptors are found in the class I group of receptors (characterized by four cysteine residues and a W-S-X-W-S motif). A subgroup of this family of receptors also has an Ig-like domain. Class II receptors are similar to those of class I in having the cluster of four cysteine residues, but they lack the W-S-X-W-S motif. The TNF receptor family and the IL-1 receptor family with their common structural motifs are also shown. (Modified and reproduced, with permission, from Taniguchi T: Cytokine signaling through nonreceptor protein tyrosine kinases. Science 1995;268:252.)

cell differentiation and to participate in establishing the morphological body plan of the organism during embryogenesis. Some members of the TGF-β family participate in the formation of cartilage and bone and in the development of the sexual organs.

Although TFG-β (and family members) perform growth factor functions, one the best observed effects of TGF-β is its *inhibition* of growth of many cell types. The *yin* of growth factors and the *yang* of TGF-β may represent one of the important mechanisms of cell cycle arrest and the development of the morphological characteristics of the forming embryo. For example, members of the TGF-β family are expressed at sites where autonomic neurons differentiate. **Bone morphogenic protein 2 (BMP2),** a member of the TGF-β family, is expressed in the dorsal aorta of the developing embryo near where sympa-

thetic ganglia form. BMP2 is also involved in expansion of sympathetic neurons. TGF-β1, in contrast, drives certain embryonic cells to form smooth muscle cells. Thus these two members of the same "growth factor family" act instructively to influence the formation of progenitor cells that perform quite different functions and generate cellular diversity. Members of the TGF-β family are participants in development across all the phylogenetic spectra.

The TGF-βs are homodimers with a molecular weight of 25,000. They are synthesized in precursor forms and secreted as latent complexes that require proteolytic processing for activation. Once TGF-β is proteolytically processed, it can affect many cell types. In addition to its role in development and differentiation, TGF-β is also an important for wound healing and downregulating some causes of inflam-

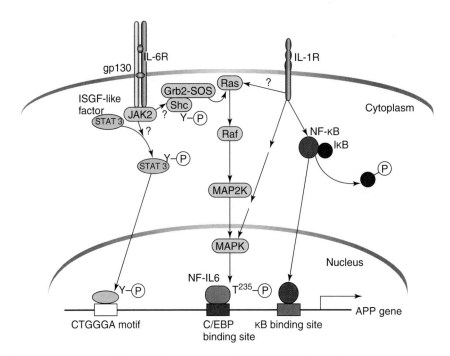

Figure 10–10. A model of two cytokine signaling pathways showing how each can stimulate both its own specific genes as well as activation of the Ras pathway. IL-6 and IL-1 not only have the ability to activate their own specific responsive genes through the STAT or NF-κB pathway, but also can stimulate the activation of Ras, leading to activation of the MAPK pathway and cell division. (Modified and reproduced, with permission, from Kishimoto T et al: Cytokine signal transduction. Cell 1994;76:259. © 1994 Cell Press.)

mation. For example, TGF-β stimulates synthesis of extracellular matrix proteins such as collagen types II and IV and fibronectin; stimulates osteogenic activity; and acts as a chematotactic factor for monocytes, fibroblasts, and astrocytes. In contrast, TGF-β suppresses proliferation and function of T- and B-lymphocytes and inhibits proliferation of endothelial and epithelial cells.

TGF-β Receptors

The TGF-β receptors represent the third type of signaling receptor class cited at the beginning of the

Figure 10–11. Many cytokines and growth-factor receptors are activated by JAKs and use the same STAT. This illustration shows that many interleukins use the same STAT molecules to activate downstream genes. Note that all STATs dimerize before entering the nucleus and binding to their responsive elements (RE) on the promoter of the gene they activate. (Abbreviations: EPO = erythropoietin; IL = interleukin; LIF = leukemia inhibitory factor; CNTF = ciliary neurotrophic factor; GH = growth factor; INF = interferon.)

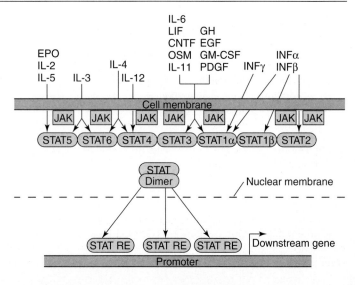

chapter. These receptors are unique because their signaling motif is a kinase that autophosphorylates serine or threonine residues on the receptor, instead of tyrosines (as is the case for RPTKs and hematopoietic cytokine receptors).

There are three major types of TGF-β receptors: type I (53 kDa), type II (70–85 kDa), and type III (200 kDa). The type III receptor is a surface proteoglycan that appears to regulate the access of TGF-β to the other two receptor types. Types I and II are single-pass transmembrane receptors that have a serine-threonine kinase domain within their cytoplasmic domain (Figure 10–12A), and both are necessary for downstream signaling. When TGF-β binds to the receptor, types I and II form a heterodimer that activates the kinase domains.

Several different experimental approaches have demonstrated the requirement of both type I and type II TGF-β receptors for the signaling event. This requirement is another important difference between TGF-β receptors and the other receptors discussed in this chapter. Experiments were performed to identify which TGF-β receptor was required to transmit the TGF-β signal (Fig. 10–12B). Cells con-

taining no TGF-β receptor were transfected with type I and II receptors individually and together. The transfected cells were then exposed to TGF-β. When either type II or type I was transfected alone, no TGF-β signal was detected when TGF-β was added. The TGF-β signal only occurred when both fully functional type I and II receptors were transfected together.

Only a few downstream substrates of the TGF-β receptor have been identified. It now appears that one of the first signals that occurs after TGF-β binds to its receptor is the activation of PKC. Cells have a number of physiologic responses to TGF-β, as mentioned above; some undoubtedly result from binding of intracellular proteins to the activated receptor. However, the precise binding and activation events have not been clearly established. TGF-β apparently regulates the expression of proteins that inhibit cell cycle activity in many cells.

Although type I and II receptors are required for signaling, there is considerable heterogeneity in the structure of these receptors in different cell types, which may account for the diversity of responses elicited by this cytokine.

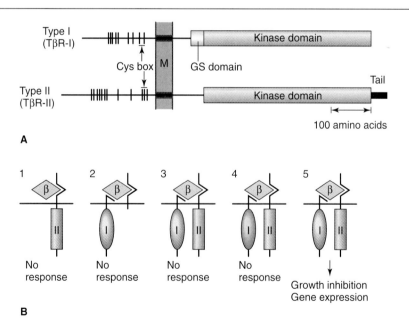

Figure 10–12. A model of TGF-β type I and II receptors and the mechanisms of dimerization and signaling. (A) Arrangement of the two receptor types. Both contain an extensive kinase domain in the cytoplasmic tail that is rich in serine and threonine residues. The type I receptor also contains a GS box (GSGSG) proximal to the kinase domain whose function is unknown. There are several cysteine-rich areas in the extracytoplasmic region. (B) Experiments that demonstrated that both type I and II receptors are required for signaling to occur. Fully competent type I and II receptors alone failed to generate a signal. If one of the receptors was mutagenized and the other normal a signal failed to occur. Only when both receptors were present and competent could a TFG-β signal be generated. (Modified and reproduced, with permission, from Massague J et al: The TGF-β family and its composite receptors. Trends Cell Biol 1994;4:176.)

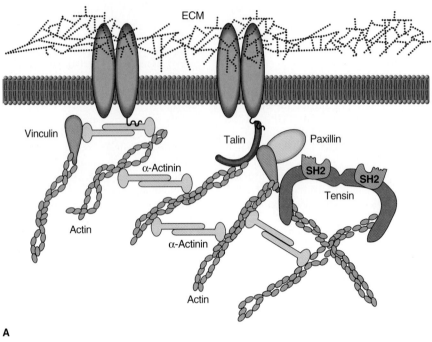

A

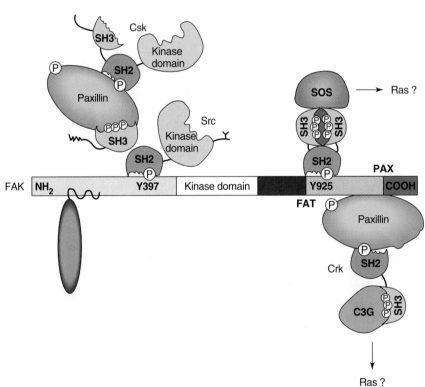

B

SIGNALING THROUGH INTEGRIN RECEPTORS

THE ECM-INTEGRIN-CYTOSKELETON CONNECTION

Integrins are the cell surface receptors that mediate cell attachment to the extracellular matrix. As described in Chapter 8, these receptors are involved in cell-cell and cell-matrix interactions and are an integral part of many cellular functions, including embryonic development, tumor cell growth and metastasis, apoptosis, coagulation, and cell migration to sites of inflammation. Recall that the integrins are noncovalently linked dimers composed of α and β subunits derived from among 16 α and 8 β subunit families. At least 20 different integrins have been identified. Although most integrins are involved in the formation of cellular connections with extracellular matrix molecules, some are essential for the formation of connections between *cells*. These are the so-called **intracellular adhesion molecules (ICAMs).**

Both receptor clustering and ligand occupancy are crucial for activation of intracellular integrin responses. Integrin receptor engagement and clustering lead to the formation of focal adhesion plaques (often referred to as focal adhesions). These plaques are where integrins form a link to intracellular cytoskeletal complexes containing bundles of actin filaments. These supramolecular complexes play an important part in modulating cell adhesion and in regulating changes in cell shape that are essential for locomotion and spreading (see Chapter 8).

The Structure & Components of the Adhesion Plaques

Like the cytokine receptors, the cytoplasmic domains of integrin subunits have no intrinsic catalytic activity. Rather, they function by coupling with cytoplasmic proteins that form complexes containing both cytoskeletal and signaling proteins. It is important to emphasize that integrins link extracellular matrix proteins on the outside of the cell to cytoskeletal proteins and actin filaments on the cytoplasmic face (ie, the inside) of the cell. A proposed model of this arrangement is shown in Figure 10–13. The precise molecular interactions have not been unequivocally established, but the model shown is likely a reasonable facsimile of this supramolecular complex.

SUMMARY

In this chapter we have considered a large group of polypeptide molecules collectively known as cytokines that function as information-bearing molecules. The receptors of these cytokines fall into two main groups: those that have a tyrosine kinase domain built into the receptor and those that use *cytoplasmic* tyrosine kinases to activate the receptor.

In addition, we considered a third group, the TGF-β receptors, which have a serine-threonine kinase domain as a part of their polypeptide structure. The signaling cascade is less well understood for TGF-β.

Each member of the large subgroup of cytokines known as growth factors has its own cognate receptor, which contains a tyrosine kinase as part of its polypeptide structure. When the receptor is activated (ie, its tyrosines phosphorylated), intracellular molecules are recruited to the receptor and become activated. As a result, a signaling cascade is initiated. Growth factor signaling involves activation of a critical membrane-associated GTPase, Ras, which specifically activates the kinase Raf-1. Raf-1 brings the growth factor signal to a junction kinase that can initiate the steps toward cell proliferation, cytoskeletal changes, or altered gene expression that leads to cell differentiation.

Two families of intracellular soluble tyrosine kinases were discussed, the Src family and the JAK family. Members of the Src family are predominantly associated with the signaling pathway leading to cell division, whereas JAK family members are involved with stimulating gene expression of differentiated cells. The JAK family is found mostly in cells of the

---

Figure 10–13. A model showing how signaling occurs through integrins. (A) The transmembrane integrins are linked to molecules on the outside of the cell (the extracellular matrix [ECM]), and their cytoplasmic domains associate with such cytoskeletal proteins as vinculin, talin, α-actinin, and paxillin, which link them to f-actin (actin filaments). In this assembly, intracellular proteins cluster to form a densely packed complex known as a focal adhesion. These assemblies of structural proteins stabilize adhesion plaques and regulate cell shape, morphology, and motility. These structures are also the site where integrin-induced changes in cell behavior are mediated. The cartoon shows a possible arrangement of the various molecules in the focal adhesion complex. (B) The presence of SH2 domains in signaling molecules and how they may dock onto the cytoplasmic tyrosine kinase known as FAK (focal adhesion kinase). Src family members associate with the FAK as they do with the adapter protein Grb2. Possible pathways leading to Ras activation are shown. The cartoon emphasizes the importance of clustered structural proteins and provides a visual concept of how these molecules could be interacting in an integrin-induced signaling cascade, which would alter cellular morphology and behavior. (Modified and reproduced, with permission, from Clark EA, Brugge JS: Integrins and signal transduction pathways: the road taken. Science 1995;268:235.)

hematopoietic, immune, and nervous system. The receptors that activate JAKs are different from the growth-factor receptors in that tyrosine kinase is not a part of their polypeptide structure. However, like growth-factor receptors, JAKs are activated by being phosphorylated on their cytoplasmic domains. Tyrosine phosphatases are critical to attenuating the signal. The PTPs and PSPs are quite numerous, and their activity is as carefully regulated as that of the protein kinases.

One subfamily of growth factors, known as transforming growth factor-β (TGF-β) acts both a growth inhibitor of cells and as a stimulator of cell growth and differentiation. Finally, special receptors known as integrins permit cells to respond to their extracellular matrices. Taken together, the examples presented in this chapter demonstrate the molecular language of how cells receive and process the information that controls their behavior.

REFERENCES

Blumer KJ, Johnson GL: Diversity in function and regulation of MAP kinase pathways. Trends Biol Sci 1994; 19:236.

Claesson-Welsh L: Platelet-derived growth factor receptor signals. J Biol Chem 1994;269:32023.

Davis RJ: The mitogen-activated protein kinase signal transduction pathway. J Biol Chem 1993;268:14553.

Erpel T, Courtneidge SA: Src family protein tyrosine kinases and cellular signal transduction pathways. Curr Opin Cell Biol 1995;7:176.

Felder CC: Muscarinic acetylcholine receptors: signal transduction through multiple effectors. FASEB J 1995; 9:619.

Howe LR et al: Activation of the MAP kinase pathway by the protein kinase raf. Cell 1992;71:335.

Hunter T et al: Receptor protein tyrosine kinases and phos-

phatases. Cold Spring Harbor Symp Quant Biol 1992; 57:25.

Ihle JN: Cytokine receptor signalling. Nature 1995;377: 591.

Marshall MS: Ras target proteins in eukaryotic cells. FABEB J 1995;9:13118.

Seger R, Krebs EG: The MAPK signaling cascade. FASEB J 1995;9:726.

Shenolikar S: Protein serine/threonine phosphatases—new avenues for cell regulation. Annu Rev Cell Biol 1994; 10:55.

Stoddard BL et al: Receptors and transmembrane signaling. Cold Spring Harbor Symp Quant Biol 1992;62:1.

Vojtek AB et al: Mammalian ras interacts directly with the serine/threonine kinase raf. Cell 1993;74:205.

Appendix A: Microscopy

Table A–1. Basic methods of tissue preparation for microscopy.*

Method and Purpose	Types and Procedures	Limitations and Associated Artifacts
Fixation: Preserves structural organization of cells, tissues, and organs of interest. Prevents bacterial and enzymatic digestion, insolubilizes tissue components to prevent diffusion, and protects against damage from subsequent steps in tissue processing.	**Chemical Fixation:** Common approach. Chemical fixatives used individually or in mixtures. Best results achieved by rapid penetration of living tissue with fixative. Small tissue pieces may be fixed by **immersion.** Entire organs may be fixed by **perfusion** (fixative pumped through vessels serving the tissue of interest).	Fixative-induced changes in chemical composition and fine structure may produce staining artifacts. Structural changes include denaturing and cross-linking proteins.
	Freezing (Physical Fixation): May be used for light or electron microscopy. Tissue embedded in cryoprotectant (glycerin). Rapid freezing at low temperatures reduces ice crystal formation and associated artifacts. Allows tissue to be sectioned (or fractured) without dehydration or clearing. Faster than chemical fixation. Avoids dissolving lipids and denaturing fixative-sensitive proteins (eg, enzymes, antigens).	Frozen specimens do not last as long as chemically fixed specimens. Obtaining serial frozen sections is very difficult.
Dehydration (substitution): Eases penetration of tissue by clearing agent. Prepares fixed tissue for infiltration with embedding medium.	Replaces water in tissue with organic solvent; commonly, **ethanol.** Fixed tissue immersed in series of alcohol-water mixtures with increasing alcohol concentration, to 100% alcohol.	Alcohol may denature proteins of interest. Water loss causes uneven shrinkage of components with different water content. May create unnatural spaces between cells and tissue layers.
Clearing: Prepares fixed tissue for infiltration. Dehydrating agent replaced with clearing agent.	Dehydrated tissue immersed in series of clearing agent-alcohol mixtures with increasing clearing agent concentration, or placed directly into clearing agent. **Xylene** (paraffin solvent) commonly used for light microscopy. **Propylene oxide** (plastic solvent) commonly used for EM.	Clearing agents may denature proteins of interest. Some components shrink unevenly as their proteins denature.
Infiltration: Prepares cleared tissue for embedding.	Cleared tissue is immersed in a series of clearing agent-embedding medium mixtures with increasing embedding medium concentrations, at medium-high temperature. Evaporating clearing agent is replaced by embedding medium.	Heat may denature proteins of interest. Bubbles left behind during poor infiltration.
Embedding: Prepares infiltrated tissue for sectioning. Makes tissue firm and prevents crushing or other tissue disruption during sectioning. Permits thin, uniform sectioning.	Infiltrated tissue positioned in mold filled with embedding medium, which hardens into a block. Block is attached to a chuck that holds it in microtome for sectioning. *For light microscopy,* paraffin commonly used, other media are celloidin, plastics, and polyethylene glycol (water soluble) wax. *For EM,* plastics and epoxy resins (eg, **Epon** and **Araldite**) are common. Require a catalyst to harden (polymerize) after infiltration. Harder embedding media allow thinner sectioning, a requirement for EM.	The improved sectioning allowed by embedding has limitations associated with dehydration, clearing, and infiltration.

(continued)

Table A–1 (cont'd).

Method and Purpose	Types and Procedures	Limitations and Associated Artifacts
Sectioning: Most tissues too thick and opaque for microscopic analysis of internal structure. Thin slices allow light or electrons to penetrate specimen and form image.	*For light microscopy,* standard rotary **microtome** with steel blade will cut 3–8-μm sections of specimens embedded in paraffin, celloidin, or polyethylene glycol. Glass or diamond knives will cut 1–5-μm sections of plastic-embedded tissue. Frozen sections, 5–25 μm, are cut with a freezing microtome or in a **cryostat** (standard microtome in a refrigerated chamber). *For EM,* an **ultramicrotome** with a glass or diamond knife will cut very thin sections (0.08–0.1 μm or up to 0.5 μm for high-voltage EM). Ultramicrotomes include stereomicroscope to observe cutting.	Sections typically provide only a two-dimensional image of a three-dimensional structure. Dull knife can crush or pinch tissue. Chatter (wavelike variations in section thickness) results from knife vibration during sectioning. Burr on knife can tear tissue.
Mounting: Eases handling and decreases damage to specimen during examination.	*For light microscopy,* sections placed on **glass slides,** often precoated with thin layer of albumin, gelatin, or polylysine to improve attachment. After staining, sections covered with glass coverslips to preserve them for repeated examination. *For EM,* specimens mounted on **copper grids.** Electron beam cannot penetrate glass.	Tissue sections may develop folds, making some regions appear to have more cells and stain darker. For grid-mounted specimens, only portions lying between crossbars will be visible.
Staining: Most tissue substructure is indistinguishable even at high magnification. Stains, ligands with specific binding affinities and optical properties, and radiolabels are used to localize and distinguish cell and tissue components. Knowledge of specificities of such substances provides additional information about structure and composition.	**For light microscopy:** Once sections are on slide, paraffin is dissolved. Tissue may be rehydrated before staining. Plastic sections stained without removing plastic. Most stain affinities based on reciprocal acid–base characteristics of stain and tissue components. Acidic stains (eg, eosin) bind basic (ie, **acidophilic**) structures and compounds (eg, cytoplasmic proteins). Basic stains (eg, hematoxylin) bind acidic (ie, **basophilic**) tissue components (eg, nucleic acids in ribosomes). Stain mixtures reveal multiple cell components. Hematoxylin and eosin (H&E), most common stain mixture for light microscopy, distinguishes nucleus from cytoplasm.	Acid-base boundaries may not correspond to boundaries between structures. Multiple staining procedures may be needed to characterize a particular cell or tissue component. Because colors are artifacts of staining, it is best to focus more on tissue component structure than color.
	For TEM: Most stains (contrasting agents) for TEM chosen for electron-absorbing or -scattering ability and affinity for particular cell components. **Heavy metal salts,** such as lead citrate and uranyl acetate, are common. The fixative osmium tetroxide interacts with lipids to form electron-dense precipitate and doubles as a stain for cell membranes.	TEM stains stop electrons from penetrating. TEM images are shadows of heavy metal deposits. Actual tissue structures not seen.
	For SEM: SEM specimens not stained per se. First subjected to **critical point drying,** to prevent artifacts related to surface tension., After dehydration, specimens soaked in liquid miscible with CO_2 or Freon and put in critical point chamber. Chamber is heated to a critical temperature (31 °C), raising pressure to a critical 73 atm, at which the gas and liquid phases exist without surface tension and liquid escapes specimen without altering structure. Specimen is then mounted on a stub and sputter-coated (sprayed) with fine mist of heavy metal particles (eg, gold) before viewing.	SEM reveals surface architecture in exquisite detail, but heavy metal coating prevents electrons from penetrating to reveal internal structure.

*Reproduced, with permission, from Paulsen DF. *Basic Histology: Examination & Board Review.* Appleton & Lange. 1996.

Table A–2. Special methods of tissue preparation for microscopy.*

Method and Purpose	Types and Procedures	Limitations
Cryofracture and Freeze Etching: Permit EM examination of tissues without prior fixation and embedding and thus without related artifacts. Allow verification of results obtained by conventional EM techniques.	Tissue frozen at very low temperatures and fractured with sharp blade (cryofracture). Specimen kept in vacuum while ice sublimates, lowering ice level from specimen surface to reveal more structures (freeze etching). Etched tissue sprayed at an angle with gold particles to give shadowed effect and then coated with a layer of fine carbon particles to form a replica. Tissue and replica returned to atmospheric pressure, tissue dissolved in strong acid, and replica mounted on grid. EM of replica produces shadowed-relief image and provides limited pseudo-three-dimensional view of cell and tissue components.	Image produced is entirely a controlled artifact. None of the original tissue is seen. Resolution is limited by particle size and thickness of coating.
Radioautography (auto-radiography): Allows localization of radioactive elements in cells or tissues. Especially useful in tracking radiolabeled precursors and molecules into which they are incorporated from one part of tissue or cell to another.	Tissue incubated with radiolabeled precursors before fixation, eg, ^{3}H-thymidine for DNA, ^{3}H-uridine for RNA, ^{3}H- or ^{14}C-leucine for protein. Sections mounted on slide, cleared of embedding medium, covered with photographic emulsion, and left in dark. Emulsion exposed (silver bromide reduced to elemental silver) in areas in contact with radiolabel; when developed, black grains (light microscopy) or curling particle tracks (EM) appear over labeled structures. Number of grains or tracks in emulsion proportionate to radiolabel present. For light microscopy, sections often counterstained to reveal tissue architecture.	Radiation exits labeled tissue component in various directions. Some labeled structures may not expose overlying emulsion, and silver grains over one structure may have been exposed by radiation from neighbor.

*Reproduced, with permission, from Paulsen DF. *Basic Histology: Examination & Board Review.* Appleton & Lange. 1996.

Appendix B: Amino & Nucleic Acids

Figure B–1. Deoxyribonucleic acid (DNA) nucleotides. DNA nucleotides connected in a single row form a molecule of single stranded DNA. (Reproduced from Seashore MR, Wappner RS. *Genetics in Primary Care & Clinical Medicine.* Appleton & Lange, 1996.)

Table B–1. L-α-Amino acids present in proteins.*

Name	Symbol	Structural Formula	pK$_1$	pK$_2$	pK$_3$
With Aliphatic Side Chains			α-COOH	α-NH$_3^+$	R Group
Glycine	Gly [G]	H—CH—COO$^-$; $^+$NH$_3$	2.4	9.8	
Alanine	Ala [A]	CH$_3$—CH—COO$^-$; $^+$NH$_3$	2.4	9.9	
Valine	Val [V]	(H$_3$C)$_2$CH—CH—COO$^-$; $^+$NH$_3$	2.2	9.7	
Leucine	Leu [L]	(H$_3$C)$_2$CH—CH$_2$—CH—COO$^-$; $^+$NH$_3$	2.3	9.7	
Isoleucine	Ile [I]	CH$_3$—CH$_2$—CH(CH$_3$)—CH—COO$^-$; $^+$NH$_3$	2.3	9.8	
With Side Chains Containing Hydroxylic (OH) Groups					
Serine	Ser [S]	CH$_2$(OH)—CH—COO$^-$; $^+$NH$_3$	2.2	9.2	about 13
Threonine	Thr [T]	CH$_3$—CH(OH)—CH—COO$^-$; $^+$NH$_3$	2.1	9.1	about 13
Tyrosine	Tyr [Y]	See below.			
With Side Chains Containing Sulfur Atoms					
Cysteine	Cys [C]	CH$_2$(SH)—CH—COO$^-$; $^+$NH$_3$	1.9	10.8	8.3
Methionine	Met [M]	CH$_2$(S—CH$_3$)—CH$_2$—CH—COO$^-$; $^+$NH$_3$	2.1	9.3	
With Side Chains Containing Acidic Groups or Their Amides					
Aspartic acid	Asp [D]	$^-$OOC—CH$_2$—CH—COO$^-$; $^+$NH$_3$	2.0	9.9	3.9
Asparagine	Asn [N]	H$_2$N—C(=O)—CH$_2$—CH—COO$^-$; $^+$NH$_3$	2.1	8.8	
Glutamic acid	Glu [E]	$^-$OOC—CH$_2$—CH$_2$—CH—COO$^-$; $^+$NH$_3$	2.1	9.5	4.1
Glutamine	Gln [Q]	H$_2$N—C(=O)—CH$_2$—CH$_2$—CH—COO$^-$; $^+$NH$_3$	2.2	9.1	

(continued)

Table B–1 (cont'd).

Name	Symbol	Structural Formula	pK$_1$	pK$_2$	pK$_3$
With Side Chains Containing Basic Groups			α-COOH	α-NH$_3^+$	R Group
Arginine	Arg [R]		1.8	9.0	12.5
Lysine	Lys [K]		2.2	9.2	10.8
Histidine	His [H]		1.8	9.3	6.0
Containing Aromatic Rings					
Histidine	His [H]	See above.			
Phenylalanine	Phe [F]		2.2	9.2	
Tyrosine	Tyr [Y]		2.2	9.1	10.1
Tryptophan	Trp [W]		2.4	9.4	
Imino Acids					
Proline	Pro [P]		2.0	10.6	

*Modified and reproduced from Murray RK et al. *Harper's Biochemistry,* 24 ed. Appleton & Lange. 1996, p. 25.

Figure B–2. Ribonucleic acid (RNA) nucleotides. The main function of RNA molecules, which are made from DNA templates, is to direct the synthesis of proteins. (Reproduced from Seashore MR, Wappner RS. *Genetics in Primary Care & Clinical Medicine.* Appleton & Lange, 1996.)

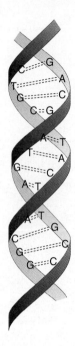

Figure B–3. DNA double helix. Hydrogen bonds hold together two complementary molecules of single-stranded DNA, which wrap around each other to form the double-stranded, helical molecule. An individual's genome consists of their entire complement of DNA. (Reproduced from Seashore MR, Wappner RS. *Genetics in Primary Care & Clinical Medicine.* Appleton & Lange, 1996.)

Table B–2. Classification of the L-α-amino acids based on their relative hydrophilicity (tendency to associate with water) or hydrophobicity (tendency to avoid water in favor of a more nonpolar environment).[1]

Hydrophobic	Hydrophilic	
Alanine	Arginine	Histidine
Isoleucine	Asparagine	Lysine
Leucine	Aspartic acid	Serine
Methionine	Cysteine	Threonine
Phenylalanine	Glutamic acid	
Proline	Glutamine	
Tryptophan	Glycine	
Tyrosine		
Valine		

[1]Reproduced with permission, from Murray RK et al: *Harper's Biochemistry,* 24th ed. Appleton & Lange. 1996, p. 27.

Index

NOTE: A *t* following a page number indicates tabular material and an *f* following a page number indicates a figure.

B

Band III, 137
Basal bodies, 134–135
Basal lamina, 127, 149, 153, 156
Basal membrane, 149
Basal surface, 34
Basement membrane, 3
 types of, 4f
Basolateral surface, 34
Bassen-Kornzweig syndrome, 66t
Belt desmosome, 34
Beta-adrenergic receptor, structure
 of, 36f
Beta-oxidation, 49
Bifunctional enzyme deficiency,
 characteristics of, 53t
Bimolecular leaflet, 22
Biochemical oscillator, 109
Biosynthetic pathway, 79
Blood group antigens, 16, 19
Blood transfusion, cell surface
 antigens and, 16
Bone morphogenic protein 2
 (BMP2), 207, 209f
Bradykinin, arachidonic acid release
 and, 26
Broad beta disease, 65t
Bulk flow, 71
Bullous pemphigoid, 154
Bundling proteins, 137

C

Cadherins, 151–152
 cell adhesion and, 152f
 types of, 152t
Cadherin zipper, 152
Caenorhabditis elegans, cell
 development and, 2
Calcineurin, 186
Calcium
 cell-cell adhesion and, 152, 165
 central pores and, 35
 endoplasmic reticulum lumen
 and, 56
 intracellular release channels for,
 189
 mobilization of, 186–187
 muscle contraction and, 145–146
 as second messenger, 169, 171f
Calcium-calmodulin-dependent
 kinases (CaM kinases),
 189
Calcium ions, apoptosis and, 114
Calcium spike, 189

Calmodulin, 141, 147, 183, 189
Calnexin, endoplasmic reticulum lumen and, 56
Calreticulin, endoplasmic reticulum
 lumen and, 56
cAMP, 169
 protein kinase A and, 184–186
Cancer
 actin cytoskeleton and, 138–139
 development of, loss of cell cycle
 regulation and, 119f
 oncogenes related to, 118t
Carbohydrate(s), energy production
 and, 96–97
Carbohydrate-linked proteins, 31
Cardiac muscle, 7f
 contractile machinery of,
 146–147
 properties of, 141t
Cardiolipin, percentage composition
 of, 18t
Cargo molecules, 67
Carrier vesicles, 67
Catastrophe, 121
Catenins, 152–153
Cathepsins, substrates of, 79t
Cations, divalent, apoptosis and,
 114
CD45 antigen, 203
Cdk-cyclin complexes
 cell cycle and, 111–112, 111f
 inhibitory proteins of, 112–113
Cell(s)
 adult human types of, 9–10t
 altered components of, diseases
 related to, 38t
 cone, 191
 differentiation of, 171
 extracellular matrix in,
 156–158
 division of, mechanisms of,
 118–121
 eukaryotic
 features of, 41t
 intermediate filaments of, 128f
 molecular motors from, 131t
 gene expression in, regulation of,
 7–12
 growth of
 contact inhibition of, 113
 unregulated, 117–118
 importance of membranes in,
 13–16
 mammalian
 communicating paradigms in,
 172–173

 phenotypes of, 2–7
 organization in tissues, 2–7
 photoreceptor, structure of, 190f
 polarized, membrane faces of, 34
 programmed death of, 114, 172
 replication of, 188
 rod, signal transduction in, 191f
 senescence and aging of,
 115–116
 sensory, signaling pathways of,
 189–192
Cell adhesion
 cadherin-mediated, 152f
 integrin-mediated, 154f
 regulation of, 165f
 neural, 164f, 165
 signal transduction and, 165–166
Cell adhesion molecules, 165
Cell-cell adherens junctions,
 151–153
Cell-cell adhesion, calcium-
 independent, 165
 association, 34
 attachment, 148
 binding, 171
 communication, 173
 contact, 113, 117
 junction, in epithelial tissue, 150f
Cell cortex, 125, 137
Cell culture, 1
Cell cycle, 107f
 control of, 116–117
 duration of, 107
 nondividing compartment of, 117
 passage of cells through, 111–122
 phases of, 106–107
 regulation of
 checkpoints in, 112, 113f
 development of cancer and,
 119f
Cell cycle engine, 109–110
Cell differentiation compartment, 117
Cell-free diagonal, 117
Cell junctions, 148–155
Cell-matrix interactions, 153
Cell nucleus. *See* Nucleus
Cell proliferation minus cell death,
 114
Cell signaling, 167–173
 nitric oxide and, 173–174
 protein kinase C and, 187–189
 protein phosphatases and, 186
 Src kinases and, 202f
Cell surface antigens, blood transfu-
 sion/graft transplantation
 and, 16

Basic Science Textbooks

Color Atlas of Basic Histology, 2/e
Berman
1998, ISBN 0-8385-0445-0, A0445-5

Jawetz, Melnick, & Adelberg's
Medical Microbiology, 20/e
Brooks, Butel, & Ornston
1995, ISBN 0-8385-6243-4, A6243-8

Concise Pathology, 3/e
Chandrasoma & Taylor
1998, ISBN 0-8385-1499-5, A1499-1

Basic Methods in Molecular Biology, 2/e
Davis, Kuehl, & Battey
1994, ISBN 0-8385-0642-9, A0642-7

Introduction to Clinical Psychiatry
Elkin
1998, ISBN 0-8385-4333-2, A4333-9

Medical Biostatistics & Epidemiology
Essex-Sorlie
1995, ISBN 0-8385-6219-1, A6219-8

Review of Medical Physiology, 18/e
Ganong
1997, ISBN 0-8385-8443-8, A8443-2

Molecular Basis of Medical Cell Biology
Fuller & Shields
1998, ISBN 0-8385-1384-0, A1384-5

Basic Histology, 8/e
Junqueira, Carniero, & Kelley
1995, ISBN 0-8385-0567-8, A0567-6

Basic & Clinical Pharmacology, 7/e
Katzung
1997, ISBN 0-8385-0565-1, A0565-0

Pharmacology
Examination & Board Review, 4/e
Katzung & Trevor
1995, ISBN 0-8385-8067-X, A8067-9

Medical Microbiology & Immunology
Examination & Board Review, 4/e
Levinson & Jawetz
1996, ISBN 0-8385-6225-6, A6225-5

Clinical Anatomy
Lindner
1989, ISBN 0-8385-1259-3, A1259-9

Pathophysiology of Disease, 2/e
An Introduction to Clinical Medicine
McPhee, Lingappa, Lange, & Ganong
1997, ISBN 0-8385-7678-8, A7678-4

Color Atlas of Basic Histopathology
Milikowski & Berman
1996, ISBN 0-8385-1382-4, A1382-9

Harper's Biochemistry, 24/e
Murray, Granner, Mayes, & Rodwell
1997, ISBN 0-8385-3611-5, A3611-9

Basic Clinical Parasitology, 6/e
Neva & Brown
1994, ISBN 0-8385-0624-9, A0624-5

Pathology
Examination & Board Review
Newland
1995, ISBN 0-8385-7719-9, A7719-6

Basic Histology
Examination & Board Review, 3/e
Paulsen
1996, ISBN 0-8385-2282-3, A2282-0

Laboratory Medicine Case Book
An Introduction to Clinical Reasoning
Raskova, Mikhail, Shea, & Skvara
1997, ISBN 0-8385-5574-8, A5574-7

Medical Immunology, 9/e
Stites, Terr, & Parslow
1997, ISBN 0-8385-0586-4, A0586-6

Correlative Neuroanatomy, 23/e
Waxman
1997, ISBN 0-8385-1477-4, A1477-7

Clinical Science Textbooks

Clinical Neurology, 3/e
Aminoff, Greenberg, & Simon
1996, ISBN 0-8385-1383-2, A1383-2

Understanding Health Policy
A Clinical Approach
Bodenheimer & Grumbach
1995, ISBN 0-8385-3678-6, A3678-8

Clinical Cardiology, 6/e
Cheitlin, Sokolow, & McIlroy
1993, ISBN 0-8385-1093-0, A1093-2

Behavioral Medicine in Primary Care
Feldman & Christensen
1997, ISBN 0-8385-0636-4, A0636-9

Fluid & Electrolytes
Physiology & Pathophysiology
Cogan
1991, ISBN 0-8385-2546-6, A2546-8

Basic and Clinical Biostatistics, 2/e
Dawson-Saunders & Trapp
1994, ISBN 0-8385-0542-2, A0542-9

(more on reverse)

Basic Gynecology and Obstetrics
Gant & Cunningham
1993, ISBN 0-8385-9633-9, A9633-7

Review of General Psychiatry, 4/e
Goldman
1995, ISBN 0-8385-8421-7, A8421-8

Principles of Clinical Electrocardiography, 13/e
Goldschlager & Goldman
1990, ISBN 0-8385-7951-5, A7951-5

Medical Epidemiology, 2/e
Greenberg, Daniels, Flanders, Eley, & Boring
1995, ISBN 0-8385-6206-X, A6206-5

Basic & Clinical Endocrinology, 5/e
Greenspan & Strewler
1997, ISBN 0-8385-0588-0, A0588-2

Occupational & Environmental Medicine, 2/e
LaDou
1997, ISBN 0-8385-7216-2, A7216-3

Primary Care of Women
Lemcke, Marshall, Pattison, & Cowley
1995, ISBN 0-8385-9813-7, A9813-5

Clinical Anesthesiology, 2/e
Morgan & Mikhail
1996, ISBN 0-8385-1381-6, A1381-1

Fundamentals of Surgery
Niederhuber
1998, ISBN 0-8385-0509-0, A0509-8

Dermatology
Orkin, Maibach, & Dahl
1991, ISBN 0-8385-1288-7, A1288-8

Rudolph's Fundamentals of Pediatrics
Rudolph & Kamei
1994, ISBN 0-8385-8233-8, A8233-7

Genetics in Primary Care & Clinical Medicine
Seashore
1995, ISBN 0-8385-3128-8, A3128-4

Clinical Thinking in Surgery
Sterns
1989, ISBN 0-8385-5686-8, A5686-9

The Principles and Practice of Medicine, 23/e
Stobo, Hellman, Ladenson, Petty, & Traill
1996, ISBN 0-8385-7963-9, A7963-0

Smith's General Urology, 14/e
Tanagho & McAninch
1995, ISBN 0-8385-8612-0, A8612-2

General Ophthalmology, 14/e
Vaughan, Asbury, & Riordan-Eva
1995, ISBN 0-8385-3127-X, A3127-6

Clinical Oncology
Weiss
1993, ISBN 0-8385-1325-5, A1325-8

CURRENT Clinical References

CURRENT Critical Care Diagnosis & Treatment, 2/e
Bongard & Sue
1997, ISBN 0-8385-1454-5, A1454-6

CURRENT Diagnosis & Treatment in Cardiology
Crawford
1995, ISBN 0-8385-1444-8, A1444-7

CURRENT Diagnosis & Treatment in Vascular Surgery
Dean, Yao, & Brewster
1995, ISBN 0-8385-1351-4, A1351-4

CURRENT Obstetric & Gynecologic Diagnosis & Treatment, 9/e
DeCherney
1997, ISBN 0-8385-1401-4, A1401-7

CURRENT Diagnosis and Treatment in Psychiatry
Ebert, Loosen, & Nurcombe
1998, ISBN 0-8385-1462-6, A1462-9

CURRENT Diagnosis & Treatment in Gastroenterology
Grendell, McQuaid, & Friedman
1996, ISBN 0-8385-1448-0, A1448-8

CURRENT Pediatric Diagnosis & Treatment, 13/e
Hay, Groothuis, Hayward, & Levin
1997, ISBN 0-8385-1400-6, A1400-9

CURRENT Emergency Diagnosis & Treatment, 4/e
Saunders & Ho
1992, ISBN 0-8385-1347-6, A1347-2

CURRENT Diagnosis & Treatment in Orthopedics
Skinner
1995, ISBN 0-8385-1009-4, A1009-8

CURRENT Medical Diagnosis & Treatment 1997, 36/e
Tierney, McPhee, & Papadakis
1997, ISBN 0-8385-1489-8, A1489-2

CURRENT Surgical Diagnosis & Treatment, 11/e
Way
1997, ISBN 0-8385-1456-1, A1456-1

LANGE Clinical Manuals

Dermatology
Diagnosis and Therapy
Bondi, Jegasothy, & Lazarus
1991, ISBN 0-8385-1274-7, A1274-8

Practical Oncology
Cameron
1994, ISBN 0-8385-1326-3, A1326-6

Office & Bedside Procedures
Chesnutt, Dewar, & Locksley
1993, ISBN 0-8385-1095-7, A1095-7

Psychiatry
Diagnosis & Treatment, 2/e
Flaherty, Davis, & Janicak
1993, ISBN 0-8385-1267-4, A126 7-2

Practical Gynecology
Jacobs & Gast
1994, ISBN 0-8385-1336-0, A1336-5

Geriatrics
Lonergan
1996, ISBN 0-8385-1094-9, A1094-0

Ambulatory Medicine
The Primary Care of Families, 2/e
Mengel & Schwiebert
1996, ISBN 0-8385-1466-9, A1466-0

Poisoning & Drug Overdose, 2/e
Olson
1994, ISBN 0-8385-1108-2, A1108-8

Internal Medicine
Diagnosis and Therapy, 3/e
Stein
1993, ISBN 0-8385-1112-0, A1112-0

Surgery
Diagnosis and Therapy
Stillman
1989, ISBN 0-8385-1283-6, A1283-9

Medical Perioperative Management
Wolfsthal
1989, ISBN 0-8385-1298-4, A1298-7

LANGE Handbooks

Handbook of Gynecology & Obstetrics
Brown & Crombleholme
1993, ISBN 0-8385-3608-5, A3608-5

HIV/AIDS Primary Care Handbook
Carmichael, Carmichael, & Fischl
1995, ISBN 0-8385-3557-7, A3557-4

Handbook of Poisoning, 12/e
Prevention, Diagnosis, & Treatment
Dreisbach & Robertson
1987, ISBN 0-8385-3643-3, A3643-2

Handbook of Clinical Endocrinology, 2/e
Fitzgerald
1992, ISBN 0-8385-3615-8, A3615-0

Clinician's Pocket Reference, 8/e
Gomella
1997, ISBN 0-8385-1476-6, A1476-9

Neonatology
Management, Procedures, On-Call Problems, Diseases, and Drugs, 3/e
Gomella
1994, ISBN 0-8385-1331-X, A1331-6

Surgery on Call, 2/e
Gomella & Lefor
1996, ISBN 0-8385-8746-1, A8746-8

Internal Medicine On Call, 2/e
Haist, Robbins, & Gomella
1997, ISBN 0-8385-4056-2, A4056-6

Obstetrics & Gynecology On Call
Horowitz & Gomella
1993, ISBN 0-8385-7174-3, A7174-4

Pocket Guide to Commonly Prescribed Drugs, 2/e
Levine
1996, ISBN 0-8385-8099-8, A8099-2

Handbook of Pediatrics, 18/e
Merenstein, Kaplan, & Rosenberg
1997, ISBN 0-8385-3625-5, A3625-9

Pocket Guide to Diagnostic Tests, 2/e
Nicoll, McPhee, Chou, & Detmer
1997, ISBN 0-8385-8100-5, A8100-8

Quick Medical Spanish, 2/e
Rogers
1997, ISBN 0-8385-8258-3, A8258-4

Pocket Guide to the Essentials of Diagnosis & Treatment
Tierney
1997, ISBN 0-8385-3605-0, A3605-1

Appleton & Lange • P.O. Box 120041 • Stamford, CT • 06912-0041 • 1-800-423-1359